CAT scan	= computerized axial tomography
CDC	= Centers for Disease Control
CNS	= central nervous system
ca.	= circa
cm	= centimeter
CF	= complement fixation
CSF	= cerebrospinal fluid
CIE	= counterimmunoelectrophoresis
DTP	= diphtheria, tetanus, pertussis
ESR	= erythrocyte sedimentation rate
ELISA	= enzyme-linked immunosorbent assay
FA	= direct fluorescent or immunofluorescent antibody test
FAO	= Food and Agriculture Organization of the United Nations
g	= gram
h	= hour
HA	= hemagglutination
HAI	= hemagglutination inhibition
IHA	= indirect hemagglutination
IFA	= indirect immunofluorescent antibody test
IF	= immunofluorescent testing
i.m.	= intramuscular
i.v.	= intravenous
IgA	= immunoglobulin class
IgE	= immunoglobulin class
IgM	= immunoglobulin class
IG	= immune globulin (serum)
IEM	= immune electron microscopy
mg	= milligram
mm	= millimeter
nm	= nanometer
RBC	= red blood cell
RIA	= radioimmunoassay
SE Asia	= Southeast Asia
TMP-SMX	= trimethoprim-sulfamethoxazole
the USA	= the United States of America
UK	= the United Kingdom
USPHS	= US Public Health Service
USSR	= Union of Soviet Socialist Republic
v.	= versus
WHO	= World Health Organization
WBC	= white blood cell
wk(s)	= week(s)
yr(s)	= year(s)

*FM 8-33
NAVMED P-5038

ARMY FIELD MANUAL
FM 8-33

NAVY PUBLICATION
NAVMED P-5038

DEPARTMENTS OF THE

ARMY AND THE NAVY

Washington, DC January 20, 1985

CONTROL OF COMMUNICABLE DISEASES IN MAN

This publication has been adopted as a joint text for the Army and Navy. It provides a central source of necessary information for the management of patients so that they are not the source of a communicable disease outbreak and survive.

By order of the Secretaries of the Army and Navy:

> JOHN A. WICKHAM, JR.
> General, United States Army
> Chief of Staff

Official:

DONALD J. DELANDRO
Brigadier General, United States Army
The Adjutant General

> LEWIS H. SEATON
> Vice Admiral, MC US Navy
> Director, Naval Medicine

DISTRIBUTION:

Army:

Active Army, USAR: To be distributed in accordance with DA Form 12-11A requirements for The Field Support Guide.
ARNG: Special list.

Navy: Special list (2,455 copies to: Department of the Navy, Naval Publications and Forms Center, 5801 Tabor Ave., Philadelphia, PA 19120).

---

*This manual supersedes FM 8-33, 3 December 1981.

Control of Communicable Diseases in Man

Fourteenth Edition, 1985

ABRAM S. BENENSON
Editor

An Official Report of the
American Public Health Association

The American Public Health Association
1015 Fifteenth Street NW
Washington, DC 20005

Interdisciplinary Books, Pamphlets & Periodicals
For the Professional & the Layman

Printed in the United States of America

Printing and Binding: The John D. Lucas Printing Co.
Typography: Byrd PrePress, Springfield, VA
Set In: Garamond

International Standard Book Number: 0-87553-130-X
International Standard Serial Number: 8755-4046

46M185; 50M785; 6M1285; 10M386

Cover Design: Four basic aspects of communicable disease control are symbolized—grain: proper nutrition; flask: research; syringe: prevention and treatment; hand and soap: sanitation.

THEODORE C. EICKHOFF, M.D.
    Professor of Medicine
    Director of Internal Medicine
    University of Colorado School of Medicine
    601 E. 19th Avenue
    Denver CO 80203
ALFRED S. EVANS, M.D., M.P.H.
    John Rodman Paul Professor of Epidemiology
    Yale University School of Medicine
    60 College Street
    New Haven CT 06510
WILLIAM S. JORDAN, Jr., M.D.
    Director, Microbiology and Infectious Diseases Program
    National Institute of Allergy and Infectious Disease
    National Institutes of Health
    Bethesda MD 20205
JONATHAN MANN, M.D.
    State Epidemiologist and Chief Medical Officer
    New Mexico Health and Environment Department
    Santa Fe NM 87504
    Currently CDC Director of the Zaire AIDS Project
JAY P. SANFORD, M.D.
    President, Uniformed Services University of the Health Sciences
    Dean, School of Medicine
    4301 Jones Bridge Road
    Bethesda MD 20814
ALEXIS SHELOKOV, M.D.
    Director of Vaccine Research, The Salk Institute
    Professor of Epidemiology
    School of Hygiene and Public Health
    The Johns Hopkins University
    615 North Wolfe Street
    Baltimore MD 21205
ROBERT E. SHOPE, M.D.
    Professor of Epidemiology
    Department of Epidemiology and Public Health
    Yale University School of Medicine
    Box 3333
    New Haven CT 06510

JAMES H. STEELE, D.V.M., M.P.H.
   Professor of Environmental Health
   The University of Texas School of Public Health
   P.O. Box 20186
   Houston TX 77025
WILLIAM D. TIGERTT, M.D.
   Editor, American Journal of Tropical Medicine and Hygiene
   15 Charles Plaza Suite 2202
   Baltimore MD 21201
FRANKLIN H. TOP, Jr, M.D., COL, MC
   Director, Walter Reed Army Institute of Research
   Walter Reed Army Medical Center
   Washington DC 20307
KENNETH WARREN, M.D.
   Director Health Sciences
   The Rockefeller Foundation
   1133 Avenue of the Americas
   New York NY 10036

LIAISON REPRESENTATIVES

F. Assaad, M.D.
   World Health Organization
J. R. H. Berrie, MB, Ch.B., DPH, DIH, FFCM
   Department of Health and Social Security, England
Philip S. Brachman, M.D.
   U.S. Public Health Service
Philip A. Brunell, M.D.
   American Academy of Pediatrics
B. W. Christmas, MD, Ch.B., DPH, FFCM, MCCM(NZ)
   Department of Health, New Zealand
Alastair J. Clayton, M.B., Ch.B.
   Department of National Health and Welfare, Canada
W. A. Langsford, M.D.
   The Australian Department of Health, Australia
Donald O. Lyman, M.D.
   Association of State and Territorial Health Officers
William F. McCulloch, DVM
   Conference of Public Health Veterinarians
Robert F. Nikolewski, COL, USAF, BSC
   U.S. Department of Defense
Daniel Reid, M.D.
   Scottish Home and Health Department, Scotland
Ronald K. St. John, M.D., M.P.H.
   Pan American Health Organization

TABLE OF CONTENTS

PREFACE TO THE FOURTEENTH EDITION

The *Control of Communicable Diseases in Man* was first published by the American Public Health Association in 1917 to present the essential facts needed to control communicable diseases of man. The periodic revisions, this the fourteenth, assure that the information and recommended practices remain abreast of the advances in our knowledge of the communicable diseases and of the changes in socioeconomic conditions. The book is intended to provide a ready source of information on how to recognize a specific disease, how to manage the patients so that the disease does not spread, and to provide guidance for treatment to preserve life and limit the spread of infection. It is not intended to replace more inclusive textbooks but to be a source of basic information on which initial action can be taken.

The events in the interval since the last edition was published bear evidence that the problems presented by communicable diseases have not been solved. The emergence of acquired immunodeficiency syndrome and of its various disease manifestations has reemphasized the need for competence in the communicable disease area and the need for maintaining surveillance of disease occurrence. To make the issue more complicated, the emerging relationship between neoplasia and specific etiological agents broadens the scope of communicable disease, and, more importantly, gives hope to preventing malignancies by applying infectious disease principles, e.g., hepatocellular carcinoma prevented by immunization against hepatitis B.

Questions may be raised about the amount of space devoted to the presentation of rare and exotic diseases. This is deliberate. Physicians in developed areas are familiar with the diseases which occur in their areas, but they have had no personal contact and usually little information about the diseases occurring in remote areas to which their patients are exposed in their increasing international travel; the jet plane assures their return within the incubation period of all infectious diseases. The inclusion of smallpox, even though it has been eradicated globally, is considered necessary; should smallpox appear again through some mischance, it is essential that there be a readily available source of information for rapid recognition and appropriate immediate action. Sources of information on these diseases may not be readily available; this book attempts to fill some of the void.

This manual considers communicable diseases globally. While it is a publication of the American Public Health Association, the presentation aims to be international. Toward this end, the numbers assigned for each disease by the World Health Organization *International Classification of Disease,* 9th Revision, Clinical Modification (ICD-9 CM) have been used; the disease nomenclatures recommended by the Council for International

xvii

Organizations of Medical Sciences (CIOMS) and the World Health Organization (WHO) in *International Nomenclature of Diseases,* Volume II, Part 2, Mycoses, 1st Edition, 1982, and Volume II, Part 3, Viral Diseases, 1st Edition, 1983, have been used so far as possible. When the recommended name is too different from that in current use, the recommended name is shown as the first synonym and marked with an asterisk. This volume is a model of international cooperation, with active participation by the WHO, the Pan American Health Organization (PAHO) and the health authorities of the major English-speaking countries.

The development of the text is a collaborative project. The members of the editorial board, selected for their expertise or that of their colleagues in the specific diseases, were assigned specific chapters for review and updating. After review and some editing by the editor and associate editor, these chapters were sent to all members of the editorial board and to the liaison representatives, who had been designated by the various health agencies in the USA (governmental and nongovernmental), WHO, PAHO, and the health departments of Australia, Canada, New Zealand, Scotland and the United Kingdom, as well as to experts on specific diseases who have given freely of their time and effort. The comments and criticisms were then considered in the preparation of the penultimate version, which was again distributed to the 28 people involved. After resolution of any disagreement, the final drafts as submitted to the printer (in the form of word-processor disks) were distributed to assure that no serious errors had been introduced.

While the orientation of the book is directed primarily toward the problems encountered by the official and nonofficial disease control agencies in the United States, the practices recommended should be applicable anywhere. An increasing number of diseases, such as influenza, must be considered on a global basis; toward this end, the WHO has established a network of international collaborating centres which can provide national authorities with the services of consultation, collection and analysis of information, assistance in the establishment of standards, production and distribution of standard and reference material, exchange of information, training and organization of collaborative research, and information dissemination regarding the incidence of specific diseases. The diseases covered by these centers are indicated in the appropriate chapters; WHO should be approached for further details about the services available.

While this manual is not intended to be a therapeutic guide, the currently best clinical management, especially of the exotic diseases, is indicated in section 9B7. Since the drugs needed for treatment of some rare or exotic diseases may not be available commercially within the United States, the Director of the Centers for Disease Control (CDC) of the U.S. Public

Health Service (USPHS) has established the CDC Drug Service to provide access to rarely used drugs on an Investigational New Drug (IND) basis. These can be obtained by calling (404) 329-3670, or at night, for emergency requests only, (404) 329-2888. The items available from this source are specified under the appropriate disease discussions. Some immunoprophylactic or immunotherapeutic agents are also available from CDC. Since several of the drugs and immunobiologics are considered "Emergency Life Saving" products, they are also dispensed from the US Quarantine Stations, located in international terminals in 9 major cities throughout the USA. The release of vaccinia immune globulin is controlled by a group of physician consultants who are situated in various parts of the country. The telephone number of the closest consultant can be obtained by contacting the quarantine officer at International Air Terminals or physicians may call the Centers for Disease Control directly at (404) 329-3145 or night calls at (404) 329-2888.

While the format of earlier editions and sometimes the original words written by the previous editors, Haven Emerson and John E. Gordon, are retained, every chapter has been carefully updated. New chapters have been added; these include acquired immunodeficiency syndrome (AIDS), malignant neoplasia, cryptosporidiosis, Kawasaki syndrome, and hymenolepiasis. As indicated above, the naming of several diseases has been changed to seek conformity with CIOMS-WHO nomenclature recommendations.

This edition again presents the composite efforts of many individuals, named or not named, in many countries; the task of adjudicating among conflicting suggestions fell to the editor, who accepts the responsibility for having rejected any suggestions which consequently will be proven to have been correct.

Purposes of the manual—The primary aim is to provide an informative text for public health workers of official and voluntary health agencies including physicians, dentists, veterinarians, sanitary engineers, public health nurses, social workers, health educators and sanitarians; and for physicians, dentists and veterinarians in private practice who are concerned with the control of communicable diseases. The book is also designed for those serving with the armed forces at home and abroad, and for health workers stationed in foreign countries. School administrators and students of medicine and public health will also find the material useful.

A second general purpose is to serve public health administrators as a guide and as a source of materials in preparing regulations and legal requirements for the control of the communicable diseases, in developing programs for health education of the public and in the administrative acts of official health agencies for management of communicable disease. The needs of field workers have been given special attention; their need for a handy reference determines the format of the manual and its pocket size.

Factual knowledge is presented briefly; opinions are advanced consistent with these facts as a basis for intelligent management of communicable disease, unhampered by local custom and not restricted to prevailing practices. The emphasis is on principle because local conditions often require variation in practices from state to state within the United States and between countries. To keep facts and opinions reasonably current, the manual is revised every five years.

Scope and Contents—The presentation is standardized. Each disease is briefly identified with regard to clinical nature, differentiation from allied or related conditions and laboratory diagnostic procedures. Infectious agent, occurrence, reservoir, mode of transmission, incubation period, period of communicability, and susceptibility and resistance are presented next. Methods of control are described under the following five headings:

A. *Preventive measures:* Applicable generally to individuals and groups when and where the particular disease may occur in sporadic, endemic or epidemic form, and whether or not the disease is an active threat at the moment, e.g., chlorination of water supplies, pasteurization of milk, control of rodents and arthropods, animal management, immunization procedures, and health education of the public.

B. *Control of patient, contacts and the immediate environment:* Those measures designed to prevent infectious matter present in the body and the environment of the infected individual from spreading the disease to other persons, arthropods or animals; and recommendations on the appropriate management of contacts to assure earliest possible treatment, to prevent disease dissemination during the incubation period, and to detect any carriers and their management to minimize disease spread. Specific treatment, if available, is outlined to minimize the period of communicability and to reduce morbidity and mortality. Recommendations for isolation have been based largely on the *CDC Guideline for Isolation Precautions in Hospitals,* by Julia S. Garner and Bryan P. Simmons and *CDC Guideline for Infection Control in Hospital Personnel* by Walter W. Williams (in one volume). While the category-specific isolation precautions have been epitomized in the enclosed definitions, reference is advisable to the original publication which can be purchased from the Superintendent of Documents, U.S. Government Printing Office, Washington, D.C. 20402.

C   *Epidemic measures:* Those procedures of emergency character designed to limit the spread of a communicable disease which has developed widely in a group or community, or within an area, state or nation. These measures are not applicable when the disease occurs sporadically among widely separated individuals or separated by considerable intervals of time.

D.   *Disaster implications:* The likelihood that the disease might constitute a major problem in a disaster or catastrophe situation and whether it would be necessary to take preventive actions.

E.   *International measures:* Such controls of international travelers, immigrants, goods, animals and animal products and their means of transport based on provisions of international health regulations, conventions, intergovernmental agreements or national laws; also any controls that may protect populations of one country against the known risk of infection from another country where a disease may be present in endemic or epidemic form.

Reporting of Communicable Diseases—The first step in the control of a communicable disease is its rapid identification, followed by notification to the local health authority that the disease exists within the particular jurisdiction. Administrative practices on the diseases to be reported and how they should be reported may vary greatly from one region to another because of different conditions and different disease frequencies. This manual presents a basic scheme of reporting, directed toward a practical working procedure rather than ideal practice. The purpose is to provide necessary and timely information to permit the institution of appropriate control measures by responsible health authorities, as well as to encourage uniformity in morbidity reporting so that data between different health jurisdictions within a country and between nations can be validly compared.

A system of reporting functions in four stages. The first is the collection of the basic data in the local community where the disease occurs. The data are next assembled at district, state or provincial level. The third stage is the aggregation of the information under national auspices. Finally, for certain prescribed diseases, report is made by the national health authority to the World Health Organization.

Consideration here is limited to the first stage of the reporting system—the collection of the basic data at the local level because it is the fundamental part of any reporting scheme and because this manual is primarily for local health workers. The basic data sought at the local level are of two kinds (see Definitions, Report of a disease).

1. *Report of Cases:* Each local health authority, in conformity with regulations of higher authority, will determine what diseases are to be reported as a routine and regular procedure, who is responsible for reporting, the nature of the report required and the manner in which reports are forwarded to the next superior jurisdiction.

   Physicians are required to report all notifiable illnesses which come to their attention; in addition, the statutes or regulations of many localities require reporting by hospital, householder, or other persons having knowledge of a case of a reportable disease. Within hospitals, a specific officer should be charged with the responsibility for submitting required reports. These may be case reports or collective reports.

   Case Reports of a communicable disease provide minimal identifying data of name, address, diagnosis, age, sex and date of report for each patient and, in some instances, suspects; dates of onset and basis for diagnosis are useful. The right of privacy of the individual must be respected.

   Collective Reports are the assembled number of cases, by diagnosis, occurring within a prescribed time and without individual identifying data, e.g., "20 cases of malaria, week ending October 6."

2. *Report of Epidemics:* In addition to the requirement for individual case reports, any unusual or group expression of illness which may be of public concern (see Definitions, Epidemic) should be reported to the local health authority by the most expeditious means, whether it is included or not in the list of diseases officially reportable in the particular locality; and whether it is a well-known identified disease or an indefinite or unknown clinical entity (see Class 4, below).

For reporting purposes, the diseases listed in this manual are distributed among the following five classes, according to the practical benefit which can be derived from reporting. These classes are referred to by number throughout the text, under section 9B1 of each disease. The purpose is to provide a scheme on the basis of which each health jurisdiction may determine its list of regularly reportable diseases.

Class 1: Case Report Universally Required by International Health Regulations or as a Disease under Surveillance by WHO.

This class can be divided into:

1. Those diseases subject to the International Health Regulations

(1969), Third Annotated Edition, 1983, WHO, Geneva; i.e, the internationally quarantinable diseases—plague, cholera, yellow fever; and

1A. Diseases under Surveillance by WHO, established by the 22d World Health Assembly—louse-borne typhus fever and relapsing fever, paralytic poliomyelitis, malaria and viral influenza.

An obligatory case report is made to the health authority by telephone, telegraph, or other rapid means; in an epidemic situation, collective reports of subsequent cases in a local area on a daily or weekly basis may be requested by the next superior jurisdiction, as, for example, in a cholera epidemic. The local health authority forwards the initial report to the next superior jurisdiction by the most expeditious means if it is the first recognized case in the local area or is the first case outside the limits of a local area already reported; otherwise, weekly by mail or telegraphically in unusual situations.

Class 2: Case Report Regularly Required Wherever the Disease Occurs

Two subclasses are recognized, based on the relative urgency for investigation of contacts and source of infection, or for starting control measures.

2A. Case report to local health authority by telephone, telegraph, or other rapid means. These are forwarded to next superior jurisdiction weekly by mail, except that the first recognized case in an area or the first case outside the limits of known affected local area is reported by telephone or telegraph; example—typhoid fever and diphtheria.

2B. Case report by most practicable means; forwarded to next superior jurisdiction as a collective report, weekly by mail; examples—brucellosis and leprosy.

Class 3: Selectively Reportable in Recognized Endemic Areas

In many states and countries, diseases of this class are not reportable. Reporting may be prescribed in particular regions, states or countries by reason of undue frequency or severity. Three subclasses are recognized; 3A and 3B are primarily useful under conditions of established endemicity as a means leading toward prompt control measures and to judge the effectiveness of control programs. The main purpose of 3C is to stimulate control measures or to acquire essential epidemiological data.

3A. Case report by telephone, telegraph, or other rapid means in specified areas where the disease ranks in importance with Class

2A; not reportable in many countries; example—tularemia and scrub typhus.

3B. Case report by most practicable means; forwarded to next superior jurisdiction as a collective report by mail weekly or monthly; not reportable in many countries; example—bartonellosis and coccidioidomycosis.

3C. Collective report weekly by mail to local health authority; forwarded to next superior jurisdiction by mail weekly, monthly, quarterly, or sometimes annually; example—phlebotomus fever and fasciolopsiasis.

Class 4: Obligatory Report of Epidemics—No Case Report Required

Prompt report of outbreaks of particular public health importance by telephone, telegraph, or other rapid means; forwarded to next superior jurisdiction by telephone or telegraph. Pertinent data include number of cases, time frame, approximate population involved and apparent mode of spread; examples—staphylococcal food poisoning, infectious keratoconjunctivitis, unidentified syndrome.

Class 5: Official Report Not Ordinarily Justifiable

Diseases of this class are of two general kinds: those typically sporadic and uncommon, often not directly transmissible from person to person (chromomycosis); or of such epidemiological nature as to offer no special practical measures for control (common cold).

Diseases are often made reportable but the information gathered is put to no practical use. This leads to deterioration in the general level of reporting, even for diseases of much importance. Better case reporting results when official reporting is restricted to those diseases for which control services are provided or potential control procedures are under evaluation, or epidemiological information is needed for a definite purpose.

ACKNOWLEDGEMENTS

Grateful acknowledgement is hereby made to all the experts, both within and without the American Public Health Associaton, and within and without the USA, who have prepared and critically reviewed sections in their area of expertise. The conscientious efforts of the Editorial Committee and of the national and international Liaison Representatives (who contributed not only their own effort but called on the experts in their various countries) provided information to make the final product of greatest value. Special recognition must be made to the participation of

Dr. James Chin, my associate editor, and especially to my research associate, Charlotte Shindledecker, who managed the nuts and bolts of digging out needed information as well as assuring that everything fit together in the end. My sincere appreciation must also be expressed to the staff of the San Diego State University Foundation for their administrative support and the forbearance of my colleagues on the faculty of the Graduate School of Public Health which made the project feasible.

ACTINOMYCOSIS

1. Identification—A chronic bacterial disease most frequently localized in jaw, thorax or abdomen; bloodborne spread with generalized disease may occur. The lesions are firmly indurated areas of purulence and fibrosis which spread slowly to contiguous tissues and, eventually, draining sinuses may be formed which penetrate to the surface. Discharges from sinus tracts may contain "sulfur granules," colonies of the infectious agent.

Diagnosis is made by demonstrating slim, nonspore-forming gram-positive bacilli, with or without branching, or "sulfur granules" in tissue or pus, and by isolating the microorganisms from samples of appropriate clinical materials not contaminated with normal flora during collection. The clinical findings and culture allow distinction between actinomycosis and actinomycetoma. (See Mycetoma).

2. Infectious agents—*Actinomyces israelii* is the usual pathogen of man; *A. naeslundii, A. odontolyticus, A.viscosus* and *Arachnia propionica (Actinomyces propionicus)* also have been reported to cause human actinomycosis. All species are gram-positive, nonacid-fast anaerobic to micro-aerophilic bacteria which may be part of the normal oral flora.

3. Occurrence—An infrequent human disease, occurring sporadically throughout the world. All races, both sexes, and all age groups may be affected; greatest frequency from 15 to 35 years of age; the ratio of males to females is approximately 2:1. Also occurs in cattle, horses and other animals.

4. Reservoir—The natural reservoir of *A. israelii* and the other agents is a colonized person. In the normal oral cavity, they grow as saprophytes in and around carious teeth, in dental plaque, and in tonsillar crypts, without apparent penetration or cellular response in adjacent tissues. Sample surveys in the USA, Sweden and other countries have demonstrated *A. israelii* microscopically in granules from crypts of 40% of extirpated tonsils, and isolation in anaerobic culture from as many as 30–48% of specimens of saliva or material from carious teeth. *A. israelii* has been found in the vaginal secretions of approximately 10% of women using intrauterine devices. No external environmental reservoir such as straw or soil has been demonstrated.

5. Mode of transmission—Presumably the agent passes by contact from person to person as a part of the normal oral flora. From the oral cavity the organism may be swallowed, inhaled or introduced into jaw tissues by injury or at the site of neglected or irritating dental defects. The source of clinical disease is endogenous. Transmission by human bite has been reported but is rare.

6. Incubation period—Irregular; probably many years after colonization in the oral tissues, and days or months after precipitating trauma and actual penetration of tissues.

7. Period of communicability—Time and manner in which *Actinomyces* and *Arachnia* spp. become a part of the normal oral flora are unknown. Except for the rare instances of human bite, not related to exposure to an infected person.

8. Susceptibility and resistance—Natural susceptibility is low. Immunity following attack has not been demonstrated.

9. Methods of control—

A. *Preventive measures:* None, except that maintenance of good dental hygiene, particularly removal of accumulating dental plaque, will reduce risk of infection around teeth.

B. *Control of patient, contacts and the immediate environment:*

1) Report to local health authority: Official report not ordinarily justifiable, Class 5 (see Preface).
2) Isolation: None.
3) Concurrent disinfection: None.
4) Quarantine: None.
5) Immunization of contacts: None.
6) Investigaton of contacts: Not profitable.
7) Specific treatment: No spontaneous recovery. Prolonged administration of penicillin in high doses is usually effective; tetracycline, erythromycin and cephalosporin antibiotics are alternative choices. Surgical drainage of abscesses is often necessary.

C. *Epidemic measures:* Not applicable, a sporadic disease.

D. *Disaster implications:* None.

E. *International measures:* None.

AIDS
ACQUIRED IMMUNODEFICIENCY SYNDROME   ICD-9 279.19
(Acquired immune deficiency syndrome)

1. Identification—Onset is usually insidious with nonspecific symptoms such as lymphadenopathy, anorexia, chronic diarrhea, weight loss, fever, and fatigue progressing until an opportunistic disease develops.

Alternatively, patients may present with a severe, life-threatening opportunistic disease. Surveillance of AIDS depends upon the detection of opportunistic diseases predictive of cell-mediated immune deficiency in the absence of a known cause for immune deficiency. These opportunistic diseases include: *Pneumocystis carinii* pneumonia, chronic enteric cryptosporidiosis, disseminated strongyloidiasis, toxoplasmosis of the CNS or pneumonia, esophageal candidiasis, disseminated or CNS cryptococcosis, disseminated atypical mycobacteriosis, pulmonary or gastrointestinal or CNS cytomegalovirus infection, chronic ulcerative mucocutaneous or disseminated herpes simplex infection, progressive multifocal leukoencephalopathy, Kaposi's sarcoma, and primary lymphoma limited to the brain. The crude case fatality rate in reported cases has been approximately 46%; the case fatality rate increases with the duration since diagnosis of the disease.

There is presently no diagnostic test specific for AIDS, although serologic tests for antibody are expected to become available soon. Several laboratory findings, such as lymphopenia, hypergammaglobulinemia, anergy to mitogens and antigens, and an inversion of the T_4-helper/T_8-suppressor T-lymphocytes resulting in a relative excess of T_8 cells may accompany clinical findings.

2. Infectious agent—The causative agent is a retrovirus designated as either human T-lymphotropic virus type III (HTLV-III) or lymphadenopathy associated virus (LAV). These are considered to be the same virus; possible cofactors remain to be identified.

3. Occurrence—The syndrome was first reported in 1981, but cases occurred in the USA as early as 1978; by December 1984, more than 7,250 cases had been reported. Although the largest number of reported cases has occurred in the USA, cases have been recorded in many other countries in Europe, Africa and the Americas among all races and social classes. Patient characteristics vary in different parts of the world. In the USA, nearly all patients fall into one of several patient categories: homosexually or bisexually active men (72%), i.v. drug abusers (17%), Haitian emigrants (4%), and patients with hemophilia (1%). Other groups at risk include sexual partners of men and women in these categories, transfusion recipients, and infants born to parents in the first category. More than 90% of cases have occurred in persons 20–49 yrs; 93% of the cases of Kaposi's sarcoma have occurred among the 72% of the patients who are homosexual or bisexual males. Among i.v. drug abusers, men and women appear to be at equal risk.

4. Reservoir—Man.

5. Mode of transmission—The transmission of AIDS in many ways is analogous to that of hepatitis B; epidemiologic evidence indicates that AIDS can be transmitted from person to person through sexual contact (predominantly homosexual intercourse), sharing unclean i.v. needles, or through transfusion of blood or blood products. Transplacental transfer may occur. By 15 December 1984, only one needle-stick infection of a health worker had been reported; thus, occupational risk to medical or laboratory personnel is very low.

6. Incubation period—Unknown. Epidemiologic evidence suggests that duration from exposure to onset of symptoms has a minimum range from about 6 months to 5 yrs with a mean of 2 yrs in transfusion-associated cases.

7. Period of communicability—Unknown. Presumed to extend from asymptomatic period through appearance of opportunistic diseases. A carrier state is possible but not confirmed.

8. Susceptibility and resistance—Unknown. Presumed to be general. Convalescent cases have not been documented. Degree of immunity is unknown.

9. Methods of control—

    A. *Preventive measures:*

        1)   Sexual contact, especially anal intercourse, should be avoided with persons known or suspected to have AIDS. Members of high-risk groups should be aware that having multiple sexual partners and sharing of drug paraphernalia increase the probability of exposure to AIDS.

        2)   The Food and Drug Administration (FDA) has prepared recommendations for manufacturers of plasma derivatives and for establishments which collect plasma or blood; these are interim measures to protect recipients of blood and blood products until the efficacy of specific laboratory tests has been established. Members of groups at increased risk for AIDS should refrain from donating plasma or blood; this includes all individuals belonging to such groups, even though many individuals are at little risk of AIDS. Centers collecting plasma or blood should inform potential donors of this recommendation.

        3)   Studies are in progress to evaluate screening procedures for their effectiveness in identifying and excluding plasma and blood which has a high probability of transmitting AIDS. These procedures include specific retrovirus laboratory tests as well as careful histories and physical examinations.

        4)   Physicians should adhere strictly to medical indications for transfusions. The use of autologous transfusions is encouraged.

5) Hemophiliacs currently using coagulation factor concentrate should strongly consider changing to heat-treated products.

B. Control of patient, contacts and the immediate environment:

1) Report to local health authority: Official report is obligatory in nearly all health jurisdictions in the USA. Official report may be required in some countries or provinces, Class 2B (see Preface).

2) Isolation: Blood/body fluid precautions. Observe precautions appropriate for other specific infections that occur in AIDS patients. If patient's hygiene is poor, a private room should be used.

3) Concurrent disinfection: Of equipment contaminated with blood, all excretions, and secretions.

4) Quarantine: None. Tissue donation: Patients and their sexual partners should not donate blood, plasma, organs for transplantation or semen for artificial insemination.

5) Immunization of contacts: None.

6) Investigation of contacts: Not justified on routine basis at this time.

7) Specific treatment: No known treatment for the underlying immune deficiency. Treatment consists of specific aggressive measures for the opportunistic diseases that result from AIDS. Experimental treatments are under investigation.

C. Epidemic measures: AIDS is currently epidemic in the USA. See 9A, above, for recommendations.

D. Disaster implications: None.

E. International measures: None.

AMEBIASIS ICD-9 006

1. Identification—An infection with a protozoan parasite that exists in two forms: the hardy, infective cyst and the more fragile, potentially pathogenic trophozoite. The parasite may act as a commensal or invade the tissues, giving rise to intestinal or extra-intestinal disease. Most infections are asymptomatic, but may become clinically important under certain circumstances. Intestinal disease varies from acute or fulminating dysentery with fever, chills, and bloody or mucoid diarrhea (amebic dysentery), to mild abdominal discomfort with diarrhea containing blood or mucus alternating with periods of constipation or remission. Amebic granulomata (ameboma), sometimes mistaken for carcinoma, may occur in the wall of the large intestine in patients with intermittent dysentery or colitis of long duration. Ulceration of the skin, usually in the perianal region, occurs rarely by direct extension from intestinal lesions. Dissemination via the bloodstream may occur, producing abscess of the liver or, less commonly, of the lung or brain.

Amebic colitis is often confused with various forms of inflammatory bowel disease such as ulcerative colitis; special care should be taken to distinguish the two diseases. Amebiasis can also mimic numerous other noninfectious and infectious diseases. Conversely, the presence of amebae may be misinterpreted as the cause of diarrhea in a person whose primary enteric illness is the result of a more serious condition.

Diagnosis is made by microscopic demonstration of trophozoites or cysts in fresh or suitably preserved fecal specimens, smears of aspirates or scrapings obtained by proctoscopy, aspirates of abscesses or sections of tissue; the presence of RBCs containing trophozoites is indicative of invasive amebiasis. Examination should be done on fresh specimens by a trained microscopist since the organism must be differentiated from nonpathogenic amebae and macrophages. Cultures on special media are not routinely used. Use of reference laboratory services may be required. Serological tests are useful adjuncts in diagnosing extra-intestinal amebiasis. X-rays or radiographic or ultrasonic and CAT scanning of liver are helpful in revealing the presence and location of an amebic liver abscess and can be considered diagnostic when associated with a high titer of specific antibodies.

2. Infectious agent—*Entamoeba histolytica,* a parasitic organism not to be confused with *E. hartmanni, E. coli,* or other intestinal protozoa.

3. Occurrence—Amebiasis is ubiquitous. Published prevalence rates vary widely from place to place. In general, rates are higher in areas with poor sanitation such as parts of the tropics, in mental institutions and among sexually promiscuous male homosexuals. In areas with good sanitation, amebic infections tend to cluster in households and institutions. The proportion of infected persons who have clinical disease is usually low.

4. Reservoir—Man; usually a chronically ill or asymptomatic cyst passer.

5. Mode of transmission—Epidemic outbreaks result mainly from ingestion of fecally contaminated water containing amebic cysts. Endemic spread is by hand-to-mouth transfer of feces, by contaminated raw vegetables, by flies, possibly by soiled hands of foodhandlers, and perhaps occasionally by water. Sexually transmitted by oral-anal contact. Patients with acute amebic dysentery pose only limited danger to others because of the absence of cysts in dysenteric stools and the fragility of trophozoites.

6. Incubation period—Variable. From a few days to several months or years. Commonly 2–4 wks.

7. Period of communicability—During the period of cyst passing, which may continue for years.

8. Susceptibility and resistance—Although susceptibility to infection is general, most persons harboring the organism do not develop disease. Susceptibility to reinfection has been demonstrated.

9. Methods of control—

    A. Preventive measures:

       1) Sanitary disposal of human feces.

       2) Protect public water supplies from fecal contamination. Sand filtration of water removes nearly all cysts and diatomaceous earth filters remove them completely. Chlorination of water as generally practiced does not always kill cysts; small quantities of water as in canteens or Lyster bags are best treated with prescribed concentrations of iodine, either liquid (8 drops of 2% tincture of iodine/quart of water or 12.5 ml/liter of a saturated aqueous solution of iodine crystals) or as water purification tablets (a tablet of tetraglycine hydroperiodide, Globaline, per quart of water). Water of undetermined quality can be made safe by boiling.

       3) Educate the general public in personal hygiene, particularly in sanitary disposal of feces and in handwashing after defecation and before preparing or eating food. Disseminate information regarding the risks involved in eating unpeeled or uncooked fruits and vegetables and in drinking water of questionable purity.

       4) Supervision by health agencies of sanitary practices of persons preparing and serving food in public eating places and general cleanliness of the premises involved. Routine examination of foodhandlers as a control measure is impractical.

       5) Control flies; protect foods against fly contamination by screening and other appropriate means.

       6) Disinfectant dips for fruits and vegetables are of unproved value in preventing transmission of *E. histolytica;* washing and keeping them dry may help; cysts are killed by desiccation and temperatures above 50°C (122°F).

       7) Use of chemoprophylactic agents is not advised.

       8) Known carriers should be indoctrinated in the need for thorough handwashing after defecation.

B. *Control of patient, contacts and the immediate environment:*

1) Report to local health authorities: In selected endemic areas; in many states and countries not reportable, Class 3C (see Preface).

2) Isolation: For hospitalized patients, enteric precautions in the handling of feces and contaminated clothing and bed linen. Exclusion of symptomatic individuals from food handling and from direct care of hospitalized and institutionalized patients. Release to return to work in a sensitive occupation when asymptomatic.

3) Concurrent disinfection: Sanitary disposal of feces.

4) Quarantine: None.

5) Immunization of contacts: Not applicable.

6) Investigation of contacts and source of infection: Household members and other suspected contacts should have adequate microscopic examination of feces. Modes of transmission should be investigated epidemiologically.

7) Specific treatment: Acute amebic dysentery is best treated with metronidazole (Flagyl®) followed by iodoquinol (Diodoquin®). Dehydroemetine (Mebadin®) followed by iodoquinol is an alternative treatment. Extra-intestinal amebiasis should be treated with metronidazole, or a combination of dehydroemetine plus chloroquine (Aralen®). Abscesses may require surgical aspiration before specific therapy is given. Asymptomatic carriers may be treated with iodoquinol or diloxanide furoate (Furamide®). Metronidazole is contraindicated during the 1st trimester of pregnancy because of possible teratogenicity; dehydroemetine is also contraindicated during pregancy. Dehydroemetine and diloxanide furoate are available from the CDC Drug Service, CDC, Atlanta (see Preface).

C. *Epidemic measures:* Any group of cases requires prompt laboratory confirmation to exclude other etiologic agents (as has frequently occurred) and epidemiologic investigation to determine source of infection and mode of transmission. If a common vehicle is indicated, such as water or food, appropriate measures to correct the situation should be taken.

D. *Disaster implications:* Disruption of normal sanitary facilities and food controls will favor an outbreak of amebiasis especially in population groups with large numbers of cyst passers.

E. *International measures:* None.

ANGIOSTRONGYLIASIS   ICD-9 128.8
(Eosinophilic meningoencephalitis, Eosinophilic meningitis)

1. Identification—A disease of the CNS due to a nematode; meninges are predominantly involved. Invasion may be asymptomatic or mildly symptomatic; more commonly characterized by severe headache, stiffness of neck and back and various paresthesias. Temporary facial paralysis occurs in 5% of patients. Low-grade fever may be present. The worm has been found in the CSF and the eye. CSF usually exhibits pleocytosis with 25–100% eosinophils; blood eosinophilia is not always present. Illness may last a few days to several months. Deaths have rarely been reported.

Differential diagnosis includes tuberculous meningitis, cerebral toxoplasmosis, coccidioidal meningitis, aseptic meningitis, syphilis, cerebral cysticercosis, paragonimiasis, echinococcosis and gnathostomiasis.

Diagnosis, especially in endemic areas, is suggested by eosinophils in the CSF; confirmation by demonstration of the worms in the CSF or at autopsy.

2. Infectious agent—*Angiostrongylus cantonensis,* a nematode (lungworm of rats). The third-stage larvae are infective to man.

3. Occurrence—The disease is endemic in Hawaii, Tahiti, many other Pacific islands, Vietnam, Thailand, Malaysia, Indonesia, Taiwan, the Philippines and Cuba. The nematode is found as far north as Japan, as far south as Brisbane, Australia, and as far west as Malagasy (Madagascar) and Egypt.

4. Reservoir—The rat.

5. Mode of transmission—Ingestion of raw or insufficiently cooked snails, slugs or land planarians, which are intermediate or transport hosts harboring infective larvae. Prawns, fish and land crabs that have ingested snails or slugs may also transport the infective larvae. Lettuce and other similar vegetables contaminated by molluscs may serve as a source of infection. The molluscs are infected by first-stage larvae excreted by an infected rodent; when third-stage larvae have developed, rodents (and man) are infected when they eat the mollusc. In the rat, the larvae migrate to the brain and mature to the adult stage; the adults migrate to the surface of the brain and through the venous system to reach their final site in the pulmonary arteries.

After mating, eggs hatch in terminal branches of the pulmonary arteries, the first-stage larvae enter the bronchial system and pass up the trachea, are swallowed and passed in the feces. In man, the cycle rarely goes beyond the CNS.

6. Incubation period—Usually 1–3 wks; it may be longer or shorter.

7. Period of communicability—Not transmitted from person to person.

8. Susceptibility and resistance—Susceptibility to infection is general. Malnutrition and debilitating diseases may contribute to an increase in severity, even to a fatal outcome.

9. Methods of control—

A. Preventive measures:

1) Rat control.
2) Boiling of snails, prawns, fish and crabs for 3–5 minutes or freezing at −15°C (5°F) for 24 hours is effective in killing the larvae.
3) Educate the general public in preparation of seafoods and both aquatic and terrestrial snails.
4) Avoid eating raw foods which have been contaminated by snails or slugs; thorough cleansing of lettuce and other greens to eliminate molluscs and their products does not always eliminate infective larvae.

B. Control of patient, contacts and the immediate environment:

1) Report to local health authority: Official report not ordinarily justifiable, Class 5 (see Preface).
2) Isolation: None.
3) Concurrent disinfection: Not necessary.
4) Quarantine: None.
5) Immunization of contacts: Not applicable.
6) Investigation of contacts and source of infection: The source of food involved and its preparation should be investigated.
7) Specific treatment: None.

C. Epidemic measures: Any grouping of several cases in a particular geographic area or institution warrants prompt epidemiologic investigation.

D. Disaster implications: None.

E. Internationsl measures: None.

ABDOMINAL ANGIOSTRONGYLIASIS   ICD-9 128.8

Since 1967, a syndrome has been recognized in Costa Rica, predominantly among children under the age of 13, consisting of a symptom-complex similar to that of appendicitis with abdominal pain and tenderness in the right iliac fossa and flank, fever, anorexia, vomiting, abdominal rigidity, a tumor-like mass in the right lower quadrant, and pain on rectal examination. There is a leukocytosis generally between 20,000 to 30,000, with eosinophils ranging from 11% to 61%. On surgery, yellow granulations are found in the subserosa of the intestinal wall and eggs and larvae of *Angiostrongylus costaricensis* are found in lymph nodes, intestinal wall, omentum, etc.; adult worms are in the small arteries, generally in the ileocecal area. The infection has been recognized in man in Central and S America. The reservoir of this parasite is a rodent (cotton rat, *Sigmodon hispidus,* or *Rattus rattus)* (among which the worm is present in southern USA); slugs are the usual intermediate hosts. The adult lives in the mesenteric arteries in the cecal area, and its eggs are carried into the intestinal wall. On embryonation, the first-stage larvae migrate to the lumen, are excreted in the feces and ingested by a slug. Within the slug, the larva develops to the third-stage which is infective to the rat or to humans. The infective larvae are found in the slug's slime (mucous) left on soil or other surfaces; when ingested by man, the infective larvae penetrate the gut wall, maturing in the lymphatic nodes and vessels. The adult worms migrate to the mesenteric arterioles of the ileocecal region where oviposition occurs. In man, most of the eggs and larvae degenerate and cause a granulomatous reaction. There is no specific treatment; surgical intervention is sometimes necessary.

ANISAKIASIS   ICD-9 127.1

1. **Identification**—A parasitic disease of the human gastrointestinal tract usually manifested by cramping abdominal pain and vomiting, resulting from the ingestion of uncooked fish containing larval nematodes of the family Anisakidae. The motile larvae may burrow into the stomach wall producing acute ulceration with nausea, vomiting and epigastric pain, sometimes with hematemesis. They may migrate upward and attach in the oropharynx causing cough. In the small intestine, they cause eosinophilic abscesses and the symptoms may mimic appendicitis or regional enteritis. Sometimes they may perforate into the peritoneal cavity and rarely may involve the large bowel.

Diagnosis is made by recognition of the 2 cm long larva invading the oropharynx, or by visualizing the larva through gastroscopic examination or in surgically removed tissue.

2. **Infectious agents**—Larval nematodes of the family Anisakidae, including the genera *Anisakis, Phocanema, Contracaecum* and *Terranova.*

3. **Occurrence**—The disease occurs in individuals who eat uncooked and inadequately treated (frozen, salted, smoked) saltwater fish or squid.

This is common in Japan (sushi and sashimi), Netherlands (herring), Scandinavia and on the Pacific coast of Latin America (ceviche). Several hundred cases have been described in Japan and in prior years the disease was frequently seen in the Netherlands. Infected fish are common in USA markets.

4. Reservoir—Anisakidae are widely distributed in nature but only certain of those parasitic in sea mammals constitute a major threat to man. The natural life cycle involves transmission of larvae by predation through small crustaceans to squid or fish, then to sea mammals, with man as an incidental host.

5. Mode of transmission—The infective larvae live in internal organs of fish; often after death of their host, they invade the body muscles of the fish. When ingested by humans and liberated by digestion in the stomach, they may penetrate the gastric or intestinal mucosa.

6. Incubation period—Gastric symptoms may develop within a few hours of ingestion. Symptoms referable to the small and large bowel occur within a few days or weeks depending on the size and location of the larvae.

7. Period of communicability—Direct transmission from person to person does not occur.

8. Susceptibility and resistance—Apparently universal susceptibility.

9. Methods of control—

    A. Preventive measures:

        1)   Avoid ingestion of inadequately cooked marine fish. Heating to 60°C (140°F) or freezing at −20°C (−4°F) for at least 60 hours kills the larvae. The latter control method is used with success in the Netherlands.

        2)   Cleaning (evisceration) of fish as soon after catching them as possible reduces the number of larvae penetrating from the internal organs into the muscles.

    B. Control of patient, contacts and the immediate environment:

        1)   Report to local health authority: Not ordinarily justifiable, Class 5 (see Preface). However, a case or cases recognized in an area not previously known to be involved, or any in an area where control measures are in effect, should be reported.

        2)   Isolation: None.

        3)   Concurrent disinfection: None.

        4)   Quarantine: None.

        5)   Immunization of contacts: None.

6) Investigation of contacts: None. Examination of others possibly exposed at the same time may be productive.
7) Specific treatment: Gastroscopic removal of larvae. Excision of lesions.

C. Epidemic measures: None.

D. Disaster implications: None.

E. International measures: None.

ANTHRAX   ICD-9 022
(Malignant pustule, Malignant edema, Woolsorters' disease, Ragpickers' disease, Charbon)

1. **Identification**—An acute bacterial disease usually affecting the skin, but may rarely involve the mediastinum or intestinal tract. In cutaneous anthrax, itching of an exposed skin surface occurs first, followed by a lesion which becomes papular, then vesiculated, and in 2–6 days develops into a depressed black eschar. The eschar is usually surrounded by mild to moderate edema, sometimes with small secondary vesicles. Pain is unusual and, if present, is due to edema or secondary infection. The lesion has been confused with human orf (see Orf Virus Disease). Untreated infections may spread to regional lymph nodes and to the bloodstream with an overwhelming septicemia. Involvement of the meninges can occur. Untreated cutaneous anthrax has a case fatality rate of from 5 to 20%, but with effective antibiotic therapy, few deaths occur. The lesion evolves through typical local changes even after the initiation of antibiotic therapy.

Initial symptoms of inhalation anthrax are mild and nonspecific, resembling a common upper respiratory infection; acute symptoms of respiratory distress, x-ray evidence of mediastinal widening, fever and shock follow in 3–5 days, with death shortly thereafter. Intestinal anthrax is rare and more difficult to recognize, except that it tends to occur in explosive outbreaks; abdominal distress is followed by fever, signs of septicemia and death in the typical case. An oropharyngeal form of primary disease has been described.

Laboratory confirmation is made by demonstration of the causative organism in blood, lesions or discharges by direct microscopic examination or by culture or inoculation of mice, guinea pigs or rabbits. The bacillus can be identified by FA techniques. Examination of paired sera by indirect microhemagglutination or ELISA may be helpful.

2. **Infectious agent**—*Bacillus anthracis.*

3. Occurrence—An infrequent and sporadic human infection in most industrial countries. Primarily an occupational hazard of workers who process hides, hair (especially from goats), bone and bone products and wool, and of veterinarians and agricultural workers who handle infected animals. Human anthrax is endemic in those agricultural regions of the world where anthrax in animals is common, including countries in Africa, Asia and the Middle East; between 1979–80, over 6600 cases and 99 deaths were reported from Zimbabwe. New areas of infection in livestock may develop through introduction of animal feed containing contaminated bone meal. Environmental changes such as floods may provoke epizootics.

4. Reservoir—The spores of *B. anthracis,* which are very resistant to adverse environmental conditions and disinfection, may remain viable in contaminated soil areas for many years after the source-animal infection has terminated. Dried or otherwise processed skins and hides of infected animals may harbor the spores for years.

5. Mode of transmission—Infection of skin is by contact with tissues of animals (cattle, sheep, goats, horses, pigs and others) dying of the disease and possibly by biting flies which had partially fed on such animals; or contaminated hair, wool, hides, or products made from them such as drums, brushes, etc; and soil associated with infected animals. Inhalation anthrax results from inhalation of spores. Intestinal anthrax arises from ingestion of contaminated undercooked meat; there is no evidence that milk from infected animals transmits anthrax. The disease spreads among grazing animals through contaminated soil and feed, and among omnivorous and carnivorous animals through contaminated meat, bone meal or other feeds. Vultures have been reported to spread the organism from one area to another. Accidental infections may occur among laboratory workers.

6. Incubation period—Within 7 days, usually 2 to 5.

7. Period of communicability—No evidence of transmission from person to person. Articles and soil contaminated with spores may remain infective for years.

8. Susceptibility and resistance—Uncertain; there is some evidence of inapparent infection among persons in frequent contact with the infectious agent; second attacks have not been documented.

9. Methods of control—

  A. Preventive measures:

  1) Immunization of high-risk persons with a cell-free vaccine prepared from a culture filtrate containing the protective antigen, available in the USA from the Michigan State Health Department, P.O. Box 30035, Lansing, Michigan,

48909, is effective in preventing cutaneous and possibly inhalation anthrax; it is recommended for veterinarians and for those handling potentially contaminated industrial raw materials.

2) Educate in personal cleanliness, in modes of anthrax transmission and in care of skin abrasions for employees handling potentially contaminated articles.

3) Dust control and proper ventilation in hazardous industries, especially those which handle raw animal fibers. Continuing medical supervision of employees, with prompt medical care of all suspicious skin lesions. Use protective clothing and adequate facilities for washing and changing clothes after work. Locate eating facilities away from places of work. Vaporized formaldehyde has been employed to terminally disinfect textile mills contaminated with *B. anthracis*.

4) Thorough washing, disinfection or sterilization of hair, wool or hides, and bone meal or other feed of animal origin prior to processing.

5) Hides of animals exposed to anthrax should not be sold nor their carcasses used as food or feed supplements.

6) Conduct postmortem examination of the first animals dying of suspected anthrax with care not to contaminate soil or the environment with blood or infected tissues. Studies of subsequent animal deaths from a similar illness should be limited to a blood specimen collected aseptically from the jugular vein. Process carcasses in rendering plants, burn them or bury deeply with anhydrous calcium oxide (quick-lime), preferably at the place of death. Decontaminate soil seeded with bodily discharges with a 5% solution of lye, or bury deeply with the carcass.

7) Promptly vaccinate all animals at risk. Treat symptomatic animals with penicillin or tetracyclines; vaccinate these animals after cessation of therapy. Treatment in lieu of vaccination may be used for animals exposed to a discrete source of infection such as a contaminated commercial feed.

8) Annual vaccination of animals in enzootic areas.

9) Control effluents and trade wastes of rendering plants handling potentially infected animals and those from factories that manufacture products from hair, wool or hides likely to be contaminated.

B. *Control of patient, contacts and the immediate environment:*

1) Report to local health authority: Case report obligatory in

most states and countries, Class 2A (see Preface). Also report to appropriate livestock or agriculture authority.

2) Isolation: Drainage/secretion precautions for duration of illness for cutaneous and inhalation anthrax.

3) Concurrent disinfection: Of discharges from lesions and articles soiled therewith. Spores require steam sterilization or burning for certain destruction. Terminal cleaning.

4) Quarantine: None.

5) Immunization of contacts: None.

6) Investigation of contacts and source of infection: Search for history of exposure to infected animals or animal products and trace to place of origin. In a manufacturing plant, inspect for adequacy of preventive measures as outlined in 9A, above.

7) Specific treatment: Penicillin is the drug of choice. Tetracyclines or other broad-spectrum antibiotics may be used.

C. *Epidemic measures:* The occasional epidemics in USA are local industrial outbreaks among employees who work with animal products, especially goat hair; outbreaks may be related to consumption of meat from infected cattle or may be an occupational hazard of animal husbandry. For appropriate control measures, see 9A, above.

D. *Disaster implications:* None, except in case of floods in previously infected areas.

E. *International measures:* Sterilization of imported bone meal before use as animal feed. Disinfection of wool, hair, hides and other products when indicated and practicable; formaldehyde, ethylene oxide and cobalt irradiation have been used.

ARENAVIRAL HEMORRHAGIC FEVER   ICD-9 078.7
(Argentine H.F., Bolivian H.F., Junin virus H.F., Machupo virus H.F.)

1. Identification—Acute febrile viral illnesses, duration 7–15 days. Onset is gradual with malaise, headache, retro-orbital pain, conjunctival injection, sustained fever and sweats, followed by prostration. An exanthem appears on the thorax and flanks 3–5 days after onset; later there may be petechiae, accompanied by edema of the face, neck, and upper thorax. An enanthem with petechiae on the soft palate is frequent. Severe infections result in epistaxis, hematemesis, melena, hematuria, and gingival hemorrhage; encephalopathies with intention tremors are frequent.

Bradycardia and hypotension with clinical shock are common findings, and leukopenia and thrombocytopenia are characteristic. Moderate albuminuria is present with many cellular and granular casts and vacuolated epithelial cells in the urine. Relapses may occur. Case fatality rates range from 5 to 30%, greatest among older patients.

Diagnosis is made by isolation of virus from blood or throat washings, and serologically by titer rises of IFA or neutralizing antibodies. Laboratory studies require a high level of biosecurity (P4).

2. Infectious agents—The Junin virus of the Tacaribe group of arenaviruses for the Argentine disease, and the closely related Machupo virus for the Bolivian disease.

3. Occurrence—First described in Argentina in 1955 in rural areas among laborers in corn fields. Occurs from March to October (autumn and winter) with a peak in May or June; mainly between ages 15–44 yrs; 5 times as frequent in males as in females. About 300–600 cases are reported each year. A similar disease was subsequently described in a series of epidemics in small villages of Bolivia; no cases have been reported since 1974.

4. Reservoir—In Argentina, wild rodents of corn fields *(Calomys laucha* and *C. musculinus)* are vertebrate hosts; a related species, *C. callosus,* in Bolivia.

5. Mode of transmission—Airborne transmission by dust contaminated with infected rodent excreta may occur. Saliva and excreta of infected rodents contain the virus. Infection through abraded skin may be possible. Laboratory infections occur. There is no evidence of arthropod transmission.

6. Incubation period—Commonly 7 to 16 days.

7. Period of communicability—Probably not often directly transmitted from person to person although this has occurred in the Bolivian disease.

8. Susceptibility and resistance—All ages appear susceptible but immunity of unknown duration follows infection. Subclinical infections are rare.

9. Methods of control—

    A.   *Preventive measures:* Specific rodent control has been successful in Bolivia. In Argentina, crop rotation with addition of soy beans to classical maize cultivation has been found to reduce reservoir rodent populations.

    B.   *Control of patient, contacts and the immediate environment:*

        1)   Report to local health authority: In selected endemic areas;

in most countries not a reportable disease, Class 3A (see Preface).

2) Isolation: Strict isolation during the acute febrile period.
3) Concurrent disinfection: Of sputum and respiratory secretions, and blood-contaminated materials.
4) Quarantine: None.
5) Immunization of contacts: None.
6) Investigation of contacts: None.
7) Specific treatment: The use of specific immunoglobulins given within 8 days of onset for the treatment of Argentine disease may be effective.

C. *Epidemic measures:* Rodent control.

D. *Disaster implications:* None.

E. *International measures:* None.

ARTHROPOD-BORNE VIRAL DISEASES
(Arboviral diseases)

Introduction

A large number of arboviruses are known to produce clinical and subclinical infection in man, and the number is growing rapidly. There are four main clinical syndromes: (1) an acute CNS disease ranging in severity from mild aseptic meningitis to encephalitis with coma, paralysis and death; (2) acute benign fevers of short duration, many resembling dengue fever with and without an exanthem, although on occasion some may give rise to a more serious illness with CNS involvement or hemorrhages; (3) hemorrhagic fevers, which include acute febrile diseases with extensive hemorrhagic involvement, external or internal, frequently serious, and associated with capillary leakage, shock and significantly high case fatality rates. All of them may cause liver damage but in yellow fever hepatic damage is most severe and is accompanied by frank jaundice; and (4) polyarthritis and rash, with or without fever and of variable duration, benign or with arthralgic sequelae lasting several weeks to months. These clinical features form the basis of presentation in this book.

Most of these infections are zoonoses, accidentally acquired by man through an arthropod vector, with man an unimportant host in the cycle. In the presence of viremia and a suitable vector, a few may become epidemic with man the principal source of vector infection. Most of the viruses are mosquito-borne, several are tick-borne and others are phlebotomine-borne (sandfly). A few are transmitted by *Culicoides* spp. (midges, gnats). Laboratory infections occur, some by aerosols.

Although the agents differ, common epidemiologic factors in the transmission cycles, relating chiefly to the vector, characterize these diseases and are, therefore, important in control. Consequently, the selected diseases under each clinical syndrome are arranged in four groups: mosquito-borne, tick-borne, phlebotomine-borne and unknown. Diseases of major importance are described individually or in groups with similar clinical and epidemiological features.

Viruses believed to be associated with human disease are listed in the accompanying table with type of vector, the predominant character of recognized disease and the geographical distribution. In some instances, observed cases are too few to be certain of the usual clinical reaction. Some have been recognized only through laboratory-acquired exposure. None is included where evidence of human infection is based solely on serological survey; otherwise the number would be much greater. Those which cause diseases covered in subsequent chapters are marked on the table by an asterisk; some of the less important or less well-studied are not discussed in the text.

Approximately 90 viruses presently classified as arboviruses produce disease in man. Most of these are further classified by antigenic relationships, morphology and replicative mechanisms into families and genera, of which Togaviridae and Flaviviridae are the best known. These two genera contain agents causing predominantly encephalitis and agents causing predominantly other febrile illnesses. Togaviridae are mosquito-borne; flaviviruses include both mosquito-borne and tick-borne agents and some agents without recognized vectors. Viruses of the family Bunyaviridae and several other groups produce principally febrile diseases. Several human pathogens for which no common antigens have been demonstrated necessarily remain in a "not classified" category.

DISEASES IN MAN CAUSED BY ARTHROPOD-BORNE VIRUSES

Virus Group	Name of Virus	Vector	Disease in Man	Where Found
TOGAVIRIDAE *Alphavirus*				
	*Chikungunya	Mosquito	Fever, arthralgia, hemorrhagic fever	Africa, SE Asia, Philippines
	*Eastern equine encephalomyelitis	Mosquito	Encephalitis	Americas
	*Mayaro (Uruma)	Mosquito	Fever, arthritis, rash	S America
	Mucambo	Mosquito	Fever	S America
	*Onyong-nyong	Mosquito	Fever, arthralgia	Africa
	*Ross River	Mosquito	Arthritis, rash	Australia, S Pacific
	Semliki Forest	Mosquito	Encephalitis	Africa
	Sindbis	Mosquito	Fever, arthritis, rash	Africa, India, SE Asia, Philippines, Australia, USSR, Europe
	*Venezuelan equine encephalomyelitis	Mosquito	Fever, encephalitis	Americas
	*Western equine encephalomyelitis	Mosquito	Encephalitis	Americas
FLAVIVIRIDAE *Flavivirus*				
	*Banzi	Mosquito	Fever	Africa
	Rio Bravo (Bat salivary gland)	Unknown	Encephalitis, aseptic meningitis	USA, Trinidad

FLAVIVIRIDAE
Flavivirus (cont.)

Bussuquara	Mosquito	Fever	S America
*Dengue 1, 2, 3 and 4	Mosquito	Fever, rash, hemorrhagic fever	Throughout tropics
Ilheus	Mosquito	Fever, encephalitis	S & Central America
*Japanese encephalitis	Mosquito	Encephalitis	Asia, Pacific Is.
Kedougou	Mosquito	Fever	Africa
*Kunjin	Mosquito	Fever	Australia, Sarawak
*Kyasanur Forest disease	Tick	Hemorrhagic fever, meningoencephalitis	India
*Louping ill	Tick	Encephalitis	UK
*Murray Valley encephalitis	Mosquito	Encephalitis	Australia, New Guinea
Negishi	Unknown	Encephalitis	Japan
*Omsk hemorrhagic fever	Tick	Hemorrhagic fever	USSR
*Powassan	Tick	Encephalitis	Canada, USA
*Rocio	Mosquito	Encephalitis	Brazil
*Spondweni	Mosquito	Fever	Africa
*St.Louis	Mosquito	Encephalitis	Americas
*Tick-borne encephalitis			
*European subtype	Tick	Encephalitis	Europe
*Far Eastern subtype	Tick	Encephalitis	Europe, Asia
Usutu	Mosquito	Fever	Africa
Wesselsbron	Mosquito	Fever	Africa, Asia

*Asterisked Groups and Viruses are discussed in the text. See index for page numbers.

DISEASES IN MAN CAUSED BY ARTHROPOD-BORNE VIRUSES (Continued)

Virus Group	Name of Virus	Vector	Disease in Man	Where Found
FLAVIVIRIDAE				
Flavivirus (cont.)	*West Nile	Mosquito	Fever, encephalitis rash, hepatitis	Africa, Indian Subcontinent, Middle East, Europe
	*Yellow Fever	Mosquito	Hemorrhagic fever	Africa, S & Central America
	*Zika	Mosquito	Fever	Africa, SE Asia
BUNYAVIRIDAE				
Group C*	Apeu	Mosquito	Fever	S America
	Caraparu	Mosquito	Fever	S America
	Itaqui	Mosquito	Fever	S America
	Madrid	Mosquito	Fever	Panamá
	Marituba	Mosquito	Fever	S America
	Murutucu	Mosquito	Fever	S America
	Nepuyo	Mosquito	Fever	S and Central America
	Oriboca	Mosquito	Fever	S America
	Ossa	Mosquito	Fever	Panamá
	Restan	Mosquito	Fever	Trinidad
Bunyamwera Group	*Bunyamwera	Mosquito	Fever	Africa
	Germiston	Mosquito	Fever, rash	Africa
	Ilesha	Unknown	Fever	Africa
	Wyeomyia	Mosquito	Fever	S America, Panamá

Group	Virus	Vector	Disease	Distribution
Bwamba Group	*Bwamba	Mosquito	Fever, rash	Africa
California Group	*California encephalitis	Mosquito	Encephalitis	USA
	Guaroa	Mosquito	Fever	S America, Panamá
	Inkoo	Mosquito	Fever	Scandinavia
	*Jamestown Canyon	Mosquito	Encephalitis	USA
	*LaCrosse	Mosquito	Encephalitis	USA, Canada
	*Snowshoe hare	Mosquito	Encephalitis	USA, Canada
	Tahyna	Mosquito	Fever	Europe, Africa
	Trivittatus	Mosquito	Encephalitis	USA
Guama group	Catu	Mosquito	Fever	S America
	Guama	Mosquito	Fever	S America
Sandfly fever group* (Phlebotomus fever)	Alenquer	Unknown	Fever	S America
	Candiru	Unknown	Fever	S America
	Chagres	Phlebotomine	Fever	Central America
	SF-Naples type	Phlebotomine	Fever	Europe, Africa, Asia
	Punta Toro	Phlebotomine	Fever	Panamá
	Rift Valley fever	Mosquito	Fever, hemorrhage, encephalitis, retinitis	Africa
Simbu group	SF-Sicilian type	Phlebotomine	Fever	Europe, Africa, Asia
	*Oropouche	Culicoides	Fever, meningitis	S America
	Shuni	Mosquito, Culicoides	Fever	Africa
Nairovirus	*Nairobi sheep disease	Tick	Fever	Africa, India
	*Dugbe	Tick	Fever	Africa

*Asterisked Groups and Viruses are discussed in the text. See index for page numbers.

DISEASES IN MAN CAUSED BY ARTHROPOD-BORNE VIRUSES (Continued)

Virus Group	Name of Virus	Vector	Disease in Man	Where Found
Crimean-Congo hemorrhagic group	*Crimean-Congo hemorrhagic fever	Tick	Hemorrhagic fever	Europe, Africa Asia, Middle East
Unclassified	*Bhanja	Tick	Fever, encephalitis	Africa, Europe, Asia
	Tataguine	Mosquito	Fever, rash	Africa
REOVIRIDAE (ORBIVIRUSES)				
Changuinola group	*Changuinola	Phlebotomine	Fever	Central America
Kemerovo group*	Kemerovo	Tick	Fever	Europe
	Lipovnik	Tick	Fever	Europe
	Tribec	Tick	Fever	Europe
Colorado Tick fever	*Colorado Tick fever	Tick	Fever	USA
Ungrouped	Orungo	Mosquito	Fever	Africa
RHABDOVIRIDAE				
Vesicular stomatitis group	*Vesicular stomatitis, Indiana & New Jersey	Phlebotomine	Fever	Americas
	Chandipura	Mosquito	Fever	India, Africa
	Piry	Mosquito	Fever	S America
ORTHOMYXO-VIRIDAE	Thogoto	Tick	Meningitis, hepatitis	Africa, Europe
NOT CLASSIFIED	Bangui	Unknown	Fever, rash	Africa
	Nyando	Mosquito	Fever	Africa
	*Quaranfl	Tick	Fever	Africa

*Asterisked Groups and Viruses are discussed in the text. See index for page numbers.

ARTHROPOD-BORNE VIRAL ARTHRITIS AND RASH

ICD-9 066.3

(Ross River disease*, Epidemic polyarthritis and rash, Ross River fever)

1. **Identification**—A self-limited disease characterized by arthritis, primarily in the small joints of the extremities, which lasts from 2 days to 8 months. In many patients arthritis is followed in 1–10 days by a maculopapular rash, sometimes pruritic and rarely vesicular, which may cover much of the skin surface. Petechiae and enanthem are rare. Fever is often absent. Lymphadenopathy, paresthesias and tenderness of palms and soles are present in a small percentage of cases.

Serologic tests show a rise in titer to alphaviruses; the virus may be isolated from the blood of acutely ill patients in mosquitoes or suckling mice.

2. **Infectious agent**—Ross River virus, an alphavirus.

3. **Occurrence**—Major outbreaks have occurred in the Murray Valley, Northern Territory, and Queensland, Australia and sporadic cases in the coastal regions of Australia and New Guinea. In 1979 a major outbreak occurred in Fiji and has spread to other Pacific islands, including Tonga and the Cook Islands, with 15,000 cases in American Samoa in 1979–80.

4. **Reservoir**—Unknown. Possibly wild rodents and marsupials. Transovarian transmission in *Aedes vigilax* has been demonstrated in the laboratory, making an insect reservoir a possibility.

5. **Mode of transmission**—Transmitted by *Culex annulirostris, Ae. vigilax* and other *Aedes* spp. of mosquitoes.

6. **Incubation period**—Ten to 11 days.

7. **Period of communicability**—No evidence of transmission from person to person.

8. **Susceptibility and resistance**—Recovery is universal and followed by lasting immunity; second attacks are unknown. Inapparent infections are common, especially in children, among whom the disease is rare.

9. **Methods of control**—

   A. *Preventive measures:* The general measures applicable to mosquito-borne viral encephalitides (9A, 1–5 and 9A8).

   B. *Control of patient, contacts and the immediate environment:*

1) Report to local health authority: In selected endemic areas; in many countries not a reportable disease, Class 3B (see Preface).
2) Isolation: Protect patients from mosquitoes.
3) Concurrent disinfection: None.
4) Quarantine: None.
5) Immunization of contacts: None.
6) Investigation of contacts: Place of residence of patient during the 2 weeks prior to onset. Search for unreported or undiagnosed cases; check febrile or asymptomatic family members for serological testing.
7) Specific treatment: None.

C. *Epidemic measures:* Same as for arthropod-borne viral fevers (see Dengue, 9C).

D. *Disaster implications:* None.

E. *International measures:* None. WHO Collaborating Centres (see Preface).

ARTHROPOD-BORNE VIRAL ENCEPHALITIDES
I. Mosquito-borne   ICD-9 062
EASTERN EQUINE ENCEPHALITIS* (EASTERN EQUINE ENCEPHALOMYELITIS VIRUS DISEASE*), WESTERN EQUINE ENCEPHALITIS* (WESTERN EQUINE ENCEPHALOMYELITIS VIRUS DISEASE*), LACROSSE ENCEPHALITIS (LACROSSE VIRUS DISEASE*), CALIFORNIA ENCEPHALITIS* (CALIFORNIA ENCEPHALITIS VIRUS DISEASE*), JAPANESE ENCEPHALITIS* (JAPANESE ENCEPHALITIS VIRUS DISEASE*), MURRAY VALLEY ENCEPHALITIS*, ST. LOUIS ENCEPHALITIS* (ST. LOUIS VIRUS DISEASE*) AND ROCIO VIRUS DISEASE*

1. **Identification**—A group of acute inflammatory diseases of short duration involving parts of the brain, spinal cord and meninges. Signs and symptoms are similar but vary in severity and rate of progress. Most infections are asymptomatic; mild cases often occur as febrile headache or aseptic meningitis. Severe infections are usually marked by acute onset, headache, high fever, meningeal signs, stupor, disorientation, coma, spasticity, tremors, occasionally convulsions (especially in infants) and spastic, but rarely flaccid, paralysis. Case fatality rates range from 0.3–60%, those with Japanese (JE), Murray Valley (MV) and eastern equine (EEE)

encephalitis viral infections being highest. Neurological sequelae occur with variable frequency depending on age and infecting agent; they tend to be most severe in infants or persons infected with JE and EEE viruses. Seizure disorder may follow LaCrosse infection. Mild leukocytosis is usual; leukocytes in CSF range from 50–500/mm³, occasionally ≧1,000 in infants.

The diseases require differentiation from the tick-borne encephalitides; encephalitic and nonparalytic poliomyelitis; rabies; mumps meningoencephalitis; lymphocytic choriomeningitis; aseptic meningitis due to enteroviruses; herpes encephalitis; postvaccinal or postinfection encephalitides; and bacterial, mycoplasmal, protozoal, leptospiral and mycotic meningitides or encephalitides. Venezuelan equine, Rift Valley fever, and West Nile viruses, producing primarily arthropod-borne viral fever (see Arthropod-borne viral fevers), are sometimes responsible for encephalitis.

Specific identification is made by demonstrating specific IgM in acute phase serum or CSF, or antibody rises between early and late specimens of serum by neutralization, CF, HI, FA, ELISA or other serological tests. Cross reactions may occur within a virus group. Virus may sometimes be isolated by inoculation of suckling mice or tissue culture with the brain tissue of fatal cases, rarely with blood or CSF after symptoms have appeared; histopathological changes are not specific for individual viruses.

2. Infectious agents—Each disease is caused by a specific virus in one of three groups: EEE and western equine encephalomyelitis (WEE) in the alphaviruses; JE, MV encephalitis, St. Louis (SLE) and Rocio in the flaviviruses; LaCrosse, California encephalitis, Jamestown Canyon and snowshoe hare viruses in the California group of bunyaviruses.

3. Occurrence—EEE is recognized in eastern and northcentral USA and adjacent Canada, in scattered areas of Central and S America and in the Caribbean Islands; WEE in western and central USA, Canada and Argentina; JE in western Pacific Islands from Japan to the Philippines and in many areas of eastern Asia from Korea to Indonesia, China and India; MV in parts of Australia and New Guinea; SLE in most of USA, Ontario (Canada) and also in Trinidad, Jamaica, Panamá, and Brazil; Rocio virus disease in Brazil; LaCrosse virus disease is acquired from forest- and tire-breeding mosquitoes in the USA and Canada. Cases occur in temperate latitudes in summer and early fall, and are commonly limited to areas and years of high temperature and many mosquitoes.

4. Reservoir—LaCrosse virus overwinters in *Aedes* eggs; the true reservoir or means of winter carry-over for other viruses is unknown, possibly in birds, rodents, bats, reptiles, amphibians or surviving mosquito eggs or adults, probably differing for each virus.

5. Mode of transmission—By the bite of infective mosquitoes. Most important vectors are: for EEE in the USA and Canada, probably *Culiseta* *melanura* from bird to bird and one or more *Aedes* and *Coquillettidia* spp. from birds or animals to man; for WEE in western USA and Canada, *Culex tarsalis;* for JE, *C. tritaeniorhynchus, C. vishnui* complex, and also *C. gelidus* in tropics; for MV, probably *C. annulirostris;* for SLE in USA, *C. tarsalis,* the *C. quinquefasciatus* complex, and *C. nigripalpus;* for LaCrosse, *Ae. triseriatus.* Mosquitoes acquire the infection from wild birds or rodents (LaCrosse virus), but pigs are important for JE. LaCrosse virus is transovarially and venereally transmitted in *Ae. triseriatus.*

6. **Incubation period**—Usually 5–15 days.

7. **Period of communicability**—Not directly transmitted from person to person. Virus is not usually demonstrable in the blood of man after onset of disease. Mosquitoes remain infective for life. Viremia in birds usually lasts 2–5 days but may be prolonged in bats, reptiles and amphibia, particularly if interrupted by hibernation. Horses develop active disease with the 2 equine viruses and with JE, but viremia is rarely present in high titer or for long periods; therefore, man and horses are uncommon sources of mosquito infection.

8. **Susceptibility and resistance**—Susceptibility to clinical disease is usually highest in infancy and old age; inapparent or undiagnosed infection is more common at other ages. Susceptibility varies with virus; e.g, LaCrosse and WEE are usually diseases of children while SLE is usually a mild infection in young children. Infection results in homologous immunity. In highly endemic areas adults are largely immune to local strains by reason of mild and inapparent infection; susceptibles are mainly children.

9. **Methods of Control**—

   A. *Preventive measures:*

      1) Destroy larvae and eliminate breeding places of known or suspected vector mosquitoes.
      2) Kill mosquitoes by space and residual spraying of human habitations. (See Malaria, 9A1).
      3) Screen sleeping and living quarters; use mosquito bed nets.
      4) Avoid exposure to mosquitoes during hours of biting, or use repellents. (See Malaria, 9A4).
      5) In endemic areas, house domestic animals away from living quarters, e.g., pigs in JE endemic areas.
      6) Educate the public as to mode of spread and control.
      7) Mouse brain inactivated vaccine against JE encephalitis for children is used in Japan, Korea and Taiwan; tissue culture vaccines are used in China. For those under continued intensive exposure, EEE vaccine, inactivated, dried, is available from the CDC, Atlanta (see Preface). A Japanese-

made vaccine against JE may become available from the same source for travelers to the endemic areas.

8) Passive protection of accidentally exposed laboratory workers by human or animal immune serum.

B. *Control of patient, contacts and the immediate environment:*

1) Report to local health authority: Case report obligatory in most states of the USA and in some other countries, Class 2A (see Preface). Report under the appropriate disease; or as encephalitis, other forms; or as aseptic meningitis, with etiology or clinical type specified when known.

2) Isolation: None; virus is not usually found in blood, secretions or discharges during clinical disease. Enteric precautions are appropriate until enterovirus meningo-encephalitis (q.v.) is ruled out.

3) Concurrent disinfection: None.

4) Quarantine: None.

5) Immunization of contacts: None.

6) Investigation of contacts and source of infection: Search for missed cases and the presence of vector mosquitoes; test for viremia in both febrile and asymptomatic family members; primarily a community problem (see 9C, below).

7) Specific treatment: None.

C. *Epidemic measures:*

1) Identification of infection among horses or birds and recognition of human cases in the community have epidemiological value by indicating frequency of infection and areas involved. Immunization of horses probably does not limit spread of the virus in the community.

2) Fogging or spraying from aircraft with suitable insecticides has shown promise for aborting urban epidemics of SLE.

D. *Disaster implications:* None.

E. *International measures:* Insecticide spraying of airplanes arriving from recognized areas of prevalence. WHO Collaborating Centres (see Preface).

II. Tick-borne   ICD-9 063
FAR EASTERN TICK-BORNE ENCEPHALITIS (RUSSIAN SPRING-
SUMMER ENCEPHALITIS), CENTRAL EUROPEAN TICK-BORNE
ENCEPHALITIS, LOUPING ILL, POWASSAN VIRUS ENCEPHALITIS

1. **Identification**—A group of diseases clinically resembling mosquito-borne encephalitides, except that the Far Eastern tick-borne subtype is often associated with focal epilepsy, flaccid paralysis, particularly of the shoulder girdle and other residua. Central European tick-borne encephalitis (diphasic milk fever or diphasic meningoencephalitis) has a longer course, averaging 3 weeks; the initial febrile stage is not associated with symptoms referable to the CNS; a 2nd phase of fever and meningoencephalitis follows 4–10 days after apparent recovery; fatality and severe residua are less frequent than for the Far Eastern tick-borne disease. Louping ill in man also has a diphasic pattern and is relatively mild.

Specific identification is made by demonstration of specific IgM in acute phase serum or CSF, or by serological tests of paired sera, or by isolation of virus from blood during acute illness by inoculation of suckling mice or tissue culture. Common serological tests do not differentiate members of this group, but do distinguish the group from most other similar diseases.

2. **Infectious agents**—A complex within the flaviviruses; minor antigenic differences exist, more with Powassan than others, but viruses causing these diseases are closely related.

3. **Occurrence**—Disease of the CNS caused by this virus complex is distributed spottily over much of the USSR, other parts of eastern and central Europe, Scandinavia and the UK. In general, the Far Eastern subtype has a more eastern or Asian distribution; diphasic meningoencephalitis predominates in Europe, while louping ill is present in Scotland, northern England, and Ireland. Powassan virus is present in Canada and the USA, the virus but not the disease is found in the USSR. Seasonal incidence depends on activity of the tick vectors. *Ixodes persulcatus* is usually active in spring and early summer, while *I. ricinus* continues activity into late summer or early autumn. Areas of highest incidence are those where man has intimate association with large numbers of infected ticks, generally in rural or forested areas but also in some urban populations. Local epidemics of central European tick-borne encephalitis have occurred among persons consuming raw milk from goats or sheep, thus the name diphasic milk fever. The age pattern varies widely in different regions and is influenced by opportunity for exposure to ticks, consumption of milk from infected animals, or by previously acquired immunity. Laboratory infections are common, some with serious sequelae, others fatal.

4. **Reservoir**—The tick or a combination of tick and mammal appears

to be the true reservoir; transovarian tick passage of some USSR viruses has been demonstrated. Sheep and deer are the hosts most involved in louping ill. Rodents and sometimes other mammals and birds, rarely man, give rise to tick infections in Europe and Asia.

5. Mode of transmission—By the bite of infective ticks, or by consumption of milk from certain infected animals. *Ixodes persulcatus* is the principal vector in eastern USSR and *I. ricinus* in western USSR and other parts of Europe; the latter is also the vector of louping ill of sheep in Scotland. *I. cookei* is the principal vector in eastern Canada and USA. Larval ticks usually ingest virus by feeding on rodents, sometimes other mammals and birds. Adult ticks may acquire infection from man. Raw milk may be a vehicle for diphasic meningoencephalitis.

6. Incubation period—Usually 7–14 days.

7. Period of communicability—Not directly transmitted from person to person. A tick infected at any stage remains infective for life. Viremia in a variety of vertebrates may last for several days; in man up to 7–10 days.

8. Susceptibility and resistance—Both sexes and all ages are susceptible. Infection, whether inapparent or overt, leads to immunity.

9. Methods of control—

   A.   *Preventive measures:*

     1) See Rickettsioses, Tick-borne, 9A1 and 2, for measures against ticks.

     2) Inactivated virus vaccines have been used extensively in central Europe and the USSR with reported safety and effectiveness.

     3) Boil or pasteurize milk of susceptible animals in areas where diphasic meningoencephalitis occurs.

   B.   *Control of patient, contacts and the immediate environment:*

     1) Report to local health authority: In selected endemic areas; in most countries not a reportable disease, Class 3B (see Preface).

     2) Isolation: None, after tick removal.

     3) Concurrent disinfection: None.

     4) Quarantine: None.

     5) Immunization of contacts: None.

     6) Investigation of contacts and source of infection: Search for missed cases, presence of tick vectors and animals excreting virus in milk.

     7) Specific treatment: None.

   C.   *Epidemic measures:* See Rickettsioses, Tick-borne, 9C.

D. **Disaster implications:** None.

E. **International measures:** WHO Collaborating Centres (see Preface).

ARTHROPOD-BORNE VIRAL FEVERS
I. Mosquito-borne
Yellow fever and Dengue are presented as separate chapters.

A. VENEZUELAN EQUINE ENCEPHALOMYELITIS VIRUS DISEASE
ICD-9 066.2

(Venezuelan equine encephalitis, Venezuelan equine fever)

1. **Identification**—Clinical manifestations of infection are influenza-like, with an abrupt onset of severe headache, chills, fever, myalgia, retro-orbital pain, and nausea and vomiting. Conjunctival and pharyngeal injection are the only physical signs. Most infections are relatively mild with symptoms lasting 3–5 days. Some cases may have a diphasic fever course; after a few days of fever, particularly in children, CNS involvement may appear, ranging from somnolence to frank encephalitis with disorientation, convulsions, paralysis, coma and death. During the 1971 Texas outbreak, 3 of 40 cases studied had severe CNS involvement with sequelae of personality change and/or paralysis.

Diagnosis is suspected on clinical and epidemiological grounds (presence of an equine epizootic exposure in infected area), and confirmed by virus isolation or rise in antibody titer. Virus can be isolated in tissue culture from blood and from nasopharyngeal washings during the first 72 hours of symptoms; acute and convalescent sera 10 days apart reveal a rising antibody titer. Laboratory infections occur unless proper containment facilities are used.

2. **Infectious agent**—An alphavirus, with epizootic and enzootic serotypes.

3. **Occurrence**—Endemic in northern S America, Trinidad, Central America and Panamá, Mexico and Florida. Appear as epizootics principally in northern and western S America; the one in 1970–71 spread through Central America into the USA.

4. **Reservoir**—A rodent-mosquito cycle maintains the enzootic subtypes. Epizootic subtypes are transmitted in a cycle involving horses, which

serve as the major source of virus to provide large scale infection of mosquitoes which in turn infect man.

5. Mode of transmission—By the bite of an infected mosquito. Viruses of the complex have been isolated from a number of genera including *Culex (Melanoconion), Aedes, Mansonia, Psorophora, Haemagogus, Sabethes* and *Anopheles.* Laboratory infections by aerosols are common.

6. Incubation period—Usually 2–6 days, can be as short as 1 day.

7. Period of communicability—Human cases are infectious for mosquitoes for at least 72 hours; the mosquitoes probably transmit virus throughout life. Person-to-person transmission may occur but has not been demonstrated. Virus is present in the pharyngeal secretions and is stable when aerosolized.

8. Susceptibility and resistance—Susceptibility is general. Mild infections and subsequent immunity occur frequently in endemic areas.

9. Methods of control—

    A.   Preventive measures:

        1)   General mosquito control procedures.
        2)   Avoid forested endemic areas, especially at dusk and dawn.
        3)   An investigational attenuated virus vaccine (TC-83) for Venezuelan equine encephalomyelitis has been used effectively to protect laboratory workers and other adults at high risk. (Available in USA from the CDC, Atlanta, see Preface). This vaccine proved to be effective in protecting horses during the 1970–71 epizootic; control of infection in horses effectively prevented additional human cases.

    B.   Control of patient, contacts and the immediate environment:

        1)   Report to local health authority: In selected endemic areas; in most countries not a reportable disease, Class 3B (see Preface).
        2)   Isolation: Blood/body fluid precautions. In a screened room or in quarters treated with a residual insecticide for at least 5 days after onset or until afebrile.
        3)   Concurrent disinfection: None.
        4)   Quarantine: None.
        5)   Immunization of contacts: None.
        6)   Investigation of contacts: Search for unreported or undiagnosed cases.
        7)   Specific treatment: None.

    C.   Epidemic measures:

1) Immunize horses and/or restrict their movement from the affected area.
2) Community survey to determine density of vector mosquitoes, their breeding places and effective control measures.
3) Establish an intensive appropriate mosquito control program.
4) Use repellents for those exposed to mosquitoes.
5) Identify the disease among horses and prevent mosquito feeding.

D. *Disaster implications:* None.

E. *International measures:* Vaccinate animals and restrict their movement from epizootic areas to areas free of the disease.

B. BUNYAMWERA VIRUS   ICD-9 066.3
DISEASE (BUNYAMWERA FEVER), BWAMBA VIRUS DISEASE (BWAMBA FEVER), CHIKUNGUNYA VIRUS DISEASE (CHIKUNGUNYA FEVER), MAYARO VIRUS DISEASE (MAYARO FEVER, URUMA FEVER), O'NYONG-NYONG, RIFT VALLEY FEVER, WEST NILE FEVER, GROUP C VIRUS DISEASE (GROUP C VIRAL FEVERS), OROPOUCHE VIRUS DISEASE (OROPOUCHE FEVER), AND OTHERS.

1. Identification—A group of febrile illnesses usually lasting a week or less, many of which are dengue-like (see table for mosquito-borne viruses). Usual onset is with headache, malaise, arthralgia or myalgia and occasionally nausea and vomiting; generally some conjunctivitis and photophobia. Fever may or may not be diphasic (saddleback). Rashes are common in West Nile, Mayaro, chikungunya and o'nyong-nyong disease. Hemorrhages sometimes occur in chikungunya virus disease in SE Asia and India; leukopenia is common; convalescence frequently prolonged. Meningoencephalitis occasionally complicates West Nile, Kunjin and Oropouche virus infections. Rift Valley fever cases may develop encephalitis, hemorrhage, or retinal damage and blindness. Several group C viruses are reported to produce weakness in the lower limbs; rarely fatal, except in cases with encephalitis or hemorrhage from Rift Valley fever. Epidemics of chikungunya, o'nyong-nyong, Rift Valley fever, and Oropouche may involve thousands of patients.

Serological tests differentiate other fevers of viral or unknown origin, but chikungunya, o'nyong-nyong, and other alphaviruses are difficult to distinguish from one another. Specific diagnosis is possible by virus isolation from blood during the febrile period by inoculation of suckling mice or tissue culture. Laboratory infections occur with many of these viruses.

2. **Infectious agents**—Each disease is due to an independent virus of the same name as the disease. West Nile, Banzi, Kunjin, Spondweni, and Zika viruses are flaviviruses; the closely related chikungunya and o'nyong-nyong along with Mayaro are alphaviruses. Group C bunyaviruses are Apeu, Caraparu, Itaqui, Madrid, Marituba, Murutucu, Nepuyo, Oriboca, Ossa and Restan. Oropouche is a Simbu group bunyavirus; Rift Valley fever is in the sandfly fever group. Others in smaller groups are listed in the preceding table.

3. **Occurrence**—West Nile virus is present in Egypt, Israel, India, France and probably is widespread in parts of Africa and the northern Mediterranean area. Chikungunya virus is found in Africa, India, SE Asia and the Philippine Islands; Rift Valley, o'nyong-nyong, Bwamba and Bunyamwera fevers thus far have been identified only in Africa. Mayaro and group C virus diseases occur in tropical S America, Panamá and Trinidad; Oropouche virus disease is found in Trinidad and Brazil; Kunjin virus in Australia. Seasonal incidence depends on vector prevalence. Occurrence is primarily rural or forest, though occasionally Rift Valley fever, Oropouche and chikungunya occur in explosive urban or suburban outbreaks.

4. **Reservoir**—Unknown for some viruses in the group. Most appear to be tropics-dependent and to require a continuous vertebrate-mosquito cycle. Oropouche virus may be transmitted by *Culicoides*. Birds are a source of mosquito infection for West Nile; sheep and other domestic ruminants for Rift Valley, and rodents for group C viruses.

5. **Mode of transmission**—In most instances by bite of an infective mosquito; for chikungunya, *Aedes aegypti* and possibly others; West Nile, *Culex univittatus* in Egypt and *C. pipiens molestus* in Israel; o'nyong-nyong, *Anopheles* spp.; Mayaro, *Mansonia* and *Haemagogus* spp.; Bunyamwera, *Aedes* spp.; group C viruses, species of *Aedes* and *Culex (Melanoconion)*. For Rift Valley in sheep and other animals, *Aedes caballus*, *Ae. circumluteolus* and *Ae. theileri; Ae. lineatopennis* may be infected transovarially and account for maintenance of virus over periods of several years; most human infections are associated predominantly with handling of infective material of animal origin during necropsy and butchering. *Culex pipiens* was implicated in a 1977 epidemic of Rift Valley fever in Egypt with 600 deaths.

6. **Incubation period**—Usually 3–12 days.

7. **Period of communicability**—Not directly transmitted from person to person. Infected mosquitoes probably transmit virus throughout life. Viremia, essential to vector infection, is present for many of these viruses during early clinical illness in man.

8. **Susceptibility and resistance**—Susceptibility appears general, in both sexes and throughout life. Inapparent infections and mild but

undiagnosed disease are common. Infection leads to immunity; susceptibles in highly endemic areas are mainly young children.

9. Methods of control—

A. *Preventive measures:*

1) The general measures applicable to mosquito—borne viral encephalitides (9A1–5 and 9A8). For Rift Valley, precautions in care and handling of infected animals and their products, as well as human acute-phase blood.

2) An experimental inactivated tissue culture vaccine is used for Rift Valley; live and inactivated vaccines are used for sheep, goats and cattle.

B. *Control of patient, contacts and the immediate environment:*

1) Report to local health authority: In selected endemic areas; in most countries not a reportable disease, Class 3B (see Preface). For Rift Valley fever, notify WHO, FAO, and OIE.

2) Isolation: Blood and body fluid precautions. Keep patient in screened room or in quarters treated with an insecticide for at least 5 days after onset or until afebrile. Blood of hemorrhagic Rift Valley fever cases is infectious.

3) Concurrent infection: None.

4) Quarantine: None.

5) Immunization of contacts: None.

6) Investigation of contacts: Determine place of residence of patient during fortnight before onset. Search for unreported or undiagnosed cases.

7) Specific treatment: None.

C. *Epidemic measures:*

1) Community survey to determine density of vector mosquitoes, to identify their breeding places and to promote their elimination.

2) Use mosquito repellents for persons exposed because of occupation or otherwise to bites of vectors.

3) Identification of the disease among sheep and other animals (Rift Valley) and serological survey of birds (West Nile) or rodents (group C viruses) have epidemiological value by indicating frequency of infection and areas involved.

4) Immunize sheep, goats, and cattle against Rift Valley fever.

D. *Disaster implications:* None.

E. *International measures:* For Rift Valley fever, vaccinate animals and restrict their movement from enzootic areas to those
free from disease, and do not butcher sick animals; for others,
none except enforcement of international agreements designed
to prevent transfer of mosquitoes by ships, airplanes and land
transport. WHO Collaborating Centres (see Preface).

II. Tick-borne   ICD-9 066.1
COLORADO TICK FEVER AND OTHER TICK-BORNE FEVERS

1. **Identification**—Colorado tick fever is an acute febrile, often
diphasic, dengue-like disease with infrequent rash. A brief remission is
usual, followed by a second bout of fever lasting 2–3 days; neutropenia and
thrombocytopenia almost always occur on the 4th–5th day of fever.
Characteristically a moderately severe disease but rarely severe in children,
with occasional encephalitis, myocarditis, or tendency to bleed. Deaths are
rare. Bhanja can cause severe neurological disease and death.

Laboratory confirmation of Colorado tick fever is made by isolation of
virus by inoculation of suckling mice or cell cultures with erythrocytes or
demonstration of antigen in erythrocytes by IF; CF and neutralizing
antibodies do not appear for 2 weeks or longer. Clinical manifestations of
other types and diagnostic methods vary only slightly except that serum
is used for virus isolation.

2. **Infectious agents**—The viruses of Colorado tick fever and Nairobi
sheep disease (Ganjam), and the Kemerovo, Tribec-Lipovnik, Quaranfil,
Bhanja and Dugbe viruses.

3. **Occurrence**—Known areas of Colorado type are in western Canada
and in Washington, Oregon, Idaho, Montana, California, Nevada, Utah,
Wyoming, Colorado, New Mexico and S Dakota in the USA. Virus has
been isolated from *Dermacentor andersoni* ticks in British Colombia. Most
frequent in adult males, but also affects children and women; seasonal
incidence parallels the period of greatest tick activity; endemic in
occurrence and common in much of the affected area. Geographic
distribution of other types is shown in the introductory table.

4. **Reservoir**—For Colorado type, small mammals, ground squirrels,
porcupine, chipmunk and *Peromyscus* spp. Also ticks, principally *D.
andersoni.*

5. **Mode of transmission**—To man by bite of an infective vector tick.
In Colorado type, immature ticks *(D. andersoni)* acquire infection by
feeding on infected viremic animals; they remain infected through the
various moults and transmit virus to man by feeding as adult ticks.

6. **Incubation period**—Usually 4–5 days.

7. **Period of communicability**—Not directly transmitted from person to person, except by transfusion. The wildlife cycle is maintained by ticks, which remain infective throughout life. Virus is present in man during the course of the fever and, in Colorado tick fever, from 2–16 weeks or more after onset.

8. **Susceptibility and resistance**—Susceptibility apparently is universal. Second attacks are rare. Experimental reinfection is unsuccessful.

9. **Methods of control**—

    A. *Preventive measures:* Control of ticks and rodent hosts. (See Rocky Mountain spotted fever, 9A1 and 9A2).

    B. *Control of patient, contacts and the immediate environment:*

        1) Report to local health authority: In endemic areas (USA); in most states and countries not a reportable disease, Class 3B (see Preface).

        2) Isolation: Blood and body fluid precautions. No blood donations for 4 months.

        3) Concurrent disinfection: None; remove ticks from patients.

        4) Quarantine: None.

        5) Immunization of contacts: None.

        6) Investigation of contacts and source of infection: Identification of tick-infested areas.

        7) Specific treatment: None.

    C. *Epidemic measures:* Not applicable.

    D. *Disaster implications:* None.

    E. *International measures:* WHO Collaborating Centres (see Preface).

III. Phlebotomine-borne

SANDFLY FEVER	ICD-9 066.0
(Phlebotomus fever, Pappataci fever)	
CHANGUINOLA VIRUS DISEASE	ICD-9 066.0
(Changuinola fever)	
VESICULAR STOMATITIS VIRUS DISEASE	ICD-9 066.8
(Vesicular stomatitis fever, VSV)	

1. **Identification**—A 3–4 day fever clinically resembling influenza but without inflammation of the respiratory tract. Headache, with fever of

38.3°–39.5°C (101°–103°F), sometimes higher, retrobulbar pain on motion of the eyes, injected sclerae, malaise, nausea, and pain in the limbs and back are characteristic. Leukopenia is usual on the 4th–5th day after onset of fever. Symptoms may be alarming, but death is unknown. Diagnosis is suspected by the clinical picture and the occurrence of multiple similar cases. Complete recovery may be preceded by prolonged mental depression.

Diagnosis may be confirmed by titer rise in serological tests or by isolation of virus from blood in newborn mice or in cell culture; for VSV infections, from throat swabs and vesicular fluid.

2. Infectious agents—The sandfly fever group of viruses; at least five related immunological types (Naples, Sicilian, Candiru, Chagres and Punta Toro) have been isolated from man and differentiated. In addition, Changuinola virus and vesicular stomatitis virus of the Indiana type, both of which produce febrile disease in man, have been isolated from *Lutzomyia* spp.

3. Occurrence—In those parts of Europe, Africa and Asia where the vector exists; also in Central and S America, where closely related viral agents are present. A disease of subtropical and tropical areas with long periods of hot, dry weather; in general, in a belt extending around the Mediterranean and eastward into Burma and China. Seasonal, between April and October, and prone to appear as a disease of troops and travelers from nonendemic areas.

4. Reservoir—Principal reservoir is the man-sandfly complex; an animal reservoir is suspected, but not yet demonstrated except that arboreal rodents and nonhuman primates may harbor New World sandfly fever viruses and possibly vesicular stomatitis virus. Rodents (gerbils) have been implicated in harboring Old World sandfly viruses. Transovarian transmission of some viruses has been demonstrated in phlebotomines.

5. Mode of transmission—By bite of an infective sandfly. The vector of the classical viruses is a small hairy, blood-sucking midge, *Phlebotomus papatasii*, the common sandfly, which bites at night and has a limited flight range. Sandflies of the genus *Sergentomyia* also have been found to be infected and may be vectors. Members of the genus *Lutzomyia* or *Brumptomyia* are involved in Central and S America.

6. Incubation period—Up to 6 days, usually 3–4 days, rarely less.

7. Period of communicability—Virus is present in the blood of an infected person at least 24 hours before and 24 hours after onset of fever. Phlebotomines become infective about 7 days after biting an infected person and remain so for their normal life span of about 1 month.

8. Susceptibility and resistance—Susceptibility is essentially universal; homologous acquired immunity is possibly lasting. Relative resistance of native populations in sandfly areas is probably attributable to infection early in life.

9. **Methods of control—**

    A.   *Preventive measures:* Control of sandflies is the important consideration. (See Leishmaniasis, Cutaneous, 9A1).

    B.   *Control of patient, contacts and the immediate environment:*

         1)   Report to local health authority: In selected endemic areas; in most countries not a reportable disease, Class 3C (see Preface).

         2)   Isolation: None; prevent access of sandflies to infected individuals for the first few days of illness by very fine screening or mosquito bed nets (10–12 mesh/cm or 25–30 mesh/inch, aperture size not more than 0.085 cm or 0.035 inch) and by spraying quarters with insecticide.

         3)   Concurrent disinfection: None; destruction of sandflies in the dwelling.

         4)   Quarantine: None.

         5)   Immunization of contacts: Not currently available.

         6)   Investigation of contacts and source of infection: In Old World, search for breeding areas of sandflies around dwellings, especially in rubble heaps, masonry cracks, and under stones.

         7)   Specific treatment: None.

    C.   *Epidemic measures:*

         1)   Community use of insecticides to destroy sandflies in and about human habitations.

         2)   Educate public on conditions leading to infection, and importance of preventing bites of sandflies by use of repellents while in infected areas, particularly after sundown.

    D.   *Disaster implications:* None.

    E.   *International measures:* WHO Collaborating Centres (see Preface).

ARTHROPOD-BORNE VIRAL HEMORRHAGIC FEVERS

Mosquito-borne viral hemorrhagic fevers: Dengue hemorrhagic fever and Chikungunya hemorrhagic fever are presented separately. The tickborne diseases are presented here.

I. CRIMEAN-CONGO HEMORRHAGIC FEVER   ICD-9 065.0

(Central Asian hemorrhagic fever)

1. **Identification**—Sudden onset with fever, malaise, weakness, irritability, headache, severe pain in limbs and loins, and marked anorexia. Vomiting, abdominal pain, and diarrhea occur occasionally. Flush on face and chest, and conjunctival injection develop early. Hemorrhagic enanthem of soft palate, uvula and pharynx and a fine petechial rash spreading from the chest and abdomen to the body are generally associated with the disease; occasionally large purpuric areas are observed. There may be some bleeding from gums, nose, lungs, uterus and intestine, but in large amount only in serious or fatal cases. Hematuria and albuminuria are common but usually not massive. Fever is constantly elevated for 5–12 days and falls by lysis. Convalescence is prolonged. Other findings are leukopenia with lymphopenia more marked than neutropenia. Thrombocytopenia is common. The reported case fatality rate ranges from 2–50%. In the USSR, there are estimated to be 5 infections for each hemorrhagic case.

Diagnosis is made by isolation of virus from blood by inoculation of cell cultures or suckling mice. Serological diagnosis is by ELISA, IFA, gel diffusion precipitation, CF or plaque reduction neutralization test. Specific IgM may be present during the acute phase; some sera show nonspecific neutralization with certain strains.

2. **Infectious agent**—The Crimean-Congo hemorrhagic fever virus, a Nairovirus.

3. **Occurrence**—Observed in the steppe regions of the western Crimea, on the Kersch peninsula, in Kazakstan and Uzbekistan, in the Rostov-Don and Astrakhan regions of USSR, as well as in Yugoslavia, Bulgaria, Iraq, the Arabian Peninsula, Pakistan and China. Most patients are agricultural workers in fallow lands, dairy workers or medical personnel. Seasonal occurrence is from June to September, the period of vector activity. Virus or antibodies in man have been observed in several areas of central and east Africa; hemorrhagic fever cases have been reported from S Africa.

4. **Reservoir**—In nature, believed to be hares, birds and *Hyalomma* spp. of ticks in USSR; reservoir hosts remain undefined in Africa but *Hyalomma*

and *Boophilus* ticks and insectivores and rodents may be involved. Domestic animals (sheep, goats and cattle) may act as amplifying hosts during epizootics.

5. Mode of transmission—By bite of infective adult *Hyalomma marginatum* or *H. anatolicum.* Immature ticks are believed to acquire infection from the animal hosts. Nosocomial transmission from patients to medical workers after exposure to blood and secretions has been important in recent outbreaks; infection is also associated with butchering infected animals.

6. Incubation period—Three to 12 days.

7. Period of communicability—Usually not directly transmitted from person to person; however, nosocomial infections occur after exposure to blood and secretions. An infected tick probably remains so for life.

8. Susceptibility and resistance—Immunity for at least 1 year.

9. Methods of control—

    A.   *Preventive measures:* See Rocky Mountain spotted fever, 9A, for preventive measures against ticks. No available vaccine.

    B.   *Control of patient, contacts and the immediate environment:*

        1)   Report to local health authority: In selected epidemic areas; in most countries not a reportable disease, Class 3B (see Preface).

        2)   Isolation: Blood and body fluid precautions.

        3)   Concurrent disinfection: Bloody discharges may be infective; decontaminate by heat or chlorine disinfectants.

        4)   Quarantine: None.

        5)   Immunization: None.

        6)   Investigation of contacts and source of infection: Search for missed cases and the presence of infective animals and possible vectors.

        7)   Specific treatment: Convalescent serum is reported to be useful.

    C.   *Epidemic measures:* See Rocky Mountain spotted fever, 9C.

    D.   *Disaster implications:* None.

    E.   *International measures:* WHO Collaborating Centres (see Preface).

II. OMSK HEMORRHAGIC FEVER   ICD-9 065.1
KYASANUR FOREST DISEASE   ICD-9 065.2

1. Identification—These two diseases have marked similarities. Onset is sudden, with headache, fever, pain in lower back and limbs, and severe prostration; often associated with conjunctivitis, diarrhea and vomiting by the 3rd–4th day. A papulovesicular eruption on the soft palate is an important diagnostic sign. Usually there is no involvement of the CNS; a mild meningoencephalitis may occur in Kyasanur Forest Disease (KFD). Severe cases are associated with hemorrhages but with no cutaneous rash. Bleeding occurs from gums, nose, gastrointestinal tract, uterus and lungs (but rarely from the kidneys), sometimes for many days and, when serious, results in shock and death; shock may also occur without manifest hemorrhage. Estimated case fatality rate is from 1–10%. Leukopenia and thrombocytopenia are marked. Febrile period ranges from 5 days to 2 weeks, at times with a secondary rise in the 3rd wk. Convalescence tends to be slow and prolonged.

Diagnosis is made by isolation of virus from blood in suckling mice or tissue cultures as long as 10 days following onset, or by serological tests.

2. Infectious agents—The Omsk hemorrhagic fever (OHF) and KFD viruses are closely related; they belong to the tick-borne encephalitis-louping ill complex of flaviviruses and are similar antigenically to the other viruses in the complex.

3. Occurrence—In the Kyasanur Forest of the Shimoga and Kanara districts of Karnataka, India, principally in young adult males exposed in the forest during the dry season from January to June. In 1983, there were 1142 cases with 104 deaths, the largest epidemic ever reported. OHF formerly occurred in rural workers and children exposed to infected ticks in the steppe regions of the Omsk Oblast in Siberia, but recently only in the Novosibirsk region. Seasonal occurrence in each area coincides with vector activity. Laboratory infections are common with both viruses.

4. Reservoir—In KFD, probably rodents, shrews and monkeys; in OHF, rodents, muskrats, and possibly ticks, since transovarian passage has been reported for other viruses of this complex.

5. Mode of transmission—By bite of infective ticks (especially nymphal stages), probably *Haemaphysalis spinigera* in KFD. In the OHF, infective ticks possibly are *Dermacentor pictus* and *D. marginatus;* recent data implicate direct transmission from muskrat to man and from contaminated water to man, suggesting that ticks may not be the principal vectors.

6. Incubation period—Usually 3–8 days.

7. Period of communicability—Not directly transmitted from person to person. Infected ticks remain so for life.

8. Susceptibility and resistance—All ages and sexes are probably susceptible; previous infection leads to immunity.

9. Methods of control—See Tick-borne Encephalitis, and Rocky Mountain spotted fever, sections 9. A formalinized mouse brain virus vaccine has been reported for OHF; an experimental vaccine has been used to prevent KFD in endemic areas of India.

ASCARIASIS
ICD-9 127.0
(Roundworm infection, Ascaridiasis)

1. Identification—A helminthic infection of the small intestine generally associated with few or no symptoms. Live worms, passed in stools or occasionally from the mouth or nose, are often the first recognized sign of infection. Some patients have pulmonary manifestations (pneumonitis, Löffler's syndrome) caused by larval migration and characterized by wheezing, coughing, fever, blood eosinophilia and pulmonary infiltration. Heavy parasite burdens may aggravate nutritional deficiency. Serious complications, sometimes fatal, include bowel obstruction by a bolus of worms, particularly in children; or obstruction of a hollow viscus such as bile duct, pancreatic duct and appendix by one or more adult worms.

Diagnosis is made by identifying eggs in feces or adult worms passed from the anus, mouth or nose. Intestinal worms may be visualized by radiologic techniques; pulmonary involvement may be confirmed by identifying *Ascaris* larvae in the sputum or gastric washings.

2. Infectious agent—*Ascaris lumbricoides,* the large intestinal roundworm of man; *A. suum,* a similar parasite of pigs, occasionally develops in man.

3. Occurrence—Common and worldwide, with greatest frequency in moist tropical countries where prevalence often exceeds 50%. The prevalence and intensity of infection is usually highest in children between 3–8 years. The distribution of *Ascaris* in the USA is limited to the southeastern states.

4. Reservoir—Infected persons; ascarid eggs in soil.

5. Mode of transmission—By ingestion of infective eggs from soil contaminated with human feces or uncooked produce contaminated with soil containing infective eggs, but not directly from person to person or from fresh feces. Heavy infections in children are frequently the result of ingesting soil. Contaminated soil may be carried long distances on feet or footwear into houses and conveyances; transmission of infection by dust is also possible. Eggs reach the soil in the feces and then undergo development (embryonation); at summer temperatures they become infective after about 2 weeks and may then remain infective for several months or years in favorable soil. The ingested embryonated eggs hatch in the intestinal lumen, the larvae penetrate the gut wall and reach the lungs by way of the circulatory system. Larvae grow and develop in the lungs; 9–10 days after infection they pass into the alveoli, ascend the trachea, and are swallowed to reach the small intestine, where they grow to maturity, mate and begin egg-laying 45–60 days after ingestion. Eggs passed by gravid females are discharged in feces.

6. Incubation period—Feces contain fertile eggs about 2 months after ingestion of embryonated eggs.

7. Period of communicability—As long as mature fertilized female worms live in the intestine. Few adult worms live more than 8 months; maximum life span is less than 18 months. The female worm can produce up to 200,000 eggs a day. Under favorable conditions embryonated eggs can remain viable in soil for years.

8. Susceptibility and resistance—Susceptibility is general.

9. Methods of control—

    A. Preventive measures:

        1) Provide adequate facilities for proper disposal of feces and prevent soil contamination in areas immediately adjacent to houses, particularly in children's play areas.

        2) In rural areas, construct privies which prevent dissemination of ascarid eggs through overflow, drainage, or otherwise. Treating human feces by composting for later use as fertilizer may not kill all eggs.

        3) Educate all people in the use of toilet facilities.

        4) Encourage satisfactory hygienic habits on the part of children; in particular, train to wash their hands before eating and handling food.

        5) In endemic areas, food should be protected from dirt, and food that has been dropped on the floor should not be eaten unless rewashed or reheated.

    B. Control of patient, contacts and the immediate environment:

        1) Report to local health authority: Official report not ordinarily justifiable, Class 5 (see Preface).

        2) Isolation: None.

        3) Concurrent disinfection: Sanitary disposal of feces.

4) Quarantine: None.
5) Immunization of contacts: None.
6) Investigation of contacts and source of infection: Determine others who should be treated. Environmental sources of infection should be sought, particularly on premises of affected families.
7) Specific treatment: Mebendazole (Vermox®), albendazole (Zentel®) are contraindicated in pregnancy; levamisole, pyrantel pamoate (Antiminth®), piperazine hexahydrate or piperazine salts.

C. *Epidemic measures:* Survey for prevalence in highly endemic areas, educate in environmental sanitation and in personal hygiene, and provide treatment facilities.

D. *Disaster implications:* None.

E. *International measures:* None.

ASPERGILLOSIS   ICD-9 117.3

1. Identification—A variety of clinical syndromes can be produced by several *Aspergillus* species: Patients with asthma and allergy to the aspergilli may develop bronchial damage and intermittent bronchial plugging, a condition called "allergic bronchopulmonary aspergillosis." Saprophytic endobronchial colonization in patients with bronchitis or bronchiectasis may cause clumps of hyphae to form within ectatic bronchi, or a large mass of hyphae may fill a previously existing cavity (fungus ball or aspergilloma); an *Aspergillus* species may appear as a concomitant organism in a bacterial lung abscess or empyema. Pneumonic aspergillosis may occur, particularly in patients receiving cytotoxic or immunosuppressive therapy; it may disseminate to the brain, kidneys and other organs and is usually fatal; invasion of blood vessels with thrombosis and infarction is characteristic of pneumonic and disseminated infection. *Aspergillus* species are the most common causes of otomycosis. The organisms may infect the implantation site of a cardiac prosthetic valve. The fungi may colonize or cause invasive infection of the paranasal sinuses. Growing on certain foods, many isolates of *A. flavus* (and occasionally other species) will produce aflatoxins or other mycotoxins; these cause disease in animals and fish and are highly carcinogenic for experimental animals, but adverse effects on man have not been proven.

Among findings that suggest a diagnosis of allergic aspergillosis are wheal and flare response to scratch or intradermal test with *Aspergillus* antigens, episodes of bronchial plugging, eosinophilia, serum precipitating antibodies against *Aspergillus,* elevated serum concentration of IgE and transient pulmonary infiltrates. Diagnosis of saprophytic endobronchial colonization is based on culture or microscopic demonstration of *Aspergillus* mycelium in sputum or in plugs of expectorated hyphae. Serum precipitins to *Aspergillus* species antigens usually are present. Chest x-ray is often diagnostic of a fungus ball. Diagnosis of invasive aspergillosis depends upon microscopic demonstration of the *Aspergillus* mycelium in infected tissue; confirmation by culture is desirable.

2. Infectious agents—*Aspergillus fumigatus, A. niger* and *A. flavus* are the most common causes of aspergillosis, though other species have also been implicated. *A. niger* or *A. fumigatus* cause most cases of fungus ball; *A. niger* is the usual cause of otomycosis.

3. Occurrence—Worldwide; uncommon and sporadic. No distinctive differences in incidence by race or sex.

4. Reservoir—Compost piles undergoing fermentation and decay are prominent reservoirs and sources of infection. Fungi are also found in hay which had been stored when damp, in decaying vegetation, in cereal grains, and in a variety of other foodstuffs stored under conditions which permit them to heat.

5. Mode of transmission—Inhalation of airborne spores.

6. Incubation period—Probably a few days to weeks.

7. Period of communicability—Not transmitted from person to person.

8. Susceptibility and resistance—The ubiquity of *Aspergillus* spp. and the usual occurrence of the disease as a secondary infection suggest a high degree of resistance by healthy persons. Susceptibility is increased by immunosuppressive or cytotoxic therapy.

9. Methods of Control—

A. Preventive measures: None which are feasible.

B. Control of patient, contacts and the immediate environment:

1) Report to local health authority: Official report not ordinarily justifiable, Class 5 (see Preface).
2) Isolation: None.
3) Concurrent disinfection: Ordinary cleanliness. Terminal cleaning.
4) Quarantine: None.
5) Immunization of contacts: None.
6) Investigation of contacts: Not ordinarily indicated.

7) Specific treatment: Amphotericin B (Fungizone®) should be tried in tissue-invasive forms. Immunosuppressive therapy should be discontinued or reduced as much as possible. Endobronchial colonization should be treated by measures to improve bronchopulmonary drainage.

C. *Epidemic measures:* Not generally applicable; a sporadic disease. Clusters of cases may occur on cancer therapy wards, in which case environmental studies should be carried out to find the source of the spores.

D. *Disaster implications:* None.

E. *International measures:* None.

BABESIOSIS   ICD-9 088.8

1. **Identification**—A rare but often severe and sometimes fatal disease of man caused by infection with a protozoan parasite of RBCs. The disease presents with fever, fatigue and hemolytic anemia lasting for several days to a few months. Asymptomatic infections occur, but their proportion is not known. Cases caused by parasite strains found in Europe have been more likely to be severe and fatal than those caused by the strains prevalent in the USA.

Diagnosis is made by identification on a blood film of the parasite within RBCs, by serologic studies (IFA), or by isolation in appropriate animals. Differentiation from *Plasmodium falciparum* on smear may be difficult in patients who have been to areas where malaria transmission occurs or who may have acquired infection by blood transfusion; if diagnosis is uncertain, manage as a case of malaria and send thick and thin smears to an appropriate reference laboratory.

2. **Infectious agents**—*Babesia microti,* and other *Babesia* species, especially *B. bovis* and *B. divergens* in Europe.

3. **Occurrence**—Recognition of infection with *B. microti* in immunologically intact hosts has been mainly in northeastern USA. Cases have been reported from Nantucket Island, Massachusetts, and from Long Island, New York; one case has been reported from Wisconsin. Human cases with other strains have been identified in California and Georgia. In Europe, human infections have been reported from Yugoslavia, France, Ireland, Scotland and the USSR, caused by *B. bovis* and *B. divergens*.

4. **Reservoir**—Presumably rodents for *B. microti* and cattle for *B. bovis* and *B. divergens*.

5. Mode of transmission—*B. microti* is transmitted during the summer months by bite of nymphal *Ixodes* ticks *(I. dammini)* carried by voles *(Microtus pennsylvanicus)* or deer mice *(Peromyscus leucopus)*. The adult tick is normally found on deer (who are not infected by the parasite). The vector of *B. bovis* and *B. divergens* in Europe appears to be *I. ricinus*.

6. Incubation period—One to 12 months reported; shorter in asplenic individuals.

7. Period of communicability—Transmission from person to person is unlikely except by blood transfusion.

8. Susceptibility and resistance—Susceptibility to *B. microti* assumed to be universal. Other members of the family Babesiidae have been known to attack immunocompromised, elderly or asplenic persons.

9. Methods of control—

A. *Preventive measures:* Control rodents around human habitation; use tick repellents; educate public in mode of transmission and the means for personal protection.

B. *Control of patient, contacts and the immediate environment:*

1) Report to local health authority: Report new suspect cases by telephone, particularly in areas not previously known to be endemic; Class 3A (see Preface).
2) Isolation: Blood/body fluid precautions.
3) Concurrent disinfection: None.
4) Quarantine: None.
5) Protection of contacts: None, but family members possibly exposed at the same time as the patient should be examined for infection and observed for fever.
6) Investigation of contacts and source of infection: Cases occurring in a new area deserve careful study. Blood donors in transfusion-related cases should be investigated promptly.
7) Specific treatment: Clindamycin in combination with quinine has been effective in experimental animal studies and in the few patients who have received this drug combination. Infection does not respond to chloroquine. Exchange transfusion may be required in asplenic patients with a high proportion of parasitized RBCs.

C. *Epidemic measures:* None.

D. *Disaster implications:* None.

E. *International measures:* None.

BALANTIDIASIS   ICD-9 007.0
(Balantidiosis; Balantidial dysentery)

1. **Identification**—A protozoan infection of the colon characteristically producing diarrhea or dysentery, accompanied by abdominal colic, tenesmus, nausea, and vomiting. Occasionally the dysentery resembles that due to amebiasis with stools containing much blood and mucus but relatively little pus. Peritoneal or urogenital invasion is rare.

Diagnosis is made by identifying the trophozoites or cysts of *Balantidium coli* in fresh feces, or trophozoites in material obtained by sigmoidoscopy.

2. **Infectious agent**—*Balantidium coli,* a large ciliated protozoan.

3. **Occurence**—Worldwide; the incidence of human disease is low. Waterborne epidemics occasionally occur in areas of poor environmental sanitation. Environmental contamination with swine feces may result in a higher incidence.

4. **Reservoir**—Swine, and possibly other animals such as nonhuman primates.

5. **Mode of transmission**—Infection is by ingestion of cysts from feces of infected hosts; in epidemics, mainly by fecally contaminated water. Sporadic transmission is by hand-to-mouth transfer of feces, through contaminated water, or through fecally contaminated food.

6. **Incubation period**—Unknown; may be only a few days.

7. **Period of communicability**—As long as the infection persists.

8. **Susceptibility and resistance**—Man appears to have a high natural resistance. In individuals debilitated from other diseases the infection may be serious and even fatal.

9. **Methods of control**—

A. *Preventive measures:*

   1) Sanitary disposal of feces.
   2) Avoid contact with hog feces.
   3) Protect public water supplies against fecal contamination. Diatomaceous earth filters remove all cysts, but ordinary water chlorination does not destroy cysts. Small quantities of water are best treated by boiling.

4) Educate and supervise foodhandlers via health agencies.
5) Educate the general public in personal hygiene.
6) Fly control; protect foods against fly contamination.

B. *Control of patient, contacts and the immediate environment:*

1) Report to local health authority: Official report not ordinarily justifiable, Class 5 (see Preface).
2) Isolation: None.
3) Concurrent disinfection: Sanitary disposal of feces.
4) Quarantine: None.
5) Immunization of contacts: Not applicable.
6) Investigation of contacts and source of infection: Microscopic examination of feces of household members and suspected contacts. Also investigate contact with hogs.
7) Specific treatment: Tetracyclines eliminate infection; metronidazole (Flagyl®) is also effective.

C. *Epidemic measures:* Any grouping of several cases in an area or institution requires prompt epidemiological investigation, especially of environmental sanitation.

D. *Disaster implications:* None.

E. *International measures:* None.

BARTONELLOSIS   ICD-9 088.0
(Oroya fever, Verruga peruana, Carrion's disease)

1. **Identification**—A bacterial infection with two markedly different clinical forms, a febrile anemia (Oroya fever) and a dermal eruption (verruga peruana). Oroya fever is characterized by irregular fever, severe anemia (macrocytic and usually hypochromic), generalized lymphadenopathy, and often delirium. Verruga peruana has a preeruptive stage characterized by shifting pain in muscles, bones, and joints; the pain, often severe, lasts minutes to several days at any one site. The dermal eruption may be miliary with widely disseminated small hemangioma-like nodules, or nodular with fewer but larger deep-seated lesions, most prominent on the extensor surfaces of the limbs. Individual nodules, particularly near joints, may develop into tumor-like masses with an ulcerated surface. Verruga peruana is often preceded by Oroya fever, with an interval of weeks to months between the two stages. The case fatality rate of untreated Oroya fever ranges from 10 to 40%; death is often

associated with *Salmonella* septicemia. Verruga peruana has a prolonged course but seldom results in death.

Diagnosis is made by demonstration of the infectious agent adherent to or within RBCs during the acute stage, in sections of skin lesions during the eruptive stage, or by blood culture on special media during either stage.

2. Infectious agent—*Bartonella bacilliformis.*

3. Occurrence—Limited to mountain valleys of Peru, Ecuador and southwest Colombia, between altitudes of 2500 to 8000 ft (750 to 2500 m) above sea level where the vector is present; no special predilection for age, race or sex.

4. Reservoir—An infected person with the agent present in the blood. In endemic areas the asymptomatic carrier rate may reach 5%. No known animal reservoir.

5. Mode of transmission—By bite of sandflies of the genus *Phlebotomus;* species not identified for all areas; *Phlebotomus verrucarum* important in Peru. These insects feed only from dusk to dawn. Blood transfusion, particularly during the Oroyo fever stage, may transmit infection.

6. Incubation period—Usually 16–22 days, but occasionally 3–4 months.

7. Period of communicability—Not directly transmitted from person to person, other than by transfused blood. Man is infectious for the sandfly for a long period; the infectious agent may be present in blood weeks before and up to several years after actual illness. Duration of infectivity of the sandfly is unknown.

8. Susceptibility and resistance—Susceptibility is general but the disease is milder in children than in adults. Inapparent infections and carriers are known. Recovery from untreated Oroya fever almost invariably gives permanent immunity to this form; the verruga stage may recur.

9. Methods of control—

    A.   *Preventive measures:*

        1)   Control of sandflies. (See Leishmaniasis, Cutaneous).
        2)   Avoid known endemic areas after sundown; otherwise apply insect repellent to exposed parts of the body.

    B.   *Control of patient, contacts and the immediate environment:*

        1)   Report to local health authority: In selected endemic areas; in most countries not a reportable disease, Class 3B (see Preface).
        2)   Isolation: Blood/body fluid precautions. The infected

individual should be protected from bites of phlebotomines (see 9A, above).

3) Concurrent disinfection: None.
4) Quarantine: None.
5) Immunization of contacts: None.
6) Investigation of contacts and source of infection: Identification of sandflies, particularly in localities where the infected person was exposed after sundown during the preceding 3-8 wks.
7) Specific treatment: Penicillin, streptomycin, chloramphenicol, and tetracyclines are all effective in reducing fever and bacteremia. Chloramphenicol or ampicillin is the drug of choice; they work directly against *Bartonella,* but more importantly also against the frequent secondary salmonellosis.

C. *Epidemic measures:* Intensification of case finding and systematic spraying of houses with a residual insecticide.

D. *Disaster implications:* Only if refugee centers are established in an endemic locus.

E. *International measures:* None.

BLASTOMYCOSIS   ICD-9 116.0
(North American blastomycosis, Gilchrist's disease)

1. Identification—Blastomycosis is a granulomatous mycosis, primarily of the lungs or skin. Pulmonary blastomycosis may be acute or chronic. Acute infection is rarely recognized but presents with the sudden onset of fever, cough and a pulmonary infiltrate on chest x-ray. The pulmonary infiltrate may progress to cavitation and fibrosis. Infection resolves spontaneously after 1–3 weeks of illness. During or after the period of resolving pneumonia, some patients exhibit extrapulmonary infection. An indolent onset evolving into the chronic disease is more common. Cough and chest aching may be mild or absent so that patients may present with infection already spread to other sites, particularly skin, and less often to bone, prostate or epididymis. Skin lesions begin as erythematous papules which become verrucous, crusted or ulcerated. Most commonly, lesions are located on the face and distal extremities. Weight loss, weakness and low-grade fever are often present. The course of untreated disseminated or chronic pulmonary blastomycosis is eventual progression and, usually, death.

Direct microscopic examination of unstained smears of sputum and material from lesions shows characteristic "broad based" budding forms of the fungus, which can be cultured. Serological test results can be misleading because of cross reactions with histoplasmosis; CF tests are often negative in cases with active disease. However, the immunodiffusion test for blastomycosis is specific; positive reactions are indicative of disease.

2. Infectious agent—*Blastomyces dermatitidis (Ajellomyces dermatitidis)*, a dimorphic fungus that grows as a yeast in the tissues and in enriched culture media at 37°C (98.6°F), and as a mold at room temperature (25°C/77°F).

3. Occurrence—Uncommon. Occurs sporadically in central and southeastern USA, Canada, Africa, India, Israel and Saudi Arabia. Rare in children; more frequent in males than in females. Disease in dogs is frequent; it has also been reported in cats, a horse, a captive African lion and a sea lion.

4. Reservoir—Probably soil.

5. Mode of transmission—Conidia, typical of the mold or saprophytic growth form, probably are inhaled in spore-laden dust.

6. Incubation period—Indefinite; probably a few weeks or less to months.

7. Period of communicability—Not transmitted directly from man or animals to man.

8. Susceptibility and resistance—Unknown. Inapparent pulmonary infections are probable but of undetermined frequency. No information on immunity; the rarity of the natural disease and of laboratory-acquired infections suggests man is relatively resistant.

9. Methods of control—

    A. Preventive measures: Unknown.

    B. Control of patient, contacts and the immediate environment:

        1) Report to local health authority: Official report not ordinarily justifiable, Class 5 (see Preface).

        2) Isolation: None.

        3) Concurrent disinfection: Sputum, discharges and all contaminated articles. Terminal cleaning.

        4) Quarantine: None.

        5) Immunization of contacts: None.

        6) Investigation of contacts: Not profitable.

        7) Specific treatment: Amphotericin B (Fungizone®), is the present drug of choice. Ketoconazole appears to be less

effective than amphotericin B but is useful in patients not
severely ill.

C.   *Epidemic measures:* Not applicable, a sporadic disease.

D.   *Disaster implications:* None.

E.   *International measures:* None.

BOTULISM, INFANT   ICD-9 008.49

1. **Identification**—A form of botulism, first recognized as a distinct
clinical entity in 1976; it has been confirmed only in infants under 1 year
of age. Illness typically begins with constipation, followed by lethargy,
listlessness, poor feeding, ptosis, difficulty in swallowing, loss of head
control, hypotonia and generalized weakness (the "floppy" baby), and, in
some cases, respiratory insufficiency and arrest. Infant botulism has a wide
spectrum of clinical severity ranging from mild illness to sudden infant
death; preliminary studies suggest that it causes an estimated 5% of the
cases of Sudden Infant Death Syndrome (SIDS). The case fatality rate of
hospitalized cases in the USA is 3%; without access to hospitals with
pediatric intensive care units, more would die.

In contrast to classical foodborne botulism (see Foodborne Intoxication,
Botulism), which is an intoxication due to ingestion of preformed botulinal
toxin, infant botulism results from colonization of the intestine by the
botulinal bacillus with subsequent in vivo toxin production.

The diagnosis is established by identification of *Clostridium botulinum*
organisms and/or toxin in patients' feces or in autopsy specimens. With few
exceptions, toxin has not been detected in the sera of patients.
Electromyography may be useful in corroborating the clinical diagnosis.

2. **Infectious agent**—*Clostridium botulinum,* a spore-forming obligate
anaerobic bacillus. Of its seven toxigenic types, A-G, most cases of infant
botulism have been caused by types A or B, a few resulted from type F
or type B/F toxin.

3. **Occurrence**—Probably worldwide. As of January 1985, about 500
hospitalized cases have been reported from four continents: Australia,
Europe, and N and S America. The actual incidence and distribution of
infant botulism remains to be determined.

4. **Reservoir**—Spores are ubiquitous in soil; they are frequently
recovered from agricultural products.

5. **Mode of transmission**—By ingestion of botulinal spores. Possible

sources of spores for infants are multiple, including foods and dust. Honey, a food item often fed to infants, frequently contains *C. botulinum* spores.

6. Incubation period—Unknown, since it cannot be determined precisely when the infant ingested the botulinal spores.

7. Period of communicability—Despite excretion of *C. botulinum* toxin and organisms at high levels (ca. 10^6 organisms/g) in patients' feces for weeks to months after onset of illness, no instances of secondary person-to-person transmission have been documented.

8. Susceptibility and resistance—All patients hospitalized to date have been between 2 weeks and 9 months of age; 94% were 6 months of age or less and the median age at onset was 13 weeks. Cases of infant botulism have occurred in all major racial and ethnic groups. Adults with special bowel problems leading to unusual gastrointestinal flora might be susceptible to "infant type" botulism.

9. Methods of control—

A. *Preventive measures: C. botulinum* spores are ubiquitous. However, identified sources such as honey should not be fed to infants.

B. *Control of patient, contacts and the immediate environment:*

1) Report to local health authority: Case report obligatory in order to rule out foodborne botulism, Class 2A (see Preface).

2) Isolation: Not required, but handwashing is indicated after handling soiled diapers.

3) Concurrent disinfection: Of feces and articles soiled therewith. In communities with a modern adequate sewage disposal system, feces can be discharged directly into sewers without preliminary disinfection. Terminal cleaning.

4) Quarantine: None.

5) Immunization of contacts: Not applicable.

6) Investigation of contacts and source of infection: Search for other cases to rule out foodborne botulism.

7) Specific treatment: Meticulous supportive care is essential. Botulinal antitoxin (an equine product) is not used because of the hazard of sensitization and anaphylaxis. The role of antibiotics, if any, has yet to be established.

C. *Epidemic measures:* None.

D. *Disaster implications:* None.

E.   International measures: None.

BRUCELLOSIS   ICD-9 023
(Undulant fever, Malta fever, Mediterranean fever, Bang's disease).

   1. Identification—A systemic bacterial disease with acute or insidious onset, characterized by continued, intermittent or irregular fever of variable duration, headache, weakness, profuse sweating, chills, arthralgia, depression, weight loss and generalized aching. Localized suppurative infections may occur; subclinical and unrecognized infections are frequent. The disease may last for several days, months, or occasionally for a year or more. Orchitis, vertebral osteomyelitis and prepatellar bursitis are characteristic features. Genitourinary involvement is reported in 2-20% of cases, with orchitis and epididymitis most common. The case fatality rate without treatment is <2%; higher for *Brucella melitensis* infections. Recovery is usual but disability is often pronounced. Part or all of the original syndrome may reappear as relapses, especially on re-exposure. A neurotic symptom complex is sometimes attributed to chronic brucellosis.
   Laboratory diagnosis is made by appropriate isolation technique of the infectious agent from blood, bone marrow or other tissues, or from discharges of the patient. Serological tests in experienced laboratories are valuable, especially when paired sera show a rise in antibody titer. Interpretation of serologic tests in chronic and recurrent cases is especially difficult since titers are usually low. Tests measuring IgG antibody may be useful, particularly in chronic cases since active infection is associated with rise in IgG antibody. Specific serologic techniques are needed for *B. canis* antibodies.

   2. Infectious agents—*Brucella abortus,* biotypes 1–7 and 9; *B. melitensis,* biotypes 1–3; *B. suis,* biotypes 1–4; and *B. canis.*

   3. Occurrence—Worldwide, especially in Mediterranean countries of Europe and north and east Africa; India, central Asia, Mexico, Central and S America. The sources of infection and the responsible organism vary according to geographic area. Predominantly an occupational disease of those working with infected animals or their tissues, especially farm workers, veterinarians and abattoir workers, hence more frequent among males. Sporadic cases and outbreaks occur among consumers of unpasteurized milk or milk products (especially cheese) from cows, sheep and goats. Isolated cases of infection with *B. canis* occur in animal handlers from contact with dogs, especially beagles. Reported incidence in the USA is about 150–250 cases annually; worldwide, the disease is often unrecognized and unreported.

4. **Reservoir**—Of human infection in the USA, cattle and swine; goats and sheep outside the USA. May occur in dogs, coyotes and caribou. *B. canis* is a problem in laboratory dog colonies and kennels; a small percentage of pet dogs and a higher proportion of strays have positive *B. canis* antibody titers.

5. **Mode of transmission**—By contact with tissues, blood, urine, vaginal discharges, aborted fetuses and especially placentas (through breaks in the skin), and by ingestion of raw milk or dairy products (cheese) from infected animals. Airborne infection of animals occurs in pens and stables and of man in laboratories and abattoirs. In the USA, approximately 20% of cases have no known animal contact; a small number of cases result from accidental self-inoculation of strain 19 *(Brucella)* vaccine; the same risk is present when Rev-I vaccine is handled.

6. **Incubation period**—Highly variable and difficult to ascertain; usually 5–30 days, occasionally several months.

7. **Period of communicability**—No evidence of communicability from person to person.

8. **Susceptibility and resistance**—Severity and duration of clinical illness are subject to wide variation. Duration of acquired immunity is uncertain.

9. **Methods of control**—Ultimate control of human brucellosis rests on the elimination of the disease among domestic animals.

A. Preventive measures:

1) Educate farmers and workers in slaughter houses, packing plants and butcher shops as to the nature of the disease and the risk in the handling of carcasses or products of potentially infected animals, and the proper operation of abattoirs to reduce exposure.

2) Search for infection among livestock by serological testing and by ring test of cow's milk; eliminate infected animals by segregation and/or slaughter. Infection among swine usually requires slaughter of the herd. Immunize young goats and sheep with live attenuated Rev-I strain of *B. melitensis;* calves and sometimes adult animals with strain 19, *B. abortus;* recommended in areas of high prevalence.

3) Pasteurize milk and dairy products from cows, sheep or goats. Boiling milk is effective when pasteurization is impossible.

4) Educate the public not to drink untreated milk or eat products made from unpasteurized or otherwise untreated milk.

5) Care in handling and disposal of placenta, discharges and fetus from an aborted animal. Disinfect contaminated areas.

B. *Control of patient, contacts and the immediate environment:*

1) Report to local health authority: Case report obligatory in most states and countries, Class 2B (see Preface).
2) Isolation: Draining/secretion precautions if there are draining lesions; otherwise none.
3) Concurrent disinfection: Of purulent discharges.
4) Quarantine: None.
5) Immunization of contacts: None.
6) Investigation of contacts and source of infection: Trace infection to the common or individual source, usually infected domestic goats, swine or cattle, or unpasteurized milk or dairy products from cows and goats. Test suspected animals, remove reactors.
7) Specific treatment: Tetracycline, tetracycline plus streptomycin or other aminoglycosides, TMP-SMX (Bactrim®, Spectra®) and possibly rifampin (RIF) alone or in combination with other antibiotics. Tetracycline should be avoided, if possible, in children less than 7 years old. Tetracycline plus streptomycin is probably associated with fewer relapses and may enhance treatment efficacy in more seriously ill patients or those with abscesses. In severely ill patients, steroids may be administered to decrease systemic toxicity. Relapses occur in about 5% of treated patients and are not due to resistant organisms; they should be retreated with the original regimen. Arthritis may occur in recurrent cases and may benefit from the use of corticosteroids.

C. *Epidemic measures:* Search for common vehicle of infection, usually unpasteurized milk or milk products from an infected herd. Recall incriminated products, stop production and distribution unless pasteurization is instituted.

D. *Disaster Implications:* None.

E. *International measures:* Control of domestic animals and animal products in international trade and transport. WHO Collaborating Centres (see Preface).

CANDIDIASIS   ICD-9 112
(Moniliasis, Thrush, Candidosis)

1. Identification—A mycosis usually confined to the superficial layers of skin or mucous membranes and presenting clinically as oral thrush, intertrigo, vulvovaginitis, paronychia or onychomycosis. Ulcers or pseudomembranes may be formed in the esophagus, gastrointestinal tract or bladder. Hematogenous dissemination may produce lesions in other organs such as kidney, spleen, lung, liver, endocardium, eye, meninges, brain, or around a prosthetic cardiac valve.

Diagnosis requires evaluation of both laboratory and clinical evidence of candidiasis. The single most valuable laboratory test is microscopic demonstration of pseudohyphae and/or yeast cells in infected tissue or fluid. Cultural confirmation is important, but isolation from sputum, bronchial washings, stool, urine, mucosal surfaces, skin or wounds is not proof of a causal relationship to the disease present.

2. Infectious agents—*Candida albicans, C. tropicalis* and occasionally other species of *Candida. Torulopsis (Candida) glabrata* is distinguished from other causes of candidiasis by not forming pseudohyphae in tissue.

3. Occurrence—Worldwide. The fungus *(C. albicans)* is often part of the normal human flora; infection depends on site and also upon many local and systemic factors.

4. Reservoir—Man.

5. Mode of transmission—By contact with excretions of mouth, skin, vagina, and especially feces from patients or carriers; from mother to infant during childbirth; and by endogenous spread. Disseminated candidiasis may originate from mucosal lesions, unsterile narcotic injections, percutaneous intravenous catheters and indwelling catheters in the bladder.

6. Incubation period—Variable, 2–5 days for thrush in infants.

7. Period of communicability—Presumably for duration of lesions.

8. Susceptibility and resistance—The frequent isolation of a *Candida* spp. from sputum, throat, feces or urine in the absence of clinical evidence of infection suggests a low level of pathogenicity or a widespread immunity. Oral thrush is a common, usually benign condition of the first few weeks of life. Clinical disease occurs when host defense is low. Local factors contributing to superficial candidiasis include interdigital intertrigo and paronychia on hands excessively exposed to water as with housewives or bartenders, or intertrigo in moist skin folds of obese individuals. Repeated skin or mucosal eruptions are common. Prominent among systemic factors predisposing to candidiasis are general debilitation, diabetes mellitus, therapy with broad-spectrum antibiotics and supraphysiologic doses of adrenal corticosteroids, parenteral hyperalimentation, and certain immune deficiencies (see AIDS). Most adults and older children have a delayed dermal hypersensitivity to the fungus and possess humoral antibodies.

9. **Methods of control—**

A. *Preventive measures:*

1) Detect and treat vaginal thrush during 3rd trimester of pregnancy to prevent neonatal thrush.
2) To prevent systemic spread, early detection and local treatment of thrush in mouth, esophagus or urinary bladder of those with predisposing systemic factors (8, above).

B. *Control of patient, contacts and the immediate environment:*

1) Report to local health authority: Official report not ordinarily justifiable, Class 5 (see Preface).
2) Isolation: None.
3) Concurrent disinfection: Of secretions and contaminated articles.
4) Quarantine: None.
5) Immunization of contacts: None.
6) Investigation of contacts: Not profitable in sporadic cases.
7) Specific treatment: Ameliorating underlying causes of candidiasis often facilitates cure, e.g., removal of indwelling venous catheters. Topical nystatin is useful in many forms of superficial candidiasis; oral clotrimazole (Mycelex®) troches have been effective for treatment of nystatin-unresponsive oral thrush. Intravenous amphotericin B (Fungizone®) with or without 5-fluorocytosine is the drug of choice for visceral or invasive candidiasis; oral 5-fluorocytosine is a possible alternative in milder cases, provided the isolated organism is susceptible. For persistent recurrence of vaginal thrush, preventive measures include discontinuing antimicrobial therapy, when possible, and oral contraceptives, and treatment of sexual partner(s) with topical nystatin or treatment of presumed bowel reservoir with oral nystatin. Ketoconazole is effective in candidiasis of the skin, mucous membranes or esophagus.

C. *Epidemic measures:* Epidemics are largely limited to thrush in newborn nurseries. Concurrent disinfection and terminal cleaning should be practiced with care comparable to that used for epidemic diarrhea in hospital nurseries (see Diarrhea, I9C).

D. *Disaster implications:* None.

E. *International measures:* None.

CAPILLARIASIS

Three types of nematodes of the superfamily Trichuroidea, genus *Capillaria,* produce disease in man.

I. CAPILLARIASIS DUE TO   ICD-9 127.5 *CAPILLARIA PHILIPPINENSIS* (Intestinal capillariasis)

1. **Identification**—A clinical syndrome first described on Luzon, Philippines, in 1963. Clinically, the disease is an enteropathy with massive protein loss and a malabsorption syndrome which lead to progressive weight loss and extreme emaciation. Fatal cases are characterized by the presence of large numbers of parasites in the small intestine together with ascites and pleural transudate. Case fatality rates of 10% have been reported. Subclinical cases also occur, but usually become symptomatic in time.

Diagnosis is made on clinical findings plus the identification of eggs, or larval or adult parasites in the stool. The eggs resemble those of *Trichuris trichiura.* Jejunal biopsy may reveal the worms in the mucosa.

2. **Infectious agent**—*Capillaria philippinensis.*

3. **Occurrence**—Intestinal capillariasis is endemic in the northern Philippine Islands; it has been found in Thailand and one case has been reported from Japan. It has reached epidemic proportions on Luzon where more than 1,500 cases have been seen. In some villages one-third of the population was found to be infected. Males between the ages of 20 and 45 yrs appear to be particularly at risk.

4. **Reservoir**—Unknown; thought to be aquatic birds. Fish may serve as intermediate hosts.

5. **Mode of transmission**—The life cycle and mode of transmission remain uncertain. Infective larvae develop in the intestine of freshwater fish which ingest eggs; monkeys fed these fish become infected and the parasite matures within the intestine. A history of ingestion of raw or inadequately cooked small fish eaten whole is frequently obtained.

6. Incubation period—Unknown in man; in monkey studies, about a month or more.

7. Period of communicability—Not transmitted directly from person to person.

8. Susceptibility and resistance—Susceptibility appears to be general in those geographic areas in which the parasite is prevalent. Attack rates are often high.

9. Methods of control—

A. Preventive measures:

    1) Uncooked fish should not be eaten in known endemic areas.

    2) Provide adequate facilities for the disposal of feces.

B. Control of patient, contacts and the immediate environment:

    1) Report to local health authority: Case report by most practicable means. Class 3B (see Preface).

    2) Isolation: None.

    3) Concurrent disinfection: None. Sanitary disposal of feces.

    4) Quarantine: None.

    5) Immunization of contacts: None.

    6) Investigation of contacts: Fecal examination of all members of family group and others with common exposure to raw or undercooked fish, with treatment of infected individuals.

    7) Specific treatment: Mebendazole (Vermox®) is the drug of choice. Thiabendazole (Mintezol®) modifies the disease, but prolonged therapy is necessary.

C. Epidemic measures: Prompt investigation of cases and contacts with treatment of cases as indicated. Education on the need to cook all fish.

D. Disaster implications: None.

E. International measures: None.

II. CAPILLARIASIS DUE TO *CAPILLARIA HEPATICA*
(Hepatic capillariasis)

ICD-9 128.8

1. Identification—An uncommon and occasionally fatal disease in humans due to the presence of adult *Capillaria hepatica* in the liver. The picture is that of an acute or subacute hepatitis with marked eosinophilia resembling the picture of visceral larva migrans.

Diagnosis is made by demonstrating eggs or the parasite in a liver biopsy or at necropsy.

2. Infectious agent—*Capillaria hepatica (Hepaticola hepatica).*

3. Occurrence—Since its first recognition in 1924 about 25 cases of human disease have been reported from N America, India, Turkey, Czechoslovakia, Italy, Africa, Hawaii, Mexico and Brazil.

4. Reservoir—Primarily an infection of rats (as many as 86% infected in some reports) and other rodents, but also seen in a large variety of domestic and wild mammals. The adult worms live and produce eggs in the liver.

5. Mode of transmission—The adult worms produce fertilized eggs which remain in the liver until the death of the animal. When infected liver is eaten, the eggs are freed by digestion, reach the soil in the feces and develop to the infective stage in 2 to 4 weeks. When a suitable host ingests these embryonated eggs, they hatch in the intestine, the larvae migrate through the wall of the gut and are transported via the portal system to the liver where they mature and produce eggs. "Spurious infection" of humans may be detected when eggs are found in the stool after infected liver, raw or cooked, has been eaten; since these eggs are not embryonated, infection cannot be established.

6. Incubation period—Three to 4 weeks.

7. Period of communicability—Not directly transmitted from person to person.

8. Susceptibility and resistance—Susceptibility is universal.

9. Methods of control—

  A. Preventive measures:

    1) Avoid ingestion of dirt directly (pica), from contaminated food, water or hands.
    2) Protect water supplies and food from soil contamination.

  B. Control of patient, contacts and the immediate environment:

    1) Report to local health authority: Official report not ordinarily justifiable, Class 5 (see Preface).
    2) Isolation: None.
    3) Concurrent disinfection: None.
    4) Quarantine: None.
    5) Immunization of contacts: None.
    6) Investigation of contacts: Not applicable.

7) Specific treatment: Mebendazole (Vermox®) or thiabendazole (Mintezol®) is probably effective.

C. *Epidemic measures:* Not applicable.

D. *Disaster implications:* None.

E. *International measures:* None.

PULMONARY CAPILLARIASIS ICD-9 128.8

A pulmonary disease manifested by fever, cough and asthmatic breathing, caused by *Capillaria aerophila (Thominx aerophila),* a nematode parasite of cats, dogs and other carnivorous mammals. Pneumonitis may be severe and heavy infections may be fatal. The worms live in tunnels in the epithelial lining of the trachea, bronchi and bronchioles; fertilized eggs are sloughed into the air passages, coughed up, swallowed and discharged from the body in the feces. In the soil, larvae develop in the egg and remain infective for a year or longer. Infection is acquired by humans, mostly children, by ingesting infective eggs in soil or in soil-contaminated food or water. Eggs may appear in the sputum in 4 weeks; symptoms may appear earlier or later. Human cases have been recorded from USSR (8 cases), Morocco and Iran (1 each); animal infection has been reported in N and S America, Europe, Asia and Australia.

CARDITIS, COXSACKIE ICD-9 074.2
(Viral carditis, Enteroviral carditis)

1. Identification—An acute or subacute myocarditis or pericarditis which occurs as the only manifestation, or may occasionally be associated with other manifestations, of infection with enteroviruses, especially Group B coxsackievirus.

The myocardium is particularly affected in neonates, in whom fever and lethargy may be followed rapidly by heart failure with pallor, cyanosis, dyspnea, tachycardia and enlargement of heart and liver. Heart failure may be progressive and fatal, or recovery may take place over a few weeks; some cases run a relapsing course over months and may show residual heart damage. In adults, pericarditis is the most common manifestation with acute chest pain, disturbance of heart rate and rhythm, and often dyspnea. The disease may be associated with epidemic myalgia (see Myalgia, Epidemic).

A similar clinical picture can be produced infrequently by infection with other viral agents. Influenza, mumps, measles, rubella, vaccinia, varicella zoster, smallpox, arboviruses (Colorado tick fever and yellow fever), lymphocytic choriomeningitis virus and echoviruses (types 6, 7, 11 and 22) have been isolated from patients with carditis.

Specific diagnosis is made by isolation of the virus from pericardial fluid, myocardial biopsy, or postmortem heart tissue. Serologic studies and viral isolation from feces can be supportive, but are not conclusive.

2. Infectious agents—Group B coxsackieviruses (types 1–5); occasionally group A coxsackieviruses (types 1, 4, 9, 16, 23) and other enteroviruses.

3. Occurrence—An uncommon disease, mainly sporadic but increased during epidemics of Coxsackie group B virus infection. Institutional outbreaks with high fatality rates in newborns have been described in maternity units.

4. Reservoir, 5. Mode of transmission, 6. Incubation period, 7. Period of communicability, 8. Susceptibility and resistance, and 9. Methods of control—Same as Epidemic Myalgia.

CAT-SCRATCH DISEASE   ICD-9 078.3
(Cat-scratch fever, Benign lymphoreticulosis)

1. Identification—A subacute, self-limited disease characterized by malaise, granulomatous lymphadenitis and variable patterns of fever. It is often preceded by a cat scratch which produces a pustular lesion, followed by involvement of a regional lymph node, usually within 2 weeks, which may progress to suppuration. A red papule usually appears at inoculation site; in most (50-90%) cases an inoculation site is found. Recurrent and chronic forms occur. Complications such as thrombocytopenic purpura, encephalitis, osteolytic lesions, and Parinaud's syndrome have been reported.

Pasteurellosis (ICD-9 027.2), a mixed aerobic and anaerobic bacterial infection including *Pasteurella multocida,* is another condition which may result from cat scratches and animal bites.

Diagnosis is based on a consistent clinical picture and histopathological characteristics of involved lymph nodes. Pus obtained from lymph nodes is bacteriologically sterile. Skin test antigens, derived from infected human lymph nodes, are not recommended for general use because of the danger of transmitting other agents.

2. Infectious agent—Not yet established but pleomorphic gram-negative silver-staining bacilli have been described in involved lymph nodes which may prove to be the etiological agent.

3. **Occurrence**—Worldwide but uncommon. Sexes equally affected; more frequent in children and young adults. Familial clustering occurs. Majority of cases are seen during late summer, fall and winter months.

4. **Reservoir**—Unknown. Cats are carriers; there is no evidence of infection. Dog scratch or bite and monkey scratch prior to the syndrome have been reported.

5. **Mode of transmission**—Most patients (about 90%) give a history of scratch, bite, lick, or other exposure to a healthy cat (often a kitten). Minor trauma by splinters or thorns is suspected as the mode of transmission in the absence of known direct contact with animals.

6. **Incubation period**—Variable, usually 3 to 14 days from inoculation to primary lesion.

7. **Period of communicability**—Unknown. Not directly transmitted from person to person.

8. **Susceptibility and resistance**—Unknown.

9. **Methods of control**—

    A. *Preventive measures:* Thorough cleansing of cat scratches.

    B. *Control of patient, contacts and the immediate environment:*

        1)   Report to local health authority: Official report not ordinarily justifiable, Class 5 (see Preface).
        2)   Isolation: None.
        3)   Concurrent disinfection: Of discharges from purulent lesions.
        4)   Quarantine: 5) Immunization of contacts: 6) Investigation of contacts: 7) Specific treatment: None.

    C. *Epidemic measures:* Not applicable.

    D. *Disaster implications:* None.

    E. *International measures:* None.

CHANCROID   ICD-9 099.0
(Ulcus molle, Soft chancre)

1. **Identification**—An acute bacterial infection localized to the genital area and characterized clinically by single or multiple painful necrotizing ulcers at the site of inoculation, frequently accompanied by painful inflammatory swelling and suppuration of regional lymph nodes. Mini-

mally symptomatic lesions may occur on the vaginal wall or the cervix; asymptomatic infections may occur in women. Extragenital lesions have been reported.

Diagnosis is made by isolation of the organism from lesion exudate on selective media which incorporates vancomycin into chocolate, rabbit or horse blood agar enriched with fetal calf serum.

2. Infectious agent—*Haemophilus ducreyi,* the Ducrey bacillus.

3. Occurrence—More commonly seen in men with no particular differences in incidence according to age or race except as determined by sexual habits. Most common in tropical and subtropical regions of the world where the incidence may be higher than that of syphilis and may approach that of gonorrhea in men. The disease is much less common in temperate zones but may occur in small outbreaks.

4. Reservoir—Infected persons.

5. Mode of transmission—By direct sexual contact with discharges from open lesions and pus from buboes. Indirect transmission is rare. Sexual promiscuity and uncleanliness favor transmission.

6. Incubation period—From 3–5 days, up to 14 days.

7. Period of communicability—As long as the infectious agent persists in the original lesion or discharging regional lymph nodes; usually until healed, in most instances a matter of weeks.

8. Susceptibility and resistance—Susceptibility is general; no evidence of natural resistance.

9. Methods of control—

A. *Preventive measures:* Preventive measures are those of syphilis (q.v.).

B. *Control of patient, contacts and the immediate environment:*

1) Report to local health authority: Case report obligatory in many states and countries, Class 2B (see Preface).
2) Isolation: None; avoid sexual contact until all lesions are healed.
3) Concurrent disinfection: None; stress personal cleanliness.
4) Quarantine: None.
5) Immunization of contacts: None.
6) Investigation of contacts: Search for sexual contacts of 2 weeks before and after onset. Women without visible signs may be carriers. Sexual contacts without signs should receive prophylactic treatment.
7) Specific treatment: Erythromycin 500 mg four times a day

for a minimum of 10 days, or TMP-SMX (80 mg, 400 mg) 2 tablets twice a day for a minimum of 7 days; continue until lesions have resolved. Fluctuant inguinal nodes should be aspirated to prevent spontaneous rupture.

C. **Epidemic measures:** Persisting occurrence or an increased incidence are indications for more rigid application of measures outlined in 9A or 9B, above. When compliance with the treatment schedule (9B7) is a problem, consideration should be given to a single dose of TMP-SMX, (640mg, 3200 mg). Prophylactic therapy to high-risk groups with or without lesions, including prostitutes, clinic patients reporting prostitute contact, and clinic patients with darkfield-negative cultures may be required to control an outbreak.

D. **Disaster implications:** None.

E. **International measures:** See Syphilis, 9E.

CHICKENPOX-HERPES ZOSTER   ICD-9 052 & 053
(Varicella—Shingles)

1. **Identification**—Chickenpox is an acute generalized viral disease with sudden onset of slight fever, mild constitutional symptoms and a skin eruption which is maculopapular for a few hours, vesicular for 3–4 days, and leaves a granular scab. Lesions commonly occur in successive crops, with several stages of maturity present at the same time; they tend to be more abundant on covered than on exposed parts of the body; may appear on scalp, high in the axilla, on mucous membranes of the mouth and upper respiratory tract and on the conjunctiva; they may be so few as to escape observation. Mild, atypical and inapparent infections occur. Occasionally, especially in adults, the fever and constitutional disturbance may be severe. The disease is rarely fatal; the most common cause of death in adults is primary viral pneumonia; among children, it is septic complications and encephalitis. Children with acute leukemia, including those in remission after chemotherapy, are at increased risk of disseminated, fatal disease. Neonates developing varicella between ages 5 and 10 days or those whose mothers develop the disease 5 days prior to or within 2 days after delivery are at increased risk of developing severe generalized chickenpox with up to a 30% mortality rate. Infection early in pregnancy may rarely be associated with congenital malformations. Clinical chickenpox has been a frequent antecedent of Reye syndrome.

Herpes zoster is a local manifestation of recurrent, recrudescent or reactivation infection with the virus which causes chickenpox. Vesicles with an erythematous base are restricted to skin areas supplied by sensory nerves of a single or associated group of dorsal root ganglia. In the immunosuppressed, extensive skin lesions may appear outside the dermatome. Lesions may appear in crops in irregular fashion along nerve pathways, are usually unilateral and are deeper seated and more closely aggregated than chickenpox; histologically they are identical. Severe pain and paresthesia are common. Zoster occurs mainly in older adults although there is some evidence that almost 10% of children being treated for a malignant neoplasm are prone to develop herpes zoster. Intrauterine infection or varicella before 2 years of age is also associated with zoster at an early age. Occasionally a varicelliform eruption follows some days after zoster and rarely a secondary eruption of zoster after chickenpox.

Laboratory tests, such as visualization of the virus by electron microscopy, isolation of virus in tissue culture, or the demonstration of a rise in serum antibodies, are not routinely required but are useful in complicated cases or in epidemiologic studies. Multinucleated giant cells may be detected in Giemsa-stained scrapings of the base of a lesion; these are not found in vaccinia or variola lesions but do occur in herpes simplex lesions.

2. **Infectious agent**—Human (alpha) herpesvirus 3 (varicella-zoster virus, V-Z virus), a member of the *Herpesvirus* group.

3. **Occurrence**—Worldwide. Infection with human (alpha) herpesvirus 3 is nearly universal. In metropolitan communities, about 75% of the population has had chickenpox by age 15 and at least 90% by young adulthood. Zoster occurs more commonly in older people. In temperate zones chickenpox occurs most frequently in winter and early spring.

4. **Reservoir**—Man.

5. **Mode of transmission**—From person to person by direct contact, droplet, or airborne spread of secretions of respiratory tract of chickenpox cases or of the vesicle fluid of patients with herpes zoster. Indirectly through articles freshly soiled by discharges from vesicles and mucous membranes of infected persons. In contrast to vaccinia and variola, scabs from varicella lesions are not infective. Chickenpox is one of the most readily communicable of diseases, especially in the early stages of the eruption; herpes zoster has a much lower rate of transmission (the contact develops chickenpox).

6. **Incubation period**—From 2–3 wks; commonly 13–17 days; may be prolonged after passive immunization against varicella or in the immunodeficient.

7. **Period of communicability**—As long as 5 but usually 1–2 days before onset of rash, and not more than 6 days after the appearance of the first crop of vesicles. Contagiousness may be prolonged in patients with

altered immunity. Patients with herpes zoster may be sources of infection for a week after the appearance of their vesiculopustular lesions.

8. Susceptibility and resistance—Susceptibility to chickenpox is universal among those not previously infected; ordinarily a more severe disease of adults than of children. One infection confers long immunity; second attacks are rare. Infection apparently remains latent and may recur years later as herpes zoster in a proportion of older adults, sometimes in children.

Neonates whose mothers are not immune, and patients with leukemia may suffer severe, prolonged or fatal chickenpox. Adults with cancer, especially of lymphoid tissue, with or without steroid therapy, immunodeficient patients and those on immunosuppressive therapy, may have an increased frequency of severe zoster, both localized and disseminated.

9. Methods of control—

A. *Preventive measures:*

    1) Protect high-risk individuals such as nonimmune neonates and the immunodeficient from exposure.

    2) Varicella-Zoster Immune Globulin (VZIG) prepared from the plasma of normal blood donors with high antibody titer to varicella-zoster virus is effective in modifying or preventing disease if given within 96 hours after exposure. (See 9B5, below).

    3) A live attenuated varicella virus vaccine has been shown to protect children with leukemia exposed to siblings with chickenpox. An efficacy trial of this vaccine among normal children has shown a very high level of protection.

B. *Control of patient, contacts and the immediate environment:*

    1) Report to local health authority: In many states and countries, not a reportable disease; Class 3C (see Preface).

    2) Isolation: Exclusion from school for 1 week after eruption first appears or until vesicles become dry; avoid contact with susceptibles. In the hospital, strict isolation is appropriate because of the risk of serious varicella in immunocompromised susceptible patients.

    3) Concurrent disinfection: Articles soiled by discharges from the nose and throat and from lesions.

    4) Quarantine: Usually none. However, in a hospital where susceptible children with known recent exposure must remain for medical reasons, the risk of spread to steroid-treated or immunologically compromised patients may justify quarantine of known contacts for a period of from

7–21 days after exposure (up to 28 days if VZIG had been given).

5) Protection of contacts: VZIG given within 96 hours of exposure may prevent or modify disease in close contacts of cases. VZIG is available from regional offices of the American Red Cross for certain high-risk individuals exposed to chickenpox. It is indicated for newborns of mothers who develop chickenpox within 5 days prior to or within 48 hours after delivery. There is no evidence that administration of VZIG to a pregnant woman will prevent fetal infection.

6) Investigation of contacts: Of no practical importance.

7) Specific treatment: Vidarabine (Ara-A®, Vira-A®) is effective against herpes zoster if begun within 72 hours of onset in the immunocompromised patient. Acyclovir (Zovirax®) is also effective against herpes zoster.

C. **Epidemic measures:** None.

D. **Disaster implications:** Outbreaks of chickenpox may occur among children when crowded together in emergency housing situations.

E. **International measures:** None.

CHLAMYDIAL INFECTIONS

As laboratory techniques improve, the chlamydial organisms are increasingly implicated as causes of human disease. These obligate intracellular parasites, which differ from viruses and from rickettsiae but, like the latter, are sensitive to broad-spectrum antibiotics, are classified into two species: *Chlamydia psittaci,* the etiologic agent of psittacosis (q.v.), and *C. trachomatis,* including several serotypes which cause trachoma (q.v.), genital infections, chlamydial conjunctivitis (q.v.) and infant pneumonia (q.v.); others cause lymphogranuloma venereum (q.v.). Chlamydiae are now recognized as important pathogens responsible for an increasingly recognized number of sexually transmitted infections, with eye and lung infections the consequences of genital infections.

GENITAL INFECTIONS, CHLAMYDIAL   ICD-9 099.8

1. **Identification**—Sexually transmitted genital infections, manifested in males primarily as a urethritis and in females by mucopurulent cervicitis.

Clinical manifestations of urethritis are usually indistinguishable from gonorrhea and include an opaque discharge of moderate or scanty quantity, urethral itching, and burning on urination. Asymptomatic infection of men occurs; infection may be found in 1–10% of sexually active men. Possible sequelae of urethral infection include epididymitis, male infertility and Reiter's syndrome.

In the female the clinical manifestations are similar to those of gonorrhea and will present most characteristically as a mucopurulent cervicitis with papillary hypertrophy of the cervical mucosa. Complications or sequelae are salpingitis with subsequent risk of infertility or ectopic pregnancy. Less frequent manifestations are bartholinitis, urethral syndrome and perihepatitis (Fitz-Hugh-Curtis syndrome). Infection frequently is asymptomatic. Infection during pregnancy may result in conjunctival or pneumonic infection of the offspring. It is not yet clear whether these infections contribute significantly to low birth weight, prematurity, or postpartum endometritis.

Infection may be acquired concurrently with gonorrhea and persist after the gonorrhea has been successfully treated with penicillin. Because gonococcal and chlamydial cervicitis are often difficult to distinguish clinically, treatment for both organisms is recommended when one is suspected.

Diagnosis of nongonococcal urethritis (NGU) or cervicitis is usually based on the failure to demonstrate *Neisseria gonorrheae* by smear and culture; chlamydial etiology is confirmed by examination of intraurethral or endocervical swab material by micro-IF with monoclonal antibody, enzyme immunoassay, or by cell culture. The intracellular organisms are rarely recoverable from the discharge itself. For other agents, see Urethritis, Nongonococcal, below.

2. Infectious agent—*Chlamydia trachomatis*, immunotypes D to K, has been identified in approximately 35–50% of cases of NGU in the USA.

3. Occurrence—Common worldwide; in the USA, Canada, Australia and Europe recognition has increased steadily in the last 2 decades.

4. Reservoir—Man.

5. Mode of transmission—Sexual contact.

6. Incubation period—Five to 10 days or longer.

7. Period of communicability—Unknown. Relapses are probably common.

8. Susceptibility and resistance—Susceptibility is general. No acquired immunity has been demonstrated.

9. Methods of control—

A. *Preventive measures:* Health and sex education. Same as for syphilis (q.v.) with emphasis on use of a condom in sexual contacts.

B. *Control of patient, contacts and the immediate environment:*

1) Report to local health authority: Not now a reportable disease in the USA, Class 5 (see Preface).

2) Isolation: Drainage/secretion precautions for hospitalized patients. Appropriate antibiotic therapy renders discharges noninfectious.

3) Concurrent disinfection: Care in disposal of articles contaminated with urethral discharges.

4) Quarantine: None.

5) Immunization of contacts: Not applicable.

6) Investigation of contacts: Prophylactic treatment of sexual contacts is recommended. As a minimum, concurrent treatment of regular consorts is a practical approach to management. If neonates had not been given systemic treatment, chest x-ray at 3 wks is advisable to exclude subclinical chlamydial pneumonia.

7) Specific treatment: Tetracycline, 2 g/d for 7–10 days or doxycycline, 100 mg twice a day for 14 days. Erythromycin is an alternative drug and is the drug of choice when pregnancy is known or suspected, given in the same dosage and duration as tetracycline. Test of cure at conclusion of therapy is desirable if facilities exist.

C. *Epidemic measures:* None.

D. *Disaster implications:* None.

E. *International measures:* None.

URETHRITIS, NONGONOCOCCAL AND NONSPECIFIC   ICD-9 099.4
(NGU, NSU)

While chlamydiae are the most frequently isolated etiological agents in cases of gonococcus-negative urethritis, other agents are involved in a significant number of cases. *Ureaplasma urealyticum* is considered the etiological agent in approximately 10–40% of NGU cases; *Herpesvirus* type 2 and *Trichomonas vaginalis* have rarely been implicated. Because of the scarcity of laboratory facilities for demonstration of chlamydia, all cases of NGU (together with their sexual contacts) are best handled as though their infections are chlamydial, especially since many chlamydia-negative cases respond to the antibiotic therapy.

CHOLERA   ICD-9 001

1. Identification—An acute bacterial enteric disease with sudden onset, profuse watery stools, occasional vomiting, rapid dehydration, acidosis and circulatory collapse. Asymptomatic infection is much more frequent than clinical illness, especially with organisms of the El Tor biotype. Mild cases with only diarrhea are common, particularly among children. In severe untreated cases, death may occur within a few hours and the case fatality rate may exceed 50%; with proper treatment, the rate is below 1%.

Diagnosis is confirmed by culturing cholera vibrios of the serogroup 01 from feces. Visualization by darkfield or phase microscopy of the characteristic vibrio motility which is inhibited by preservative-free specific antiserum, or demonstration of a significant rise in titer of antitoxic antibodies, or of agglutinating or vibriocidal antibodies (provided vaccine has not been given) help in presumptive diagnosis. In newly infected areas, the isolated organisms should be confirmed by appropriate biochemical reactions and, if possible, by testing whether the organisms produce toxin.

2. Infectious agent—*Vibrio cholerae* serovar 01, which includes the serologically indistinguishable classical and El Tor biotypes and of either Inaba or Ogawa serotypes. The same enterotoxin is elaborated by these organisms so that the clinical pictures are similar. In any single epidemic one particular type tends to be dominant; presently the El Tor biotype is predominant, except for Bangladesh, where the classical biotype has reappeared. Rare isolations have been made of serovar O1 organisms which do not elaborate the known enterotoxin. *V. mimicus* is a closely related species which can cause diarrhea; strains from some cases elaborate an enterotoxin indistinguishable from that produced by *V. cholerae* while others do not.

Vibrios that are biochemically indistinguishable but do not agglutinate in vibrio group O1 antiserum, formerly known as non-agglutinable vibrios (NAGs) or as non-cholera vibrios (NCVs) are now included in the species *V. cholerae*. Some strains elaborate the enterotoxin but most do not. Non-01 strains have caused sporadic cases and limited outbreaks of diarrheal disease, but have not been associated with large epidemics or pandemics. In the USA, most sporadic cases follow eating raw or inadequately cooked seafood. The reporting of non-O1 *V. cholerae* infections as cholera is inaccurate and leads to confusion.

3. Occurrence—During the 19th century pandemic cholera repeatedly spread from India to most of the world. During the first half of the 20th century the disease was confined largely to Asia except for a severe epidemic in Egypt in 1947.

Since 1961, cholera has spread from Indonesia through most of Asia into eastern Europe and Africa and from north Africa to the Iberian Peninsula and into Italy in 1973. In 1977 and l978 there were small outbreaks in Japan and, for the first time, cholera occurred in the S Pacific. Disease has continued in Africa, with 13 countries reporting disease in 1983. In Asia, 11 countries reported cholera and the classical biotype predominated in Bangladesh; large outbreaks occurred in the Truk Islands in 1982 and 1983.

Except for 2 laboratory-acquired cases there was no known indigenous cholera in the Western Hemisphere between 1911 and 1973, when a case occurred in Texas with no known source. In 1978, there were sporadic *V. cholerae* 01 infections in Louisiana with 8 cases and 3 asymptomatic infections, and in 1981 an outbreak involving 16 persons occurred on a Texas floating oil rig. Indigenous cases have occurred in Queensland, Australia. Sporadic imported cases have continued to occur among travelers returning to western Europe, Canada, the USA and Australia.

4. **Reservoir**—Man; recent observations in the USA and Australia suggest presence of environmental reservoirs.

5. **Mode of transmission**—Primarily through ingestion of water contaminated with feces or vomitus of patients, or, to a lesser extent, feces of carriers; or ingestion of food which had been contaminated by dirty water, feces, soiled hands, or flies. El Tor organisms can persist in water for long periods. Raw or undercooked seafoods from polluted waters caused outbreaks or epidemics in Guam, Portugal, and Kiribati. The Louisiana outbreak was traced to eating home-prepared crabs taken from lake and estuary waters contaminated with *V. cholerae,* serotype Inaba.

6. **Incubation period**—From a few hours to 5 days, usually 2–3 days.

7. **Period of communicability**—Presumably for the duration of the stool-positive stage, usually only a few days after recovery. However, the carrier state may persist for several months. Effective antibiotics, e.g., tetracycline, shorten the period of communicability. Chronic biliary infection, lasting for years, has been observed in adults, associated with intermittent shedding of vibrios in the stool.

8. **Susceptibility and resistance**—Variable; gastric achlorhydria increases risk of disease. Clinical cholera usually is confined to the lowest socioeconomic groups. Even in severe epidemics attack rates rarely exceed 2%. Infection results in a rise in agglutinating, vibriocidal and antitoxic antibodies and increased resistance to reinfection which lasts longer against the homologous serotype. In endemic areas, most persons acquire antibodies by early adulthood.

9. Methods of control—

A. *Preventive measures:*

1) See Typhoid Fever, 9A1 through 9A6.
2) Active immunization with present vaccine is of no practical value in epidemic control or in management of contacts of cases. Whole cell vaccines have been shown to provide partial protection (50%) of short duration (3–6 months) in highly endemic areas and does not prevent asymptomatic infection. It is not ordinarily recommended; other vaccines are under study.
3) Measures that inhibit or otherwise compromise the movement of people, foods, or other goods are not justified unless specifically indicated on epidemiologic grounds.

B. *Control of patient, contacts and the immediate environment:*

1) Report to local health authority: Case report universally required by International Health Regulations (1969), Third Annotated Edition, 1983, WHO, Geneva; Class 1 (see Preface).
2) Isolation: Hospitalization with enteric precautions is desirable for severely ill patients; strict isolation is not necessary. Less severe cases can be managed on an outpatient basis with oral rehydration. Crowded cholera wards can be operated without hazard to staff and visitors when effective handwashing and basic procedures of cleanliness are practiced. Fly control should be practiced.
3) Concurrent disinfection: Of feces and vomitus and of linens and articles used by patients; by heat, carbolic acid or other disinfectant. In communities with a modern and adequate sewage disposal system, feces can be discharged directly into the sewers without preliminary disinfection. Terminal cleaning.
4) Quarantine: None.
5) Management of contacts: Surveillance of contacts for 5 days from last exposure. Mass chemoprophylaxis is not helpful, but for household contacts, chemoprophylaxis with tetracycline (1 g/d for 5 days in adults and 50 mg/kg/d for children) is recommended. Doxycycline (single dose of 200 mg for adults and 4–6 mg/kg for children) or furazolidone (Furoxone®) (100 mg every 6 hours for 3 days for adults and 5 mg/kg/d for children) may also be used. Immunization of contacts is not indicated.
6) Investigation of contacts and source of infection: Investigate possibilities of infection from polluted drinking water

or from contaminated food. A search by stool culture for unreported cases is recommended only among contacts or those exposed to a possible common source in a previously uninfected area.

7) Specific treatment: Prompt fluid therapy using adequate volumes of electrolyte solutions to correct dehydration, acidosis and hypokalemia is essential. For most patients, this can be achieved by use of an oral solution containing glucose (20 g/l) or sucrose (40 g/l), sodium chloride (3.5 g/l), sodium bicarbonate (2.5 g/l) or trisodium citrate dihydrate (2.9 g/l), and potassium chloride (1.5 g/l) in a volume matching the estimated fluid loss—5% of body weight for mild and 7% for moderate dehydration. For patients in shock, isotonic i.v. fluids are given as rapidly as possible; these should contain 25–48 meq/l of bicarbonate, acetate or lactate ions and 10–15 meq/l of K^+, such as Dacca solution (5 g NaCl, 4 g $NaHCO_3$, and 1 g KCl/l), or Ringer's lactate; the WHO "diarrhea treatment solution" (4 g NaCl, 1 g KCl, 6.5 g sodium acetate or 5.4 g sodium lactate, and 8 g glucose/l) is the preferred solution. After effective circulation has been restored by the i.v. fluids, the oral solution is used to complete rehydration (about 10% of body weight) and to maintain fluid and electrolyte balance. Tetracycline and other antimicrobial agents shorten the duration of the diarrhea and reduce the fluid loss, as well as shortening the duration of vibrio excretion.

C. *Epidemic measures:*

1) Provide effective treatment facilities.
2) Adopt emergency measures to assure a safe water supply; boil water used for drinking, cooking, or for washing dishes or food containers unless the water supply is adequately chlorinated and is protected from contamination thereafter.
3) Provide appropriate safe facilities for sewage disposal.
4) Initiate a thorough investigation designed to find the vehicle and circumstances (time, place, person) of transmission and plan control measures accordingly.
5) Assure careful supervision of food and drink. After cooking or boiling, protect against contamination by flies and unsanitary handling.
6) Control flies by limiting fly breeding, by appropriate insecticides and by screening kitchens and eating places. (See Typhoid Fever 9A3).

7) Vaccine is inappropriate in the epidemic situation.

D. *Disaster implications:* Risk of outbreaks is high in areas where cholera is endemic if large groups of people are crowded together without adequate sanitary facilities.

E. *International measures:*

1) Telegraphic notification by governments to WHO and to adjacent countries of the first imported, first transferred or first nonimported case of cholera in an area previously free of the disease.

2) Measures applicable to ships, aircraft and land transport arriving from cholera areas are specified in International Health Regulations (1969), Third Annotated Edition, 1983, WHO, Geneva.

3) International travelers: Immunization is not recommended by WHO for travel from country to country in any part of the world and is not required by the USA. However, a few countries continue to require vaccinations and vaccination certificates. International Health Regulations state that "a person on an international voyage, who has come from an infected area within the incubation period of cholera and who has symptoms indicative of cholera, may be required to submit to stool examination."

4) WHO Collaborating Centres (see Preface).

CHROMOMYCOSIS   ICD-9 117.2
(Chromoblastomycosis, Dermatitis verrucosa)

1. **Identification**—A chronic spreading mycosis of the skin and subcutaneous tissues, usually of a lower extremity. Progression to contiguous tissues is slow, over a period of years, with eventual large verrucous or even cauliflower-like masses and lymphatic stasis. Rarely a cause of death. Hematogenous spread to the brain has been reported.

Microscopic examination of scrapings or biopsies from lesions reveals characteristic brown thick-walled, rounded cells that divide by fission in two planes. Confirmation of the diagnosis should be made by biopsy, and cultures of the fungus attempted.

2. **Infectious agents**—*Phialophora verrucosa, Fonsecaea (Rhinocladiella, Phialophora) pedrosoi, F. compacta, Cladosporium carrionii,* and *Rhinocladiella aquaspersa.*

3. Occurrence—Worldwide; sporadic cases in widely scattered areas, but mainly Central America, Caribbean Islands, southern USA, S America, S Pacific Islands, Australia, Malagasy and Africa. Primarily a disease of rural barefooted agricultural workers in tropical regions, probably because of more frequent penetrating wounds of feet and limbs not protected by shoes or clothing. The disease is most common in men aged 30 to 50 yrs; women are rarely infected.

4. Reservoir—Wood, soil, and decaying vegetation.

5. Mode of transmission—Minor penetrating trauma, usually a sliver with contaminated wood or other materials.

6. Incubation period—Unknown; probably months.

7. Period of communicability—Not transmitted from person to person.

8. Susceptibility and resistance—Unknown, but rarity of disease and absence of laboratory-acquired infections suggest that man is relatively resistant.

9. Methods of control—

  A. *Preventive measures:* Protect against small puncture wounds by wearing shoes or protective clothing.

  B. *Control of patient, contacts, and the immediate environment:*

  1) Report to local health authority: Official report not ordinarily justifiable, Class 5 (see Preface).
  2) Isolation: None.
  3) Concurrent disinfection: Of discharges from lesions and articles soiled therewith.
  4) Quarantine: None.
  5) Immunization of contacts: Not applicable.
  6) Investigation of contacts: Not indicated.
  7) Specific treatment: Oral 5-fluorocytosine benefits most patients and cures some. Large lesions respond better when 5-fluorocytosine is combined with i.v. amphotericin B (Fungizone®). Oral ketoconazole may cause some improvement. Small lesions are sometimes cured by excision.

  C. *Epidemic measures:* Not applicable, a sporadic disease.

  D. *Disaster implications:* None.

  E. *International measures:* None.

CLONORCHIASIS
(Chinese or Oriental liver fluke disease)

ICD-9 121.1

1. Identification—A trematode disease of the bile ducts. Clinical complaints may be slight or absent in light infections. Symptoms result from local irritation of bile ducts by the flukes. Loss of appetite, diarrhea, and a sensation of abdominal pressure are common early symptoms. Bile duct obstruction, rarely producing jaundice, may be followed by cirrhosis, enlargement and tenderness of the liver and progressive ascites and edema. A chronic disease, sometimes of 30 years or longer duration, but not often a direct or contributing cause of death except possibly by association with cholangiocarcinoma, and often completely asymptomatic.

Diagnosis is made by finding the characteristic eggs in feces or duodenal drainage fluid; to be differentiated from those of other flukes.

2. Infectious agent—*Clonorchis sinensis,* the Chinese liver fluke.

3. Occurrence—Highly endemic in southeast China, but present throughout the country except in the northwest; occurs in Japan, Taiwan, S Korea and Vietnam, principally in the Red River delta. In other parts of the world imported cases may be recognized in immigrants from Asia. In endemic areas highest prevalence is at age 55–60 yrs.

4. Reservoir—Man, cat, dog, swine and other animals.

5. Mode of transmission—Man is infected by eating raw or undercooked freshwater fish, containing encysted larvae. During digestion, larvae are freed from cysts, and migrate via the common bile duct to biliary radicles. Eggs deposited in the bile passage are evacuated in feces. Eggs in feces contain a fully developed miracidium; when ingested by a susceptible operculate snail (i.e., *Bulimus, Semisculcospira,* etc.), they hatch in its intestine, penetrate the tissues and asexually generate larvae (cercariae) that emerge into the water. On contact with a second intermediate host (about 80 species of freshwater fish, belonging mostly to the family Cyprinidae), cercariae penetrate the host fish and encyst, usually in muscle, occasionally on the underside of scales. The complete life cycle, from person to snail to fish to person, requires at least 3 months.

6. Incubation period—Unpredictable, varies with the number of worms present; flukes reach maturity within 1 month after encysted larvae are ingested.

7. Period of communicability—Infected individuals may pass viable eggs for as long as 30 years. Not directly transmitted from person to person.

8. Susceptibility and resistance—Susceptibility is universal.

9. Methods of control—

A. Preventive measures:

1) Thorough cooking, freezing at −10°C (14°F) for at least 5 days, or storage for several weeks in a saturated salt solution for all freshwater fish.

2) In endemic areas, educate the public to the dangers of eating raw or improperly treated fish and the necessity for sanitary disposal of feces to avoid contaminating sources of food fish. Prohibit use of nightsoil in fishponds.

B. Control of patient, contacts and the immediate environment:

1) Report to local health authority: Official report not ordinarily justifiable, Class 5 (see Preface).

2) Isolation: None.

3) Concurrent disinfection: Sanitary disposal of feces.

4) Quarantine: None.

5) Immunization of contacts: Not applicable.

6) Investigation of contacts and source of infection: Of the individual case, not usually indicated. A community problem (see 9C, below).

7) Specific treatment: The drug of choice is praziquantel (Biltricide®).

C. Epidemic measures: Locate source of infected fish. Shipments of dried or pickled fish are the likely source in nonendemic areas.

D. Disaster implications: None.

E. International measures: Control of fish or fish products imported from endemic areas.

OPISTHORCHIASIS   ICD-9 121.0

Opisthorchiasis is caused by small liver flukes of cats and some other fish-eating mammals. *Opisthorchis felineus* occurs in Europe and Asia, and *O. viverrini* is endemic in SE Asia, especially Thailand. The biology of these flatworms, the characteristics of the disease and methods of control are essentially the same as those of clonorchiasis, given above. Eggs cannot be distinguished from those of *Clonorchis*.

COCCIDIOIDOMYCOSIS   ICD-9 114
(Valley fever, Desert fever, Desert rheumatism, Coccidioidal granuloma)

1. **Identification**—A systemic mycosis which begins as a respiratory infection. The primary infection may be entirely asymptomatic or resemble an acute influenzal illness with fever, chills, cough and pleural pain. About

one-fifth of clinically recognized cases (an estimated 5% of all primary infections) develop erythema nodosum, most frequently in white females and rarest in black males. Primary infection may heal completely without detectable residuals, or may leave fibrosis, calcification of pulmonary lesions, a persistent thin-walled cavity, or, most rarely, progress to the disseminated form of the disease.

Disseminated coccidioidomycosis is a progressive, frequently fatal but uncommon granulomatous disease characterized by lung lesions and abscesses throughout the body, especially in subcutaneous tissues, skin, bone, peritoneum, testes, thyroid and CNS. Coccidioidal meningitis resembles tuberculous meningitis but runs a more chronic course. An estimated 1:1000 cases of symptomatic coccidioidomycosis become disseminated. Dissemination is more common during pregnancy and in blacks and Filipinos.

Diagnosis is made preferably by demonstrating the fungus by microscopic examination or by culture of sputum, pus, urine or CSF. A positive skin test to coccidioidin or spherulin appears from 2-3 days to 3 weeks after onset of symptoms. Precipitin and CF tests are usually positive within the first 3 months of clinical disease. Serial skin and serological tests may be necessary to confirm a recent infection or indicate dissemination; skin tests are often negative in disseminated disease and serological tests may be negative in the immunocompromised.

2. Infectious agent—*Coccidioides immitis,* a dimorphic fungus. It grows in soil and in culture media as a saprophytic mold that reproduces by arthroconidia; the parasitic form in tissues and under special conditions of culture grows as spherical cells (spherules) which reproduce by endospore formation.

3. Occurrence—Primary infections are common in scattered highly endemic arid and semiarid areas of the Western Hemisphere: in USA, from California to south Texas; in northern Argentina, Paraguay, Colombia, Venezuela, Mexico, and Central America. Elsewhere dusty fomites from endemic areas can transmit infection; disease has occurred in persons who have merely traveled through endemic areas. The disease affects all ages, both sexes and all races. Infection is most frequent in summer, especially after wind and dust storms. It is an important disease among migrant workers, archeologists and military personnel from nonendemic areas who move into endemic areas.

4. Reservoir—Soil; especially in and around Indian middens and rodent burrows, in regions with appropriate temperature, moisture and soil requirements; infects man, cattle, cats, dogs, horses, burros, sheep, swine, wild desert rodents, coyotes, chinchillas, llamas, and other animal species.

5. Mode of transmission—Inhalation of the infective arthroconidia from soil and in laboratory accidents from cultures. While the parasitic form is normally not infective, accidental inoculation of infected pus or culture suspension into the skin or bone can result in granuloma formation.

6. Incubation period—One to 4 weeks in primary infection. Dissemination may develop insidiously, sometimes without recognized symptoms of primary pulmonary infection.

7. Period of communicability—Not directly transmitted from man or animal to man. *C. immitis* on casts or dressings may rarely change from the parasitic to the infective saprophytic form after 7 days.

8. Susceptibility and resistance—A general susceptibility to primary infection is indicated by the high prevalence of positive coccidioidin or spherulin reactors in endemic areas; recovery is generally followed by solid, lifelong immunity. More than half of patients with symptomatic infection are between 15 and 25 years of age; males are affected much more frequently than females, probably because of occupational exposure. Susceptibility to dissemination is 10 times greater in blacks and Filipinos.

9. Methods of control—

    A.   *Preventive measures:*

        1)   In endemic areas, plant grass, oil unpaved airfields and other dust control measures.

        2)   Individuals from nonendemic areas should preferably not be recruited to dusty occupations, such as road building. Skin testing could be used to screen out susceptibles.

    B.   *Control of patient, contacts and the immediate environment:*

        1)   Report to local health authority: Case report of recognized cases, especially outbreaks, in selected endemic areas (USA); in many countries not a reportable disease, Class 3B (see Preface).

        2)   Isolation: None.

        3)   Concurrent disinfection: Of discharges and soiled articles. Terminal cleaning.

        4)   Quarantine: None.

        5)   Immunization of contacts: None.

        6)   Investigation of contacts: Not recommended except in cases appearing in nonendemic areas, where residence, work exposure and travel history should be obtained.

        7)   Specific treatment: Amphotericin B (Fungizone®) is sometimes beneficial in severe or disseminated infections. Ketoconazole has been useful in chronic, nonmeningeal coccidioidomycosis.

    C.   *Epidemic measures:* Epidemics occur only when groups of susceptibles are infected by airborne conidia. Dust control measures should be instituted where practicable (see 9A1, above).

    D.   *Disaster implications:* Possible hazard if large groups of susceptibles are forced to move through or to live under dusty conditions in areas where the fungus is prevalent.

E.   International measures: None.

CONJUNCTIVITIS
I. CONJUNCTIVITIS, ACUTE
BACTERIAL
(Pink-eye)

ICD-9 372.03

1. **Identification**—A clinical syndrome beginning with lacrimation, irritation and hyperemia of the palpebral and bulbar conjunctivae of one or both eyes, followed by edema of lids, photophobia, and mucopurulent discharge. In severe cases, ecchymoses of bulbar conjunctiva and marginal infiltration in the cornea may occur. A nonfatal disease, the clinical course may last for 2 to 3 weeks; many patients have no more than hyperemia of the conjunctivae and slight exudate for a few days.

Confirmation of clinical diagnosis by microscopic examination of a stained smear of discharge or bacteriologic culture is required to differentiate from allergic conjunctivitis or infection by adenovirus or echovirus; inclusion conjunctivitis, trachoma, and gonococcal conjunctivitis are described separately.

2. **Infectious agents**—*Haemophilus aegyptius* (Koch-Weeks bacillus) and *Streptococcus pneumoniae* appear to be the most important; *H. influenzae* serotype b, *Moraxella lacunata,* staphylococci, streptococci, *Pseudomonas aeruginosa* and *Corynebacterium diphtheriae* may produce the disease. A gram-negative diplococcus resembling the gonococcus is responsible for epidemics with much loss of sight among young children in north Africa and the Middle East.

3. **Occurrence**—Widespread and common throughout the world, particularly in warmer climates; frequently epidemic. In the USA, infection with *H. aegyptius* is largely confined to southern rural areas extending from Georgia to California, primarily during summer and early autumn; in north Africa and the Middle East, it occurs as seasonal epidemics. Infection with other organisms occurs throughout the world, often in association with acute viral respiratory disease during cold seasons.

4. **Reservoir**—Man. Carriers of *H. aegyptius* are common in many areas during interepidemic periods.

5. **Mode of transmission**—Contact with discharges from the conjunctivae or upper respiratory tract of infected persons through contaminated fingers, clothing, or other articles, including shared eye makeup applicators, multiple dose eye medications and inadequately sterilized instruments such as tonometers. May be mechanically transmitted by eye gnats or flies in some areas, but their importance as vectors is undetermined and probably differs from area to area.

6. **Incubation period**—Usually 24 to 72 hours.

7. **Period of communicability**—During the course of active infection.

8. **Susceptibility and resistance**—Children under 5 are most often affected; incidence decreases with age. The very young, the debilitated and the aged are particularly susceptible to staphylococcal infections. Immunity after attack is low-grade and varies with the infectious agent.

9. Methods of control—

A.   *Preventive measures:* Personal hygiene, hygienic care and treatment of affected eyes.

B.   *Control of patient, contacts and the immediate environment:*

   1)   Report to local health authority: Obligatory report of epidemics; no case report, Class 4 (see Preface).

   2)   Isolation: Drainage/secretion precautions. Children should not attend school during the acute stage.

   3)   Concurrent disinfection: Of discharges and soiled articles. Terminal cleaning.

   4)   Quarantine: None.

   5)   Immunization of contacts: None.

   6)   Investigation of contacts: Usually not profitable.

   7)   Specific treatment: Local application of an ointment or drops containing tetracycline, erythromycin, chloramphenicol, gentamicin or a sulfonamide such as sodium sulfacetamide, depending on the infecting organism.

C.   *Epidemic measures:*

   1)   Prompt and adequate treatment of patients and their close contacts.

   2)   In areas where insects are suspected of mechanically transmitting infection, measures to prevent access of eye gnats or flies to eyes of sick and well persons.

   3)   Insect control, according to the suspected vector.

D.   *Disaster implications:* None.

E.   *International measures:* None.

II. CONJUNCTIVITIS, ADENOVIRVAL   ICD-9 077.2
CONJUNCTIVITIS, ENTEROVIRAL   ICD-9 077.4
HEMORRHAGIC
(Apollo 11 disease, Acute hemorrhagic conjunctivitis (AHC))

1. **Identification**—A viral infection with sudden onset of pain or the sensation of a foreign body in the eye. The disease progresses rapidly (1–2 days) to the full clinical picture of swollen eyelids, hyperemia of the conjunctivae, often with a circumcorneal distribution, seromucous dis-

charge and frequent subconjunctival hemorrhages. Epithelial punctate keratitis and anterior uveitis may be present. Both eyes are almost always involved and the hemorrhages, which commence in the region of the upper fornix, may vary in size from petechiae to large ecchymoses. Preauricular adenopathy is frequently present. Few patients experience systemic symptoms, most commonly those of an upper respiratory infection. The disease is self-limited with the ocular signs and symptoms resolving in 1–2 weeks.

Polio-like paralysis, including cranial nerve palsies, lumbosacral radiculomyelitis and lower motor neuron paralysis, commencing a few days to a month after the conjunctivitis and commonly leaving some residual weakness, has been observed in a small number of patients in large outbreaks of AHC.

Laboratory confirmation of the diagnosis is made by demonstrating a rise in neutralizing antibodies to one of the causal viruses, by isolation of the virus from conjunctival swabs or scrapings, or by detection by IF of viral antigens in conjunctival swabs or scrapings.

2. Infectious agents—Picornaviruses and adenoviruses. Several serologically distinct types have been found in association with epidemics. The most prevalent picornavirus type has been designated as enterovirus 70. A variant of coxsackievirus, particularly A24, has also caused outbreaks. Adenovirus types 3, 7, 8, 11, 19 and 37 have been associated with cases and outbreaks of AHC; Ad 11 is the one most commonly associated with AHC.

3. Occurrence—Since first recognized in Ghana in 1969 and Indonesia in 1970, a pandemic occurred in 1980–82 with spread to many tropical areas of Asia, Africa, Central and S America, the Pacific Islands, as well as parts of Florida and Mexico. Smaller outbreaks have occurred in some European countries usually associated with eye clinics. No cases have, as yet, been reported from Australia. Cases also have occurred among SE Asian refugees arriving in the USA and travelers returning to the USA from areas with AHC epidemics.

4. Reservoir—Man.

5. Mode of transmission—By direct or indirect contact with discharge from infected eyes. Person-to-person transmission is most noticeable in families, where high attack rates often occur. Large epidemics have been associated with overcrowding and low standards of hygiene.

6. Incubation period—Twelve hours to 3 days.

7. Period of communicability—Unknown, but assumed to be for the period of active disease, usually about 1 week.

8. Susceptibility and resistance—Infection can occur at all ages. Reinfections and/or relapses have been reported. The role and duration of the immune response is not yet clear.

9. Methods of control—

    A. Preventive measures: Personal hygiene; avoid overcrowding. Strict asepsis in eye clinics.

B. *Control of patient, contacts and the immediate environment:*

1) Report to local health authority: Obligatory report of epidemics; no case report, Class 4 (see Preface).
2) Isolation: Drainage/secretion precautions; desirable to restrict contact with cases while disease is active, e.g., children should not attend school.
3) Concurrent disinfection: Of conjunctival discharges and articles soiled by them. Terminal cleaning.
4) Quarantine: None.
5) Immunization of contacts: None.
6) Investigation of contacts: Locate other cases.
7) Specific treatment: None.

C. *Epidemic measures:*

1) Organize adequate facilities for the diagnosis and symptomatic treatment of cases.
2) Improve standard of hygiene and limit overcrowding wherever possible.

D. *Disaster implications:* None.

E. *International measures:* WHO Collaborating Centres (see Preface).

III. CONJUNCTIVITIS, CHLAMYDIAL   ICD-9 077.0
(Inclusion conjunctivitis, Paratrachoma, Swimming pool conjunctivitis, Neonatal inclusion blennorrhea, "Sticky eye")

1. Identification—In the newborn, an acute papillary conjunctivitis with abundant mucopurulent discharge; the acute state usually subsides spontaneously in a few weeks but disease of the eye may persist for as long as a year and may result in sequelae of mild scarring of the conjunctivae and infiltration of the cornea (micropannus). Chlamydial pneumonia (see Pneumonia, Chlamydial) will occur in some infants with concurrent nasopharyngeal infection. In children and adults, an acute follicular conjunctivitis is seen with preauricular lymphadenopathy, often with superficial corneal involvement. In adults there may also be a chronic phase with minimal discharge and symptoms which sometimes persist for a year or longer. The agent may infect the urethral epithelium in men and the cervix in women and is sometimes associated with a urethritis or cervicitis.

Neonatal inclusion conjunctivitis can often be distinguished clinically from more serious gonococcal ophthalmia neonatorum (see Gonococcal Infections) by the latter's usually shorter incubation period (1–5 days).

Laboratory confirmation is made by the demonstration of typical intracytoplasmic inclusion bodies in the epithelial cells of Giemsa-stained conjunctival or genital scrapings, by specific IF staining, or by isolation of the agent in cell culture.

2. Infectious agent—*Chlamydia trachomatis* of serovars B and D through K, excluding serovars causing lymphogranuloma venereum.

3. Occurrence—Sporadic eye cases are reported throughout the world in sexually active adults. Neonatal conjunctivitis due to *C. trachomatis* is extremely common, occurring, for example, in 2–5% of newborns in the USA.

4. Reservoir—Man.

5. Mode of transmission—The agent is transmitted during sexual intercourse; the genital discharges of infected persons are infectious. Eye infection in the newborn is by direct contact with infected birth passages. Adults become infected by the transmission of genital secretions to the eye, usually by the fingers. Outbreaks have been reported among swimmers in nonchlorinated pools presumably contaminated with genitourinary exudates. Eye-to-eye transmission may occur rarely.

6. Incubation period—Five to 12 days.

7. Period of communicability—While genital or ocular infection persists.

8. Susceptibility and resistance—There is no evidence of resistance to reinfection with the inclusion conjunctivitis agent although the severity of the disease may be decreased.

9. Methods of control—

- **A.** *Preventive measures:* Difficult to apply in view of the frequently clinically inapparent nature of the genital infections.
  1) General preventive measures are those for the venereal diseases (see Syphilis, 9A).
  2) Change to erythromycin or tetracycline ophthalmic ointments in the eyes of the newborn recommended for routine prophylaxis for gonoccocal ophthalmia neonatorum since silver nitrate or penicillin is ineffective against chlamydia.
  3) Treatment of cervical infection in pregnant women will prevent subsequent transmission to the infant. Erythromycin 250 mg four times daily for 14 days is effective.

- **B.** *Control of patient, contacts and the immediate environment:*
  1) Report to local health authority: Case report of neonatal cases obligatory in most states and many countries, Class 2B (see Preface).
  2) Isolation: Drainage/secretion precautions for the first 48 hours after starting treatment.
  3) Concurrent disinfection: Aseptic techniques and hand-washing by personnel appear to be adequate to prevent nursery transmission.
  4) Quarantine: None.
  5) Immunization of contacts: Not applicable.
  6) Investigation of contacts: All sexual consorts of adult cases

and of mothers and fathers of neonatally infected infants should be examined and treated. Since infection is common in sexually active adults with multiple contacts, they should be investigated for gonorrhea and syphilis at the same time.

7) Specific treatment: For ocular infections the tetracyclines, erythromycin or sulfonamides are effective given by mouth for 2–3 wks. Local application of chemotherapeutic agents to the eye is relatively ineffective in adults. Treatment of neonatal infection by topical tetracycline, erythromycin or sulfonamides is usually effective, but oral treatment with erythromycin 50 mg/kg/d in 4 doses for 2 wks is more reliable and eliminates the risk of chlamydial pneumonia.

C. *Epidemic measures:* Sanitary control of swimming pools; ordinary chlorination suffices. Individuals contaminating swimming pools are difficult to trace.

D. *Disaster implications:* None.

E. *International measures:* WHO Collaborating Centres (see Preface).

COXSACKIE VIRUS DISEASES ICD-9 074

The coxsackieviruses are the causal agents of a group of diseases discussed here and also epidemic myalgia, coxsackie carditis, epidemic hemorrhagic conjunctivitis, and meningitis. (See each disease under its individual listing). There is evidence suggesting their involvement in the etiology of juvenile-onset insulin-dependent diabetes.

ENTEROVIRAL VESICULAR PHARYNGITIS ICD-9 074.0
(Herpangina, Aphthous pharyngitis)
ENTEROVIRAL VESICULAR STOMATITIS WITH EXANTHEM ICD-9 074.3
(Hand, foot, and mouth disease)
ENTEROVIRAL LYMPHONODULAR PHARYNGITIS ICD-9 074.8
(Acute lymphonodular pharyngitis, Vesicular pharyngitis, Vesicular stomatitis with exanthem)

1. **Indentification**—Vesicular pharyngitis (herpangina) is an acute, self-limited, viral disease characterized by sudden onset, fever, sore throat, and small (1–2 mm) discrete, grayish papulovesicular pharyngeal lesions on an erythematous base which gradually progress to slightly larger ulcers.

These lesions, which usually occur on the anterior pillars of the tonsillar fauces, soft palate, uvula and tonsils, may be present for 4 to 6 days after the onset of illness. No fatalities reported. In one series febrile convulsions occurred in 5% of cases.

Vesicular stomatitis with exanthem differs from vesicular pharyngitis in that oral lesions are more diffuse and may occur on the buccal surfaces of the cheeks and gums and on the sides of the tongue. Papulovesicular lesions which may persist from 7 to 10 days also occur commonly as an exanthem, especially on the palms, fingers and soles; occasionally maculopapular lesions appear on the buttocks. Although usually self-limited, rare cases in infants have been fatal.

Acute lymphonodular pharyngitis also differs from vesicular pharyngitis in that the lesions are firm, raised, discrete, whitish to yellowish nodules surrounded by a 3 to 6 mm zone of erythema. They occur predominantly on the uvula, anterior tonsillar pillars and posterior pharynx, with no exanthem.

Stomatitis due to herpes simplex virus requires differentiation; it has larger, deeper, more painful ulcerative lesions commonly located in the front of the mouth. These diseases are not to be confused with vesicular stomatitis caused by the vesicular stomatitis virus, normally of cattle and horses, which in man usually occurs in dairy workers, animal husbandmen and veterinarians. Foot-and-mouth disease of cattle, sheep and swine rarely affects man except for laboratory workers handling the virus; however, man can be a mechanical carrier of the virus and the source of animal outbreaks.

Differentiation of the related but distinct Coxsackie syndromes is facilitated during epidemics. Virus may be isolated from lesions and nasopharyngeal and stool specimens in suckling mice and/or tissue culture. Serologic and virologic diagnostic procedures are not routinely available unless virus is isolated to use in the serological tests.

2. Infectious agent—Coxsackievirus, Group A: types 1–6, 8, 10 and 22 for vesicular pharyngitis; type 16 predominantly and types 4, 5, 9 and 10 less often for vesicular stomatitis; and type 10 for acute lymphonodular pharyngitis. Other enteroviruses have occasionally been associated with these diseases.

3. Occurrence—Probably worldwide for vesicular pharyngitis and vesicular stomatitis, both sporadically and in epidemics; greatest incidence is in summer and early autumn; occurs mainly in children under 10 years, but adult cases are not unusual. Isolated outbreaks of acute lymphonodular pharyngitis, predominantly in children, may occur in summer and early fall. These diseases frequently occur in outbreaks among groups of children in nursery schools, childcare centers, etc.

4. Reservoir—Man and domestic animals including dogs and swine.

5. Mode of transmission—Direct contact with nose and throat discharges and feces of infected persons (who may be asymptomatic) and by aerosol droplet spread; no reliable evidence of spread by insects, water, food or sewage.

6. Incubation period—Usually 3 to 5 days for vesicular pharyngitis and vesicular stomatitis; 5 days for acute lymphonodular pharyngitis.

7. Period of communicability—During the acute stage of illness and perhaps longer, since these viruses persist in stools for several weeks.

8. Susceptibility and resistance—Susceptibility to infection is universal. Immunity to the specific etiologic virus is probably acquired by clinical or inapparent infection; duration unknown. Second attacks may occur with Group A coxsackievirus of a different immunological type.

9. Methods of control—

A.   *Preventive measures:* Reduce person-to-person contact, where practicable, by measures such as crowd reduction and ventilation.

B.   *Control of patient, contacts and the immediate environment:*

1)   Report to local health authority: Obligatory report of epidemics; no case report, Class 4 (see Preface).
2)   Isolation: Enteric precautions.
3)   Concurrent disinfection: Of nose and throat discharges. Articles soiled therewith should be washed or discarded. Careful attention should be given to prompt handwashing when handling discharges, feces and articles soiled therewith.
4)   Quarantine: None.
5)   Immunization of contacts: None.
6)   Investigation of contacts and source of infection: Of no practical value except to detect other cases in groups of preschool children.
7)   Specific treatment: None.

C.   *Epidemic measures:* General notice to physicians of increased incidence of the disease, together with a description of onset and clinical characteristics. Isolation of diagnosed cases and all children with fever, pending diagnosis, with special attention to respiratory secretions and feces.

D.   *Disaster implications:* None.

E.   *International measures:* WHO Collaborating Centres (see Preface).

CRYPTOCOCCOSIS ICD-9 117.5
(Torulosis, European blastomycosis)

1. **Identification**—A mycosis usually presenting as a subacute or chronic meningitis. Infection of lung, kidney, prostate, bone or liver may occur. The skin may show acneiform lesions, ulcers or subcutaneous tumor-like masses. Occasionally, *Cryptococcus neoformans* may act as an endobronchial saprophyte in patients with lung disease of other origin. Untreated meningitis terminates fatally within several months.

Diagnosis of cryptococcal meningitis is aided by microscopic examination of CSF mixed with India ink. Urine or pus also may contain encapsulated budding forms. Serologic tests for antigen in serum and CSF are often helpful. Diagnosis is confirmed by histopathology or by culture (media containing cycloheximide inhibit *C. neoformans* and should not be used).

2. **Infectious agent**—*Cryptococcus neoformans (Filobasidiella neoformans)*.

3. **Occurrence**—Sporadic cases occur in all parts of the world. Males are infected twice as frequently as females, mainly adults. Infection also occurs in cats, dogs, horses, cows, monkeys and other animals.

4. **Reservoir**—Saprophytic growth in the external environment. The infectious agent can be isolated consistently from old pigeon nests and pigeon droppings and from soil in many parts of the world.

5. **Mode of transmission**—Presumably by inhalation.

6. **Incubation Period**—Unknown. Pulmonary disease may precede brain infection by months or years.

7. **Period of communicability**—Not transmitted directly from person to person, or between animals and man.

8. **Susceptibility and resistance**—All races are susceptible; however, the frequency of *C. neoformans* in the external environment and the rarity of disease suggest that man has appreciable resistance. Susceptibility is increased during corticosteroid therapy, immune deficiency disorders (especially AIDS), and in disorders of the reticuloendothelial system, particularly Hodgkin's disease and sarcoidosis.

9. **Methods of control**—

    A.   *Preventive measures:* While there have been no case clusters traced to exposure to pigeon droppings, the ubiquity of *C. neoformans* in weathered pigeon droppings suggests that removal of large accumulations should be preceded by a chemical decontamination, such as by an iodophor or 5% formalin.

    B.   *Control of patient, contacts and the immediate environment:*

1) Report to local health authority: Official report required in some jurisdictions because of possible manifestation of AIDS. Class 2A (see Preface).
2) Isolation: None.
3) Concurrent disinfection: Of discharges and contaminated dressings. Terminal cleaning.
4) Quarantine: None.
5) Immunization of contacts: None.
6) Investigation of contacts and source of infection: To exclude AIDS or other immunodeficiency as correct concurrent diagnosis.
7) Specific treatment: Amphotericin B (Fungizone®) given i.v. is effective in many cases; 5-fluorocytosine is less effective alone, but is useful in combination with low dose amphotericin B. For meningeal infection, the combination is the therapy of choice.

C. *Epidemic measures:* None.

D. *Disaster implications:* None.

E. *International measures:* None.

CRYPTOSPORIDIOSIS   ICD-9 136.8

1. **Identification**—A parasitic infection principally of the intestinal epithelium, but also may extend to the epithelium of the biliary ducts and gallbladder, and to the respiratory tract in immunodeficient individuals. Usual symptom is watery or mucoid diarrhea lasting 3 to more than 14 days, with vomiting, anorexia and abdominal pain; cough and abnormal chest x-rays occur in patients with pulmonary infections. Infection may be asymptomatic; if symptomatic, the range is from mild to severe, prolonged diarrhea with striking weight loss even in immunocompetent individuals.

Diagnosis is made by identification of oocysts in fecal smears or of the parasites by intestinal biopsy. Oocysts are very small (4–6 μ) and stain with Giemsa and acid-fast stains, best after concentration by a flotation technique. Infection with this organism has not been recognized unless looked for specifically.

2. **Infectious agent**—*Cryptosporidium* spp., a coccidian protozoan.

3. **Occurrence**—Unknown. Isolated reports of cryptosporidiosis from Africa, Australia, Dominican Republic, Europe and the USA suggest that the infection is probably worldwide. Experience in the UK suggests

sporadic endemic infection, especially of children, with localized outbreaks; both rural (zoonotic) and urban (nonzoonotic) patterns occur. Outbreaks in day-care settings have been reported from Pennsylvania, Michigan, Georgia, Minnesota, New Mexico and California in late 1984.

4. **Reservoir**—Cattle, and other domestic and wild animals.

5. **Mode of transmission**—Fecal-oral. Little is known about the likelihood of transmission by fecally contaminated water or food. The parasite rests on the surface of the intestinal cell multiplying by schizogony; development of gametocytes among these surface forms results in resistant and long-lived oocysts which pass out in the feces. Animal handlers are at a high risk of exposure.

6. **Incubation period**—Not precisely known; probably about 10 days.

7. **Period of communicability**—Oocysts, the infectious stage, appear in the stool at the onset of symptoms and can persist for several weeks after symptoms resolve; outside the body in a moist environment they may remain infective for 2–6 months.

8. **Susceptibility and resistance**—People with intact immune function may have asymptomatic or self-limited symptomatic infections. In one study in Australia, the parasite was present in 4% of gastroenteritis patients who were otherwise healthy; in the UK, it was found in 2%. Individuals with impaired immunity, especially those with acquired immune deficiency syndrome (see AIDS), may have severe diarrhea lasting several months; in one study 26% of AIDS patients suffered from cryptosporidial diarrhea.

9. **Methods of control—**

   A. *Preventive measures:*

   1) Education in personal hygiene.
   2) Sanitary disposal of feces and care in handling animal excreta.
   3) Careful handwashing of those in contact with calves or other animals with diarrhea (scours).

   B. *Control of patient, contacts, and the immediate environment:*

   1) Report to local health authority: Case report by most practicable means, Class 3B (see Preface).
   2) Isolation: For hospitalized patients, enteric precautions in the handling of feces, vomit and contaminated clothing and bed linen. Exclusion of symptomatic individuals from foodhandling and from direct care of hospitalized and institutionalized patients. Release to return to work in a sensitive occupation when asymptomatic. Stress proper handwashing.

3) Concurrent disinfection: Of feces and articles soiled therewith. In communities with modern and adequate sewage disposal system, feces can be discharged directly into sewers without preliminary disinfection. Terminal cleaning.

4) Quarantine: None.

5) Immunization of contacts: None.

6) Investigation of contacts and sources of infection: Microscopic examination of feces of household members and other suspected contacts, especially those who are symptomatic.

7) Specific treatment: No treatment has been proven to be effective. Spiramycin may be effective in some cases. If the individual is taking immunosuppressive drugs, these should be stopped if possible.

C. *Epidemic measures:* Epidemiological investigation of clustered cases in an area or institution to determine source of infection and mode of transmission; a common vehicle, such as water or raw milk, should be sought; institute applicable prevention or control measures. Control of person-to-person transmission requires special emphasis on personal cleanliness and sanitary disposal of feces.

D. *Disaster implications:* None.

E. *International measures:* None.

CYTOMEGALOVIRUS INFECTIONS

Infection with cytomegalovirus (CMV) rarely produces symptomatic disease; when it does, the manifestations vary depending on the age and immunocompetence of the individual at the time of infection.

NEONATAL CYTOMEGALOVIRUS INFECTION   ICD-9 771.1
CYTOMEGALOVIRAL DISEASE   ICD-9 078.5

1. Identification—The most severe form of disease occurs in the perinatal period, following congenital or acquired infection, with signs and symptoms of severe generalized infection, especially involving the CNS and liver. Lethargy, convulsions, jaundice, petechiae, purpura, hepatosplenomegaly, chorioretinitis, intracerebral calcifications, and pulmo-

nary infiltrates occur in varying degrees. Survivors may exhibit mental retardation, microcephaly, motor disabilities, hearing loss, and evidence of chronic liver disease. Death may occur in utero; neonatal case fatality rate is high for severely affected infants. Although neonatal CMV infection occurs in 0.3–1% of births, most of these are inapparent; however, about 10% of asymptomatic congenital infections eventually manifest some degree of neurosensory disability.

Infection acquired later in life is generally inapparent, but may cause a syndrome clinically and hematologically like mononucleosis but distinguishable from EBV mononucleosis by the absence of heterophile antibodies or by virologic or serologic tests. CMV causes up to 10% of all cases of "mononucleosis" seen among university students or hospitalized adults in the age group 25 to 35 yrs. A similar syndrome may follow blood transfusion, although many post-transfusion infections are clinically inapparent. Disseminated infection with pneumonitis and hepatitis occurs in immunodeficient or immunosuppressed patients; this is a serious manifestation of AIDS.

Diagnosis is based on isolation of the virus from urine, saliva, cervical secretions, semen, breast milk, or tissue in human fibroblast cell cultures, by demonstration of typical "cytomegalic" cells in sediments of body fluids or in organs, and by significant rises in serum antibody titers.

2. **Infectious agent**—Human (beta) herpesvirus 5 (human cytomegalovirus), a member of the betaherpesvirus subfamily of the family herpesviridae; includes several antigenically related strains.

3. **Occurrence**—Worldwide. Infection is acquired early in developing countries. The prevalence of serum antibodies in adults varies from 40% in highly developed areas to almost 100% in developing countries; it is inversely related to socioeconomic status within the USA and is higher in women than in men. In UK, prevalence of antibodies is related to race rather than to social class. In various population groups, from 8–60% of infants begin shedding virus in the urine during their 1st year of life.

4. **Reservoir**—Man is the only known reservoir of human CMV; strains found in many animal species are not infectious for man.

5. **Mode of transmission**—Intimate exposure by cutaneous or mucosal contact with infectious tissues, secretions or excretions. CMV is excreted in urine, saliva, breast milk, cervical secretions, and semen during primary or reactivated infection. The fetus may be infected in utero from either a primary or reactivated maternal infection; serious fetal infection with manifest disease at birth occurs most commonly during a mother's primary infection, but infection (usually without disease) may develop even when maternal antibody existed prior to conception. Postnatal infection occurs more commonly in infants born of mothers shedding CMV in cervical secretions at delivery; thus transmission of the virus from the infected

cervix at delivery is a common means of infection in early life. Virus can be transmitted to infants through infected breast milk, an important source of infection. Viremia may be present in asymptomatic persons and the virus may be transmitted by blood transfusion, probably associated with leukocytes. CMV is the most common cause of post-transfusion mononucleosis.

6. Incubation period—Information is inexact. Illness following transfusion with infected blood begins 3-8 wks following the transfusion. Infections acquired during birth are first demonstrable 3-12 wks after delivery.

7. Period of communicability—Virus is excreted in urine or saliva for many months and may persist or be episodic for several years following primary infection. After neonatal infection, virus may be excreted for 5–6 yrs. Adults appear to excrete virus for shorter periods, but the virus persists as a latent infection. Under 3% of healthy adults are pharyngeal excretors. Excretion recurs with immunodeficiency and immunosuppression.

8. Susceptibility and resistance—Infection is nearly universal. Fetuses, patients with debilitating diseases, those on immunosuppressive drugs, and especially organ allograft recipients (kidney, heart, bone marrow) are more susceptible to overt and severe disease.

9. Methods of control—

A. Preventive measures:

1) Care in handling diapers, and handwashing after diaper changes or toilet care; avoid kissing infected infants.

2) Women of childbearing age who work in hospitals (especially delivery and pediatric wards) and in preschools (especially those with mentally retarded populations) should observe strict standard measures of hygiene such as handwashing.

3) Wet-nurses for babies born of mothers known to be antibody-free should be checked serologically to assure freedom from infection.

4) Avoid transfusing neonates of seronegative mothers with blood from a seropositive donor.

5) Avoid transplanting organ tissues from a seropositive donor to a seronegative recipient.

B. Control of patient, contacts and the immediate environment:

1) Report to local health authority: Official report not ordinarily justifiable, Class 5 (see Preface).

2) Isolation: None. Secretion precautions may be applied

while in the hospital for patients known to be excreting virus.

3) Concurrent disinfection: Discharges from hospitalized patients and articles soiled therewith.
4) Quarantine: None.
5) Immunization of contacts: None available.
6) Investigation of contacts and source of infection: None, because of the high prevalence of asymptomatic shedders in the population.
7) Specific treatment: None.

C. *Epidemic measures:* None.

D. *Disaster implications:* None.

E. *International measures:* None.

DENGUE FEVER
(Breakbone fever)

ICD-9 061

1. **Identification**—An acute febrile disease characterized by sudden onset, fever for about 5 days and rarely more than 7 and sometimes diphasic, intense headache, retro-orbital pains, joint and muscle pains, and rash. Early general erythema occurs in some cases. A rash usually appears 3–4 days after onset of fever and is either maculopapular or scarlatiniform. Petechiae may appear on the feet or legs, in the axillae, or on the palate on the last day of fever or shortly thereafter. Dark-skinned races frequently have no visible rash. Recovery may be associated with prolonged fatigue and depression. Leukopenia, thrombocytopenia and lymphadenopathy are usual. Epidemics are explosive but the fatality rate is exceedingly low. Dengue with hemorrhagic manifestations is presented below.

Differential diagnosis includes all diseases listed under Arthropod-borne viral fevers, including Colorado tick fever, the sandfly fevers; influenza, rubella, and others.

HI, CF, ELISA and neutralization tests are diagnostic aids. Virus is isolated from blood by inoculation of mosquitoes, or by mosquito or vertebrate cell culture techniques, then identified with type-specific monoclonal antibodies.

2. **Infectious agent**—The viruses of dengue fever include immunological types 1, 2, 3, and 4; they are flaviviruses. The same viruses are responsible for dengue hemorrhagic fever, below.

3. **Occurrence**—Dengue viruses are now endemic in most countries of

tropical Asia (Sri Lanka, India, Bangladesh, Burma, Thailand, Laos, Cambodia, Vietnam, Malaysia, Singapore, Indonesia, New Guinea and the Philippines), northern Australia, and west Africa. Since 1971, epidemics of dengue fever have involved much of Polynesia and more recently, Micronesia; it appears to be endemic in Tahiti. Type 2 dengue virus is endemic on several islands of the Caribbean and in several Central and S American countries; in 1977–1978, an epidemic of type 1 virus occurred throughout the Caribbean and Central America extending into Mexico and the Rio Grande Valley in 1980. In 1981, dengue type 4 was introduced into the Caribbean and an epidemic of type 2 in Cuba caused about 400,000 cases and 158 deaths from dengue hemorrhagic fever with shock. During 1983, dengue was reported from 22 states in Mexico, as well as from El Salvador and Honduras; types 1, 2 and 4 have been involved. Epidemics can occur wherever vectors are present and virus is introduced, whether in urban or rural areas.

4. Reservoir—Man, together with the mosquito, is one; the monkey-mosquito complex may be a reservoir in western Malaysia and west Africa. Dengue virus may be transmitted transovarially at a low rate.

5. Mode of transmission—By the bite of infective mosquitoes, *Aedes aegypti, Ae. albopictus,* or one of the *Ae. scutellaris* complex, which had been infected by biting an infectious human. In Malaysia, *Ae. niveus* complex and in west Africa, *Ae. furcifer-taylori* complex mosquitoes are involved in enzootic monkey-mosquito transmission.

6. Incubation period—Three to 15 days, commonly 5–6 days.

7. Period of communicability—Not directly transmitted from person to person. Patients are usually infective for mosquitoes from the day before onset to the 5th day of disease. The mosquito becomes infective 8–11 days after the blood meal and remains so for life.

8. Susceptibility and resistance—Susceptibility is apparently universal, but children usually have a milder disease than adults. Homologous immunity is of long duration; heterologous immunity, though present, is brief and may permit mild, undiagnosed febrile illness.

9. Methods of control—

    A. Preventive measures:

        1) Community survey to determine density of vector mosquitoes, to identify breeding places, and to promote and implement plans for their elimination.

        2) Educate the public on personal measures for protection against mosquitoes, including use of repellents, air conditioning and bed nets (see Malaria, 9A3 and 9A4).

B. *Control of patient, contacts and the immediate environment:*

1) Report to local health authority: Obligatory report of epidemics; no case report, Class 4 (see Preface).
2) Isolation: Blood/body fluid precautions. Prevent access of mosquitoes to patients for at least 5 days after onset by screening the sickroom or by spraying quarters with a residual insecticide, or by a bed net.
3) Concurrent disinfection: None.
4) Quarantine: None.
5) Immunization of contacts: None. If dengue occurs near possible jungle foci of yellow fever, immunize the population for yellow fever because the urban vector for the two diseases is the same.
6) Investigation of contacts: Determine place of residence of patient during the fortnight before onset and search for unreported or undiagnosed cases.
7) Specific treatment: None.

C. *Epidemic measures:*

1) Search for and destroy *Aedes* species of mosquitoes in places of human habitation and eliminate man-made breeding sites.
2) Use mosquito repellents for persons exposed through occupation to bites of vector mosquitoes.
3) Fogging or airplane spraying with suitable insecticides have shown promise for aborting epidemics.

D. *Disaster implications:* None.

E. *International measures:* Enforce international agreements designed to prevent spread of the disease by man, monkey, and mosquito and transfer via ships, airplanes and land transport from areas where infection exists. WHO Collaborating Centres (see Preface).

DENGUE HEMORRHAGIC FEVER   ICD-9 065.4
CHIKUNGUNYA HEMORRHAGIC   ICD-9 065.4
FEVER

1. **Identification**—A severe illness endemic in most of tropical Asia, characterized by abnormal vascular permeability, hypovolemia and abnormal blood clotting mechanism(s). Recognized principally in children although adults are affected in some outbreaks. Sudden onset of high fever is accompanied by anorexia, vomiting, headache and abdominal pain. Hemorrhagic phenomena are seen frequently and include a positive

tourniquet test, easy bruisability, bleeding at venipuncture sites, a fine petechial rash, epistaxis, or gum bleeding. Gastrointestinal hemorrhage is infrequent and more usually follows a period of uncontrolled shock. The liver may be enlarged during the febrile stage which lasts 2–7 days. In some patients, after a few days of fever, their condition suddenly deteriorates with signs of circulatory failure such as cool, blotchy skin, circumoral cyanosis, rapid pulse and, in severe cases, hypotension or abnormally narrow pulse pressure, i.e., the dengue shock syndrome. In all cases, platelet counts are abnormally low; in severe cases there is an elevated hematocrit, low serum albumin, elevated transaminases, a prolonged prothrombin time and low levels of C3 complement protein. The fatality rate of cases with shock is as high as 40–50% in untreated cases; with good hospital care and fluid therapy, rates are usually <5%.

Infection with these viruses without hemorrhagic manifestations is covered above. Yellow fever, also a hemorrhagic fever, is presented separately.

Serologic tests show a rise in titer against dengue viruses, usually of the anamnestic (secondary) type (IgG) or against chikungunya virus. Primary-type antibody responses have been reported in a few cases. Virus can be isolated from blood during the acute febrile stage by inoculation of mosquitoes or tissue culture. Isolation from organs at autopsy is possible by mosquito inoculation.

2. Infectious agent—Dengue virus, types 1, 2, 3 and 4—flaviviruses. Most shock cases are seen during the second of sequential dengue infections. Chikungunya virus, an alphavirus, has been responsible for some mild cases with hemorrhagic manifestations (not hypovolemia) in Bangkok, and for some severe hemorrhagic cases in Calcutta.

3. Occurrence—Outbreaks have occurred in the Philippines, Burma, Thailand, Indonesia, Malaysia, Singapore, Vietnam, Sri Lanka, India, the S Pacific and Cuba. During 1981 in Cuba, 158 deaths occurred among 400,000 cases of type 2 dengue four years following introduction into the Caribbean of type 1 virus; one-third of the deaths occurred among those under 15 years old. Dengue hemorrhagic fever is observed almost exclusively among indigenous members of the population. Occurrence is limited to rainy seasons and areas of high *Aedes aegypti* prevalence.

4. Reservoir—Man and *Aedes aegypti.*

5. Mode of transmission—By bite of an infective *Ae. aegypti* mosquito. Viruses have been isolated from this mosquito during epidemics. Other *Aedes*, especially *Ae. albopictus*, may also be involved.

6. Incubation period—Unknown.

7. Period of communicability—No evidence of transmission from person to person.

8. Susceptibility and resistance—Pathogenesis of the hemorrhagic complication is best explained by immune enhancement of infection following sensitization of hosts to previous dengue infections; it may also relate to enhanced virulence of a particular strain, or to unusual genetic susceptibility of hosts. Modal age of attack in epidemics thus far recognized is about 3–5 yrs, with a range from 4 months to the young adult years. Prevalence of dengue antibodies in the general population is high in older children and in adults.

9. Methods of control—

A. Preventive Measures: See Dengue fever, above.

B. Control of patient, contacts and immediate environment:

1) to 6) See Dengue fever, above.

7) Specific treatment: Hypovolemic shock resulting from plasma loss from an acute increase in vascular permeability often responds to oxygen therapy and rapid replacement with fluid and electrolyte solution (lactated Ringer's solution at 10–20 ml/kg/hr) and plasma. The rate of fluid and plasma administration must be judged by estimates of loss. Blood transfusions are indicated only when severe bleeding results in a true falling hematocrit. Heparin should be used when there is specific laboratory evidence of disseminated intravascular coagulation. Aspirin is contraindicated.

C., D., and E. See Dengue fever, above.

DERMATOPHYTOSIS   ICD-9 110

(Tinea, Ringworm, Dermatomycosis, Epidermophytosis, Trichophytosis, Microsporosis)

Dermatophytosis or tinea are general terms, essentially synonymous, applied to mycotic disease of keratinized areas of the body (hair, skin and nails). Various genera and species of fungi known collectively as the dermatophytes are causative agents. The dermatomycoses are subdivided according to sites of infection.

I. TINEA CAPITIS   ICD-9 110.0
(Ringworm of the scalp and beard, Kerion, Favus)

1. **Identification**—Begins as a small papule and spreads peripherally, leaving scaly patches of temporary baldness. Infected hairs become brittle and break off easily. Occasionally boggy, raised and suppurative lesions develop, called kerions.

Favus of the scalp is a variety of tinea capitis caused by *Trichophyton schoenleinii;* it is characterized by a mousy odor and by formation of small, yellowish cuplike crusts (scutulae) which look as though they were stuck on the scalp. Affected hairs do not break off but become gray and lusterless and eventually fall out and leave baldness which may be permanent.

Tinea capitis is easily distinguished from piedra, a fungus infection of the hair occurring in S America and some countries of SE Asia and Africa. Piedra is characterized by black, hard "gritty" or white, soft pasty nodules on the hair shafts, caused by *Piedraia hortai* and *Trichosporon beigelii* respectively.

Examination of the scalp under UV light (Wood's lamp) for yellow-green fluorescence is helpful in diagnosing tinea capitis caused by *Microsporum canis* and *M. audouini; Trichophyton* species do not fluoresce. Microscopic examination of scales and hair in 10% potassium hydroxide reveals characteristic hyaline ectothrix arthrospores. The fungus should be cultured for confirmation of the diagnosis.

2. **Infectious agents**—Various species of *Microsporum* and *Trichophyton.* Identification of genus and species is important epidemiologically and to determine prognosis.

3. **Occurrence**—Tinea capitis caused by *M. audouini* formerly had been widespread, particularly in urban areas but *T. tonsurans* infections are now epidemic in urban areas in eastern USA, Puerto Rico and Mexico. *M. canis* infections occur in both rural and urban areas wherever infected cats and dogs are present and is the primary causative agent in Australia. *T. mentagrophytes* var. *mentagrophytes* and *T. verrucosum* infections occur primarily in rural areas where the disease exists in cattle, horses, rodents and wild animals.

4. **Reservoir**—Man for *M. audouinii, T. schoenleinii* and *T. tonsurans;* animals, especially dogs, cats and cattle, harbor the other organisms noted above.

5. **Mode of transmission**—Direct skin-to-skin or indirect contact, especially from the backs of theater seats, barber clippers, toilet articles or clothing contaminated with hair from infected persons or animals.

6. **Incubation period**—Ten to 14 days.

7. Period of communicability—Fungus persists on contaminated materials as long as lesions are present and viable.

8. Susceptibility and resistance—Children before the age of puberty are highly susceptible to *M. canis;* all ages are subject to *Trichophyton* infections. Reinfections are rarely if ever noted.

9. Methods of Control—

  A.   *Preventive measures:*

    1)   In the presence of epidemics or in hyperendemic areas involving non-*Trichophyton* species, heads of young children should be surveyed by UV light (Wood's lamp) before entering school. Also search for spotty alopecia and well-circumscribed lesions, especially in children with unkempt hair.

    2)   Educate the public, especially parents, to the danger of acquiring infection from infected children as well as from dogs, cats and other animals.

  B.   *Control of patient, contacts and the immediate environment:*

    1)   Report to local health authority: Obligatory report of epidemics; no individual case report, Class 4 (see Preface). Outbreaks in schools should be reported to school authorities.

    2)   Isolation: None.

    3)   Concurrent disinfection: In mild cases, daily washing of the scalp removes loose hair. In severe cases wash scalp daily and cover hair with a cap. Contaminated caps should be boiled after use.

    4)   Quarantine: Not practical.

    5)   Immunization of contacts: None.

    6)   Investigation of contacts and source of infection: Study household contacts, pets and farm animals for evidence of infection; treat if infected. Some animals, especially cats, may be inapparent carriers.

    7)   Specific treatment: Griseofulvin (GrisPEG®) by mouth for at least 4 weeks is treatment of choice for many. Topical antifungal medications such as Whitfield's ointment may be used concurrently. Systemic antibacterial agents are useful if ringworm lesions become secondarily infected by bacteria, together, in the case of kerions, with a keratolytic cream and a cotton cover for the scalp. Examine weekly and take cultures; when cultures become negative, complete recovery may be assumed.

C. *Epidemic measures:* In epidemics in schools or other institutions educate children and parents as to mode of spread, prevention and personal hygiene; enlist services of physicians and nurses for diagnosis; carry out follow-up surveys.

D. *Disaster implications:* None.

E. *International measures:* None.

II. TINEA UNGUIUM   ICD-9 110.1
(Ringworm of the nails, Onychomycosis)

1. **Identification**—A chronic fungal disease involving one or more nails of the hands or feet. The nail gradually thickens, becomes discolored and brittle, and an accumulation of caseous-appearing material forms beneath the nail, or the nail becomes chalky and disintegrates.

Diagnosis is made by microscopic examination of potassium hydroxide preparations of the nail and of detritus beneath the nail for hyaline fungal elements. Etiology should be confirmed by culture.

2. **Infectious agents**—*Epidermophyton floccosum,* various species of *Trichophyton* and rarely *Microsporum* species.

3. **Occurrence**—Common.

4. **Reservoir**—Man; rarely animals or soil.

5. **Mode of transmission**—Presumably by direct contact with skin or nail lesions of infected persons, possibly from indirect contact (contaminated floors and shower stalls). Low rate of transmission, even to close family associates.

6. **Incubation period**—Unknown.

7. **Period of communicability**—As long as an infected lesion is present.

8. **Susceptibility and resistance**—Injury to nail predisposes to infection. Reinfection is frequent.

9. **Methods of control**—

A. *Preventive measures:* Cleanliness and use of a fungicidal agent such as cresol for disinfecting floors in common use; frequent hosing and rapid draining of shower rooms.

B. *Control of patient, contacts and the immediate environment:*

1)   Report to local health authority: Official report not ordinarily justifiable, Class 5 (see Preface).

2), 3), 4), 5), 6): Not practical.

7) Specific treatment: Griseofulvin (GrisPEG®) by mouth is the treatment of choice; should be given until nails grow out (about 6 months for fingernails, 18 months for toenails).

C. *Epidemic measures, D. Disaster implications, and E. International measures:* Not applicable.

III. TINEA CRURIS   ICD-9 110.3
(Ringworm of groin and perianal region)
TINEA CORPORIS   ICD-9 110.5
(Ringworm of the body)

1. Identification—A fungal disease of the skin other than of the scalp, bearded areas and feet, characteristically appearing as flat, spreading, ring-shaped lesions. The periphery is usually reddish, vesicular or pustular and may be dry and scaly or moist and crusted. As the lesion progresses peripherally, the central area often clears, leaving apparently normal skin. Differentiation from inguinal candidiasis and tuberculoid leprosy is necessary, since treatment differs.

Presumptive diagnosis is made by taking scrapings from the advancing lesion margins, clearing in 10% potassium hydroxide and examining microscopically for segmented, branched hyaline filaments of fungus. Final identification is by culture.

2. Infectious agents—Most species of *Microsporum* and *Trichophyton;* also *Epidermophyton floccosum.*

3. Occurrence—Worldwide and relatively frequent. Males are infected more often than females.

4. Reservoir—Man, animals and soil; *T. cruris,* almost always man.

5. Mode of transmission—Direct or indirect contact with skin and scalp lesions of infected persons, lesions of animals; contaminated floors, shower stalls, benches and similar articles.

6. Incubation period—Four to 10 days.

7. Period of communicability—As long as lesions are present and viable fungus persists on contaminated materials.

8. Susceptibility and resistance—Susceptibility is widespread, aggravated by friction and excessive perspiration in axillary and inguinal regions, and when environmental temperatures and humidity are high. All ages are susceptible.

9. Methods of control—

A. *Preventive measures:* Launder towels and clothing with hot water and/or fungicidal agent; general cleanliness in showers and dressing rooms of gymnasiums, especially repeated washing of benches. A fungicidal agent such as cresol should be used to disinfect benches and floors. Frequent hosing and rapid draining of shower rooms.

B. *Control of patient, contacts and the immediate environment:*

1) Report to local health authority: Obligatory report of epidemics; no individual case report, Class 4 (see Preface). Report infections of school children to school authority.

2) Isolation: Infected children should be excluded from gymnasiums, swimming pools and activities likely to lead to exposure of others.

3) Concurrent disinfection: Effective and frequent laundering of clothing.

4) Quarantine: None.

5) Immunization of contacts: None.

6) Investigation of contacts and source of infection: Examination of school and household contacts and of household pets and farm animals; treat infections as indicated.

7) Specific treatment: Thorough bathing with soap and water, removal of scabs and crusts, and application of an effective topical fungicide such as miconazole may suffice. Griseofulvin (GrisPEG®) by mouth is effective; ketoconzaole is useful in griseofulvin-resistant ringworm, but hepatotoxicity prevents it from being the drug of choice.

C. *Epidemic measures:* Educate children and parents concerning the nature of the infection, its mode of spread and the need to maintain good personal hygiene.

D. *Disaster implications:* None.

E. *International measures:* None.

IV. TINEA PEDIS   ICD-9 110.4
(Ringworm of the foot, Athlete's foot)

1. Identification—Scaling or cracking of the skin, especially between the toes, or blisters containing a thin watery fluid are characteristic; commonly called "athlete's foot." In severe cases, vesicular lesions appear on various parts of the body, especially the hands; these dermatophytids do not contain the fungus but are an allergic reaction to fungus products.

Diagnosis is verified by microscopic examination of potassium hydroxide-treated scrapings from lesions between the toes which reveal septate branching filaments. Clinical appearance of lesions is not diagnostic.

2. Infectious agents—*Trichophyton rubrum, T. mentagrophytes* var. *interdigitale* and *Epidermophyton floccosum.*

3. Occurrence—Worldwide; a common disease. Adults more often affected than children; males more than females. Infections are more frequent and more severe in hot weather.

4. Reservoir—Man.

5. Mode of transmission—Direct or indirect contact with skin lesions of infected persons or contaminated floors, shower stalls and other articles used by infected persons.

6. Incubation period—Unknown.

7. Period of communicability—As long as lesions are present and viable spores persist on contaminated materials.

8. Susceptibility and resistance—Susceptibility is variable and infection may be inapparent. No differences in racial susceptibility. Repeated attacks are frequent.

9. Methods of control—

 A. *Preventive measures:* Those for tinea corporis, above. Educate the public to maintain strict personal hygiene; special care in drying areas between toes after bathing. Regular use of a dusting powder containing an effective fungicide on the feet and particularly between the toes. Occlusive shoes may predispose to infection and disease.

 B. *Control of patient, contacts and the immediate environment:*

  1) Report to local health authority: Obligatory report of epidemics; no individual case report, Class 4 (see Preface). Report high incidence in schools to school authorities.
  2) Isolation: None.
  3) Concurrent disinfection: Boil socks of heavily infected individuals to prevent reinfection.
  4) Quarantine: None.
  5) Immunization of contacts: None.
  6) Investigation of contacts and source of infection: None.
  7) Specific treatment: Topical fungicides such as miconazole or clotrimazole (Lotrimin®, Gyne-Lotrimin®). Expose feet to air by wearing sandals; use dusting powders. Griseofulvin (GrisPEG®) by mouth may be indicated in

severe, protracted disease, but is usually less effective than conscientious application of local fungicides.

C. *Epidemic measures:* Thoroughly clean and wash floors of gymnasiums, showers and similar sources of infection. Educate the public concerning the mode of spread.

D. *Disaster implications:* None.

E. *International measures:* None.

DIARRHEA, ACUTE ICD-9 009.2

Diarrhea is a clinical syndrome of diverse etiology, associated with loose, or watery stools and often vomiting and fever. It is a symptom of bacterial, viral and parasitic enteric agents causing cholera, shigellosis, salmonellosis, yersiniosis, giardiasis and viral gastroenteropathy. (See each disease under its individual listing). It can be caused by infection with *Escherichia coli* and *Campylobacter* strains (see below), non-cholera vibrios and *Vibrio parahaemolyticus,* other infectious diseases such as malaria and measles, and intestinal helminths as well as chemical agents. Approximately 70–80% of diarrheal episodes in people visiting treatment facilities can be diagnosed etiologically if all the newer laboratory tests are available and are utilized. Relatively few laboratories have these capabilities, however. From a practical clinical standpoint, most of these illnesses may be thought of as a single entity since the basic therapy required to prevent a fatal outcome, fluid and electrolyte replacement, is similar for all.

I. DIARRHEA CAUSED BY ICD-9 008.0
ESCHERICHIA COLI

1. Identification—Strains of *Escherichia coli* which cause diarrhea are of at least 3 types: invasive, enterotoxigenic (toxin-producing) and enteropathogenic. In addition, some serotypes produce a cytotoxin to Vero monkey cells; one serotype has been associated with hemorrhagic colitis. Invasive strains cause disease localized primarily in the colon, manifested by fever and mucoid and occasionally bloody diarrhea; pathologic changes resemble those seen with shigellosis. Enterotoxigenic strains behave more like *Vibrio cholerae* in producing a profuse watery diarrhea without blood or mucus; abdominal cramping, vomiting, acidosis, prostration, and dehydration can occur; fever may or may not be present; the symptoms usually last fewer than 3 to 5 days. Both invasive and enterotoxic strains usually cause sporadic disease, particularly in under-

developed countries, although they may cause common source outbreaks. The enteropathogenic strains generally belong to the "classical" enteropathogenic serotypes which have been associated with outbreaks of acute diarrheal disease in newborn nurseries. Although they may produce diarrhea through adherence mechanisms and elaboration of Shiga-like toxins, the pathogenic mechanisms are not well understood.

Specific diagnosis is made by isolation from stools of strains of *E. coli* that are shown by appropriate tests to be invasive, to elaborate toxins, or to be identified as an "enteropathogenic" serotype with the use of commercially available antisera. These serotypes are not always pathogenic and may be found in healthy persons.

2. Infectious agent—Enterotoxigenic (heat labile toxin-LT, heat stabile toxin-ST, or both-LT/ST), invasive, or "enteropathogenic" strains of *E. coli*.

3. Occurrence—Outbreaks may occur in nurseries and institutions and as common source foodborne or waterborne outbreaks in the community. In areas with poor sanitation, endemic diarrhea is frequently due to *E. coli*. "Traveler's diarrhea" is most commonly due to enterotoxigenic *E. coli*.

4. Reservoir—Infected persons, often asymptomatic.

5. Mode of transmission—The major mode of transmission is fecal contamination of food, water or fomites; person-to-person spread has also been demonstrated. Persons with diarrhea excrete large numbers of organisms in their stool and constitute the greatest hazard. Spread from mother to infant may occur during delivery, or by the fecal-oral route. Contaminated hands of uninfected personnel may transmit organisms to other infants. Poor handwashing after patient contact, inadequate personal toilet hygiene of carriers, and poor environmental sanitation contribute to spread of infections.

6. Incubation period—Twelve to 72 hours.

7. Period of communicability—Not known; presumably for the duration of fecal excretion, which may be several weeks.

8. Susceptibility and resistance—Infants, particularly prematures and malnourished children, are most susceptible to enteropathogenic strains. Breast-feeding may confer some protection. Immunity to enterotoxin and surface antigens of the bacteria has been demonstrated but its duration is unknown. Local secretory immunity within the intestine is probably most important.

9. Methods of control—

    A. Preventive Measures:

        1)   For general measures for prevention of fecal-oral spread of infection, see Typhoid Fever, 9A.

2) For travelers going to high-risk areas where it is not possible to obtain safe food or water, prophylactic short-term (about 2 weeks) antibiotic therapy may be considered with either TMP-SMX (160 mg–800 mg/d) or doxycycline (100 mg) orally once daily. The promotion of resistant strains is the major potential disadvantage.

3) Prevention of hospital nursery outbreaks depends primarily on adequate handwashing practices, a scrupulously clean nursery and isolation of patients with diarrhea and culturing stools to establish the etiologic agent.

    a) Breast feed if possible; encourage mother-infant hospitalization in obstetrical facilities.

    b) If breast feeding is not possible, prepare feeding formulas aseptically; fill the bottle, apply nipple, cover with a cap, sterilize, and refrigerate with nipple and caps on bottles until feeding time; if available, use disposable formula containers. Evaluate sterility by periodic bacteriologic sampling of locally prepared formulas; such sampling of commercially prepared formula is not necessary except in epidemiologic investigations.

    c) Provide nurseries for the healthy newborn and premature infants separate from those with ill infants. Provide each infant with individual equipment, including thermometer, kept at the bassinet; use no common bathing or dressing tables and no bassinet stands for holding or transporting more than one infant at a time.

    d) Provide separate isolation facilities for sick infants or older children. Isolate for at least 6 days all infants born outside the hospital or to a mother with diarrheal or respiratory illness. Control visitors to minimize spread of infection. Monitor laundry procedures to assure absence of pathogens from materials returned to the nursery.

    e) Keep systematic daily record for each infant of number and consistency of stools.

    f) Spread of infection (even in the absence of an outbreak) can be limited by housing each entire cohort of infants born during different time periods in separate areas throughout hospitalization; i.e., they should not be mixed with other cohorts from birth to the time of discharge. Personnel should not care for infants from more than one cohort.

B. *Control of patient, contacts and the immediate environment:*

1) Report to local health authority: Obligatory report of

epidemics; no individual case report, Class 4 (see Preface). Two or more concurrent cases of diarrhea requiring treatment for these symptoms in a nursery or among those recently discharged are to be interpreted as an outbreak requiring investigation.

2)   Isolation: Enteric precautions for known and suspected cases.

3)   Concurrent disinfection: Of all fecal discharges and soiled articles. In communities with a modern and adequate sewage disposal system, feces can be discharged directly into sewers without preliminary disinfection. Thorough terminal cleaning.

4)   Quarantine: Use enteric precautions and cohort methods. (9A3, above).

5)   Immunization of contacts: None.

6)   Investigation of contacts and source of infection: See 9C2, below.

7)   Specific treatment: Electrolyte fluid therapy (oral or i.v.) is the most important measure (see Cholera, 9B7). Most cases do not require any other therapy. For severe enteropathogenic infantile diarrhea, nonabsorbable antibiotics such as neomycin (100 mg/kg/d) or colistin (10 to 15 mg/kg/d) may be administered in 3 to 4 divided doses for 5 days. For the rare cases of severe diarrhea with enteroinvasive strains, oral absorbable or parenteral antibiotics such as ampicillin (50 mg/kg/d) may be given. For severe "traveler's diarrhea," early treatment with TMP-SMX (160 mg–800 mg) orally twice daily for 5 days is effective.

C.   *Epidemic measures:* For nursery epidemics (see 9B1, above), the following—

1)   All babies with diarrhea should be placed in one nursery under enteric precautions. Admit no more babies to the contaminated nursery; suspend maternity service unless a clean nursery is available with separate personnel and facilities; promptly discharge infected infants when medically possible. For the babies exposed in the contaminated nursery, provide separate medical and nursing personnel skilled in the care of communicable disease. Observe contacts for at least 2 weeks after the last case leaves the nursery; promptly remove each new case to one nursery ward used for these infants. Maternity service may be resumed after discharge of all contact babies and mothers, and thorough cleaning and terminal disinfection. Put into

practice recommendations of 9A, above, so far as feasible in the emergency.

2) Carry out a thorough epidemiologic investigation into the distribution of cases by time, place, person and exposure to risk factors to determine how transmission is occurring.

D. *Disaster implications:* None.

E. *International measures:* WHO Collaborating Centres (see Preface).

II. DIARRHEA CAUSED BY CAMPYLOBACTER
ICD-9 008.49

(Campylobacter enteritis, Vibrionic enteritis)

1. **Identification**—An acute enteric disease of variable severity characterized by diarrhea, abdominal pain, malaise, fever, nausea and vomiting. The illness is frequently self-limited within 1 to 4 days and usually lasts no more than 10 days. A prolonged illness occurs in up to 20% of patients who present for medical attention, especially adults; relapses can occur. Gross or occult blood in association with mucus and WBCs is usually present in the liquid foul-smelling stools. A typhoidal-type syndrome, reactive arthritis and rarely febrile convulsions and meningitis have been described.

Diagnosis is based on isolation of the organisms from stool using selective media, reduced oxygen tension and an incubation temperature of 43°C (109.4°F). Visualization of motile curved, spiral or S-shaped rods similar to those of *Vibrio cholerae* by phase-contrast or darkfield microscopy of stool can provide rapid presumptive evidence for *Campylobacter* enteritis.

2. **Infectious agents**—*Campylobacter jejuni (C. fetus* subsp. *jejuni)* and *C. coli* are the usual cause of *Campylobacter* diarrhea in man. A diversity of biotypes and serotypes occur which may be helpful for epidemiological purposes.

3. **Occurrence**—These organisms are an important cause of diarrheal illness in all parts of the world and in all age groups, causing 5–14% of diarrhea worldwide. *Campylobacter* may be responsible for a greater proportion of enteritis than either *Salmonellae* or *Shigellae.* Common source outbreaks have occurred, most often associated with foods, unpasteurized milk, and unchlorinated water. The largest number of cases in temperate areas occurs in the warmer months. These organisms are an important cause of "traveler's diarrhea."

4. **Reservoir**—Animals, including swine, cattle, sheep, cats, dogs, other pets, and rodents; birds, including poultry.

5. Mode of transmission—By ingestion of the organisms in food or in unpasteurized milk or water; from contact with infected pets (especially puppies and kittens), wild animals, or infected infants; and possibly from cross-contamination from these sources to foods eaten uncooked or poorly refrigerated.

6. Incubation period—The usual incubation period is 3–5 days, with a range of 1–10 days.

7. Period of communicability—Throughout the course of infection; usually from several days to several weeks. Individuals not treated with antibiotics excrete organisms for as long as 2–7 wks; a chronic carrier state is unusual. The temporary carrier state is probably of little epidemiologic importance, except in infants and others who are incontinent of stool. Among animals and poultry, a chronic carrier state becomes established so that they constitute the primary source of infection.

8. Susceptibility and resistance—Universal susceptibility when a large enough number of organisms is ingested. Immune mechanisms are not well understood.

9. Methods of control—

  A. Preventive measures:

    1) Thorough cooking of all foodstuffs derived from animal sources, particularly poultry. Avoid recontamination within the kitchen after cooking is completed.
    2) All milk should be pasteurized and all water supplies chlorinated.
    3) Recognition, control and prevention of *Campylobacter* infections among domestic animals and pets. Puppies and kittens with diarrhea are possible sources of infection. Handwashing after animal contact should be stressed.

  B. Control of patient, contacts and the immediate environment:

    1) Report to local health authority: Obligatory case report, Class 2B (see Preface).
    2) Isolation: For hospitalized patients, enteric precautions. Exclusion of symptomatic individuals from foodhandling, from care of hospitalized patients and from custodial institutions and daycare centers; exclusion of asymptomatic infected individuals is indicated only for those with questionable hygienic habits. Stress proper handwashing.
    3) Concurrent disinfection: Of feces and articles soiled therewith. In communities with a modern and adequate sewage disposal system, feces can be discharged directly

into sewers without preliminary disinfection. Terminal cleaning.

4) Quarantine: None.

5) Immunization of contacts: No immunization available.

6) Investigation of contacts and sources of infection: Useful only to detect outbreaks; outbreaks should be investigated to identify the implicated food, water or raw milk to which others may have been exposed.

7) Specific treatment: None generally indicated except rehydration and electrolyte replacement (see Cholera, 9B7). A short course of antibiotic therapy may be given for patients with severe or prolonged illness, or when prompt termination of fecal excretion of *C. jejuni* or *C. coli* is desired. Antimicrobial treatment may not shorten the duration of clinical illness. *C. jejuni* or *C. coli* organisms are susceptible in vitro to a number of antimicrobial agents, including erythromycin, tetracyclines and aminoglycosides.

C. *Epidemic measures:* Groups of cases such as in classrooms should be reported immediately to local health authority, with search for vehicle and mode of spread.

D. *Disaster implications:* A risk when mass feeding and poor sanitation coexist.

E. *International measures:* WHO Collaborating Centres (see Preface).

DIPHTHERIA   ICD-9 032

1. Identification—An acute bacterial disease of tonsils, pharynx, larynx, nose, occasionally of other mucous membranes or skin and sometimes the conjunctiva or genitalia. The characteristic lesion, caused by liberation of a specific cytotoxin, is marked by a patch or patches of an adherent grayish membrane with surrounding inflammation. The throat is moderately sore in faucial diphtheria, with cervical lymph nodes somewhat enlarged and tender; in severe cases, there is marked swelling and edema of the neck. Laryngeal diphtheria is serious in infants and young children, while nasal diphtheria is mild, often chronic and marked by one-sided nasal discharge and excoriations. Inapparent infections outnumber recognized cases. The lesions of cutaneous diphtheria are variable and may be indistinguishable from, or a component of, impetigo. Late effects of absorption of toxin,

appearing after 2–6 weeks, include cranial and peripheral motor and sensory nerve palsies and myocarditis (which might occur early), and are often severe. Case fatality rates of 5 to 10% for noncutaneous diphtheria have changed little in 50 years.

Diphtheria should be suspected in the differential diagnosis of bacterial and viral pharyngitis, Vincent's angina, infectious mononucleosis, syphilis, and candidiasis, especially if they follow antibiotic use. Administration of antibiotics for all sore throats, on the assumption that most are streptococcal, may delay diagnosis and therapy of diphtheria with a fatal result.

Diagnosis is confirmed by bacteriologic examination of lesions. If diphtheria is strongly suspected, specific treatment should be initiated with antibiotics and antitoxin while studies are pending and continued even in the face of a negative laboratory report.

2. Infectious agent—*Corynebacterium diphtheriae* of gravis, mitis, or intermedius biotype. Toxin production results when the bacteria are infected by corynebacteriophage containing the gene *tox;* toxigenic strains cause severe and fatal disease.

3. Occurrence—A disease of colder months in temperate zones, involving primarily unimmunized children under 15 years of age; often found among adults in population groups whose immunization was neglected. Formerly a prevalent disease, it has largely disappeared in those areas where effective immunization programs have been carried out. In the USA, from 1980–83 an average of 4 cases was reported annually, two-thirds of the affected persons were ≧20 years of age. In the tropics, seasonal trends are less distinct; inapparent, cutaneous and wound diphtheria cases are much more common.

4. Reservoir—Man.

5. Mode of transmission—Contact with a patient or carrier; more rarely with articles soiled with discharges from lesions of infected persons. Raw milk has served as a vehicle.

6. Incubation period—Usually 2–5 days, occasionally longer.

7. Period of communicability—Variable, until virulent bacilli have disappeared from discharges and lesions; usually 2 weeks or less and seldom more than 4 weeks. The rare chronic carriers may shed organisms for 6 months or more. Appropriate antibiotic therapy terminates shedding promptly.

8. Susceptibility and resistance—Infants born of immune mothers are relatively immune; protection is passive and usually lost before the 6th month. Recovery from clinical attack is not always followed by lasting immunity; immunity is often acquired through inapparent infection. Prolonged active immunity can be induced by toxoid. Serosurveys in the

USA indicate that more than 40% of adults lack protective levels of circulating antitoxin. Antitoxic immunity protects against systemic disease but not against local infection in the nasopharynx.

9. Methods of control—

A. *Preventive measures:*

1) The only effective control is by a community program of active immunization with diphtheria toxoid, including an adequate program to maintain immunity. It is generally administered as a triple antigen with diphtheria toxoid combined with tetanus toxoid containing an aluminum adjuvant and pertussis vaccine (DTP).

2) The following schedules are recommended for use in the USA; some countries may recommend different ages for specific doses or fewer than 4 doses in the primary series; some, as Australia, use DTP through 8 years of age.

   a) For children less than 7 years of age—
   A primary series of four doses of diphtheria toxoid with tetanus toxoid and pertussis vaccine as DTP. The first three doses are given at 4 to 8 week intervals beginning when the infant is 6–8 weeks old. While these elicit good antitoxic response which is maintained by exposure to organisms in areas of high prevalence, the 4th dose given 1 year after the 3rd dose assures greater and longer protection in developed areas with low prevalence of diphtheria. This schedule does not need to be restarted because of any delay in administering the scheduled doses. A 5th dose is usually given prior to school entry; this dose is not necessary if the 4th dose were given after the 4th birthday.

   b) For persons 7 years of age and older—
   For a previously unimmunized individual, a primary series of 3 doses of adsorbed tetanus and diphtheria toxoids (adult type, Td) is given. The first 2 doses are given at 4 to 8 week intervals and the 3rd dose 6 months to 1 year after the 2nd dose. Because adverse reactions increase with age, a highly purified toxoid at reduced concentration must be used beyond age 6.

   c) Active protection should be maintained by administering a dose of Td every 10 years thereafter. (Not in UK).

3) Special efforts should be made to assure that persons who are at higher risk to patient exposure, such as health workers, are fully immunized and receive a booster dose of Td every 10 years.

4) Educational measures to inform the public and particularly the parents of young children of the hazards of diphtheria and the necessity for active immunization.

B. Control of patient, contacts and the immediate environment:

1) Report to local health authority: Case report is obligatory in most states and countries, Class 2A (see Preface).

2) Isolation: Strict isolation for pharyngeal diphtheria, contact isolation for cutaneous diphtheria, until two cultures from both throat and nose (or skin lesions in cutaneous diphtheria) taken not less than 24 hours apart, and not less than 24 hours after cessation of antimicrobial therapy, fail to show diphtheria bacilli. Where culture is impractical, isolation may be ended after 14 days appropriate antibiotic treatment. (See 9B7, below.)

3) Concurrent disinfection: Of all articles in contact with patient, and all articles soiled by discharges of patient. Terminal cleaning.

4) Quarantine: Adult contacts whose occupations involve handling food, especially milk, or close association with unimmunized children should be excluded from that work until bacteriological examination proves them not to be carriers.

5) Management of contacts: Contacts of cases of faucial or cutaneous diphtheria previously immunized should have a booster dose of Td. Contacts intimately exposed and not previously immunized should be cultured and given an appropriate antibiotic (oral erythromycin or i.m. penicillin) and immunization started with the first dose of toxoid. Daily surveillance is advised for 7 days.

6) Investigation of contacts: The search for carriers by use of nose and throat cultures is not ordinarily useful or indicated if provisions of 9B5, above, are carried out.

7) Specific treatment: If diphtheria is strongly suspected, antitoxin (only antitoxin of equine origin is available) should be given without awaiting bacteriological confirmation. After completion of tests to rule out hypersensitivity, a single dose of 20,000 to 100,000 units is given, depending upon the duration of symptoms, area of involvement and severity of the disease. Intramuscular administration usually suffices; in severe infections both i.v. and i.m. antitoxin may be indicated. Both erythromycin and penicillin are effective against the organism, but should be administered only after cultures are taken, in conjunction with but not as a substitute for antitoxin. If a carrier state

is demonstrated: for adults, give erythromycin 1.0 g/day orally (or 40 mg/kg/d) for 7 days or 600,000 to 2 million units (for children 20 pounds or less, 300,000 units; over 20 pounds, 600,000 units) of aqueous procaine penicillin i.m. daily for 10 days; or 1.2 million units benzathine penicillin (600,000 units for children less than 60 pounds).

C. *Epidemic measures:*

1) Immunize the largest possible number of the population group involved, with emphasis on protection of infants and preschool children. Repeat immunization efforts 1 month later to provide at least 2 doses to the recipients.
2) In areas with appropriate facilities, carry out a prompt field investigation of reported cases to verify diagnosis, determine biotype and toxigenicity of *C. diphtheriae,* identify contacts, trace sources of infection and define population groups at special risk.

D. *Disaster implications:* Outbreaks can occur when social or natural conditions lead to crowding of susceptible groups, especially infants and children.

E. *International measures:* Completed primary immunization of susceptible persons traveling to or through countries where either faucial or cutaneous diphtheria is common or a booster dose of Td for those previously inoculated is advisable.

DIPHYLLOBOTHRIASIS   ICD-9 123.4
(Broad or Fish tapeworm infection)

1. Identification—An intestinal tapeworm infection of long duration. Symptoms commonly are trivial or absent. A few patients in whom the worms are attached in the jejunum develop vitamin B_{12} deficiency anemia; massive infections may be associated with diarrhea, obstruction of the bile duct or intestine, and toxic symptoms.

Diagnosis is confirmed by identification of eggs or segments (proglottids) of the worm in feces.

2. Infectious agent—*Diphyllobothrium latum,* a cestode.

3. Occurrence—The disease occurs in lake regions in subarctic, temperate and tropical zones where eating raw or partly cooked freshwater fish is popular. Prevalence increases with age. The disease is highly

endemic in Finland and Soviet Karelia. In N America, endemic foci have been found among Eskimos in Alaska and Canada. Infections in the USA are sporadic and usually come from eating uncooked fish from midwestern or Canadian lakes.

4. Reservoir—Mainly an infected person discharging eggs in feces; other hosts include dogs, bears and other fish-eating mammals.

5. Mode of transmission—Man acquires the infection by eating raw or inadequately cooked fish. Eggs produced by mature segments of the worm in the intestine are discharged in feces into bodies of fresh water in which they mature, hatch, and infect the first intermediate hosts (copepods of the genera *Cyclops* and *Diaptomus*). Susceptible species of freshwater fish (pike, perch, turbots) ingest infected copepods and become second intermediate hosts in which the worms transform into the plerocercoid (larval) stage which is infective for man and fish-eating mammals such as fox, mink, bear, cat, dog, pig, walrus and seal. The egg-to-egg cycle takes at least ll weeks.

6. Incubation period—From 3–6 wks from ingestion to passage of eggs in the stool.

7. Period of communicability—Not directly transmitted from person to person. Man and other definitive hosts continue to disseminate eggs in the environment as long as worms remain in the intestine, sometimes for many years.

8. Susceptibility and resistance—Man is universally susceptible. No apparent resistance follows infection.

9. Methods of control—

    A.   *Preventive measures:* Thorough heating (56°C/133°F for 5 minutes) of freshwater fish or freezing for 24 hours at −18°C (0°F) insures protection.

    B.   *Control of patient, contacts and the immediate environment:*

        1)   Report to local health authority: Official report not ordinarily justifiable, Class 5 (see Preface).

        2)   Isolation: None.

        3)   Concurrent disinfection: None; sanitary disposal of feces.

        4)   Quarantine: None.

        5)   Immunization of contacts: None.

        6)   Investigation of contacts: Not usually justified.

        7)   Specific treatment: Praziquantel (Biltricide®) and niclosamide (Niclocide®) are the drugs of choice.

    C.   *Epidemic measures:* None.

    D.   *Disaster implications:* None.

E. *International measures:* None.

DRACUNCULIASIS   ICD-9 125.7
(Guinea-worm infection, Dracontiasis)

1. Identification—An infection of the subcutaneous and deeper tissues by a large nematode. A blister appears, usually on a lower extremity, especially the foot, when the gravid, meter-long adult female worm is ready to discharge its larvae. Burning and itching of the skin in the area of the lesion and frequently fever, nausea, vomiting, diarrhea, dyspnea, generalized urticaria, and eosinophilia may accompany or precede vesicle formation. After the vesicle ruptures, the worm discharges larvae whenever the infected part is immersed in water. The prognosis is good unless there are multiple worms or unless a bacterial infection occurs which may produce severe crippling sequelae.

Diagnosis is made by microscopic identification of larvae or recognition of the adult worm.

2. Infectious agent—*Dracunculus medinensis,* a nematode.

3. Occurrence—In India, Africa, and the Middle East, especially in regions with dry climates. Local prevalence varies greatly; in some localities nearly all inhabitants are infected, in others few, mainly young adults.

4. Reservoir—An infected person; there are no significant animal reservoirs.

5. Mode of transmission—Larvae discharged by the parent worm into fresh water are eaten by minute crustacean copepods known as cyclops and in about 2 weeks develop into the infective stage. Man swallows the infected cyclops in drinking water from infested step-wells and ponds; larvae are liberated in the stomach or duodenum, migrate through the viscera, become adults, and the female, after mating, migrates to the subcutaneous tissues (most frequently of the legs) where she grows and develops to full maturity.

6. Incubation period—About 12 months.

7. Period of communicability—From rupture of vesicle until larvae have been completely evacuated from the uterus of the gravid worm, usually 2 to 3 weeks. In water, the larvae are infective for the cyclops for about 5 days; after ingestion by the cyclops, the larvae become infective for man after 12-14 days at temperatures >25° C (>77° F) and remain infective in the cyclops for over 1 month. Not directly transmitted from person to person.

8. Susceptibility and resistance—Susceptibility is universal. No acquired immunity; multiple and repeated infections may occur in the same person.

9. **Methods of control**—The provision of safe water to the populations at risk could lead to eradication of the disease. Foci of disease formerly present in some parts of the Middle East have been eliminated in this manner.

A. *Preventive measures:*

1) Provide potable water. Abolish step-wells and take other measures such as the use of occlusive bandages to prevent contamination of drinking water by infected persons immersing feet or other affected parts of the body.
2) Boil drinking water or filter through fine mesh cloth (such as nylon gauze with a mesh size of 100μ) to remove cyclops.
3) To kill cyclops in ponds, tanks, reservoirs and step-wells, the insecticide temephos (Abate®) is effective and safe. Chemically treat drinking water with chlorine or iodine to kill the larvae and copepods.
4) Educate the public to drink only boiled or filtered water, or water from closed or pump wells. Instruct infected persons in mode of spread of the infection and the danger in contaminating wells or other water supplies.

B. *Control of patient, contacts and the immediate environment:*

1) Report to local health authority: Official report not ordinarily justifiable, Class 5 (see Preface).
2) Isolation: None.
3) Concurrent disinfection: None.
4) Quarantine: None.
5) Immunization of contacts: None.
6) Investigation of contacts and source of infection: Obtain information as to source of drinking water at probable time of infection (about 1 year previously). Search for other cases.
7) Specific treatment: Thiabendazole (Mintezol®), niridazole (Ambilhar®), metronidazole (Flagyl®) and mebendazole (Vermox®) have been used; they help to reduce inflammation and hasten expulsion of the worm, but their efficacy is undetermined.

C. *Epidemic measures:* In hyperendemic situations, field survey to determine prevalence, to discover sources of infection and to guide control measures as described in 9A, above.

D. *Disaster implications:* None.

E. *International measures:* The World Health Assembly has adopted a resolution to eliminate dracunculiasis as a public health problem in the course of the International Drinking Water Supply and Sanitation Decade (1981–1990).

EBOLA-MARBURG VIRUS DISEASE   ICD-9 078.89
(African hemorrhagic fever, Marburg disease, Ebola disease)

1. **Identification**—Systemic febrile illnesses usually characterized by sudden onset with malaise, fever, myalgia, headache and pharyngitis, followed by vomiting, diarrhea, a maculopapular rash, renal and hepatic involvement and a hemorrhagic diathesis. Laboratory findings indicate multiple system involvement, primarily of liver, pancreas, kidney and, to a much less degree, CNS and heart. Leukopenia, thrombocytopenia and transaminase elevation are often seen. Approximately 25% of reported cases of Marburg virus infection were fatal; case fatality rates of Ebola infections in Africa have ranged from 50% to nearly 90%.

Diagnosis is made by IFA for detection of antibody, preferably IgM, and by visualization of the virus in the blood or in liver or kidney sections by electron microscopy, or by its isolation in tissue culture, guinea pigs, or monkeys, or by serologic tests on survivors. Laboratory studies should be carried out only where maximal protection against infection of the staff and of the community is available (P4 containment).

2. **Infectious agents**—Virions are 80 nm in diameter and variable in length (usually 700-900 nm but can be up to 14,000 nm); they are filamentous and may be branched or coiled. The two viruses—Ebola and Marburg—are antigenically distinct, and are not related to other known infectious agents.

3. **Occurrence**—Marburg disease has been recognized on four occasions: in 1967, 31 persons, with 7 deaths, in the Federal Republic of Germany and Yugoslavia were infected following exposure to African green monkeys *(Cercopithecus aethiops)* from Uganda; in 1975, the index fatal case of 3 diagnosed in S Africa had originated in Zimbabwe; in 1980, there were two confirmed cases in Kenya, one fatal; and in 1982, a case was diagnosed in S Africa, which had been acquired in Zimbabwe.

Ebola disease was first recognized in the western equatorial province of the Sudan and the adjacent region of Zaire in 1976; a second outbreak occurred in the same area in Sudan in 1979. A serological survey disclosed antibodies in 7% of asymptomatic individuals in the epidemic area.

4. Reservoir—The reservoirs are unknown despite extensive studies. African green monkeys have not been incriminated as a natural reservoir of Marburg virus; Ebola antibodies have been found in domestic guinea pigs but there has been no evidence of transmission to man.

5. Mode of transmission—Person-to-person transmission occurs by direct contact with infected blood, secretions, organs, semen or by the aerosol route. Nosocomial infections have been frequent; all cases died on whom contaminated syringes and needles had been used. Transmission through semen has occurred 7 weeks after clinical recovery.

6. Incubation period—The incubation period is 3–7 days in Marburg and 2–21 days in Ebola virus disease.

7. Period of communicability—As long as blood and secretions contain virus. Secondary infections with Ebola virus occurred in about 5% of case contacts in Zaire and 10–15% in Sudan, among those with greatest direct contact. Ebola virus was isolated from the seminal fluid on the 61st but not the 76th day after onset of illness in a laboratory-acquired case.

8. Susceptibility and resistance—All ages are susceptible.

9. Methods of control—Control measures in 9B, C, D and E in Lassa Fever apply, plus restriction of sexual intercourse until semen can be assumed to be free of virus.

ECHINOCOCCOSIS   ICD-9 122

This disease in man is produced by cysts of varying size which are the larval stage of the tapeworm *Echinococcus;* the adult worms are found in dogs and other carnivores. Three closely related species cause different clinical manifestations: (1) unilocular echinococcosis or cystic hydatid disease, (2) multilocular or alveolar hydatid disease, and (3) polycystic hydatid disease.

Signs and symptoms consistent with space-occupying lesions with a history of travel to endemic areas warrant inclusion of echinococcosis in the differential diagnosis. The lesions can be defined by x-ray, CT scanning and sonography. The diagnosis is supported by positive results in serological tests. Most tests are not specific and positive results should be confirmed with tests that detect antibody against "antigen 5," a genus-specific antigen isolated from unilocular hydatid fluid. Definitive diagnosis is made by microscopic identification of parasitic tissue obtained surgically, at necropsy or from sputum after the rupture of pulmonary cysts.

I. ECHINOCOCCOSIS DUE TO *ECHINOCOCCUS GRANULOSUS*
(Unilocular echinococcosis, Hydatid disease)

ICD-9 122.4

1. **Identification**—Signs and symptoms vary according to the size, number and location of the cysts. These grow slowly and eventually may exceed 10 cm in diameter in middle and older age groups. Cysts of *E. granulosus* are unilocular, have a laminated noncellular wall, are usually surrounded by a fibrous pericyst of host origin and are found frequently in the liver and lungs and less commonly in the kidney, spleen, bone, CNS and elsewhere; no organ of the body is exempt. Infection may be asymptomatic and cysts are frequently found on routine chest x-rays or at autopsy. However, in vital organs they may cause severe symptoms and death. Species identification is based on the thick laminated cyst walls, brood capsules, and the structure and measurements of the protoscolex hooks.

2. **Infectious agent**—*Echinococcus granulosus,* a small tapeworm of the dog.

3. **Occurrence**—This parasite is common where dogs are used to herd grazing animals and also have intimate contact with humans. Lebanon, Israel, Jordan, Syria, Iraq, Saudi Arabia, Greece, Sardinia, north Africa, Kenya, Asia, western Canada and Alaska, Argentina, Uruguay, southern Brazil, Peru and Chile are enzootic areas. Human cases have been completely eliminated in Iceland and greatly reduced in Cyprus, Australia and New Zealand. Infections are rarely acquired within mainland USA.

4. **Reservoir**—Definitive hosts are the dog, wolf, dingo or other Canidae infected with adult worms; the usual intermediate hosts are herbivores. In domestic life cycles, the dog is the definitive host and the sheep usually the intermediate host.

5. **Mode of transmission**—By hand-to-mouth transfer of tapeworm eggs from dog feces. Exposure occurs in handling dogs and objects soiled with dog feces and through contaminated food and water. Eggs may survive for several months in pastures, gardens and around households. Ingested eggs hatch in the intestine, the larvae migrate through the mucosa and are carried by the blood to various organs where they produce cysts. This may occur in a variety of herbivores and also man. Carnivores become infected by eating viscera containing hydatid cysts. The dog-sheep cycle is important in most areas where *E. granulosus* is endemic. In other regions the dog-cattle, dog-camel, dog-kangaroo, or dog-pig cycle predominates. In northwest Canada, the disease is maintained in a wolf-moose cycle from which sled dogs may bring the parasite to man.

6. Incubation period—Variable, from months to years, depending upon the number and location of cysts and how rapidly they grow.

7. Period of communicability—Not directly transmitted from person to person or from one intermediate host to another. Dogs begin to pass eggs of the parasite approximately 7 weeks after infection. Most infections in dogs are lost spontaneously by 6 months, but adult worms may survive as long as 2–3 years. Dogs may be infected repeatedly.

8. Susceptibility and resistance—Children are more likely to be exposed to infection through contact with infected dogs; there is no evidence that they are more susceptible to infection than are adults. Man does not harbor the adult worm.

9. Methods of control—

A. *Preventive measures:*

1) Adequate inspection of the carcasses and rigid control of slaughtering of herbivorous animals so that dogs have no access to uncooked viscera.

2) Incineration or deep burial of infected organs from dead intermediate hosts.

3) Periodic treatment of high-risk dogs; reduce their numbers in endemic areas to a level compatible with occupational requirements for dogs.

4) Educate the general public in endemic areas to the dangers of close association with dogs and of the need for controlled slaughtering of animals.

5) Field and laboratory personnel exposed to infection should observe all safety precautions and have serological examination every 6 months.

B. *Control of patient, contacts and the immediate environment:*

1) Report to local health authority: In selected endemic areas; not a reportable disease in most states and countries, Class 3B (see Preface).

2) Isolation: None.

3) Concurrent disinfection: None.

4) Quarantine: None.

5) Immunization of contacts: None.

6) Investigation of contacts and source of infection: Examination of familial associates for suspicious tumors. Check dogs kept in and about houses for infection in an attempt to determine source and practices leading to infection.

7) Specific treatment: Surgical resection of isolated cysts is the treatment of choice. Studies with mebendazole

(Vermox®) have given conflicting results; treatment with this drug should be restricted to complicated cases in whom surgery is not feasible or has failed; its use may be advisable postoperatively if spillage of cyst contents has occurred.

C. *Epidemic measures:* In highly endemic areas, destruction of wild and stray dogs. Mass anthelmintic treatment of dogs; praziquantel (Biltricide®) is drug of choice.

D. *Disaster implications:* None.

E. *International measures:* Coordinated programs by neighboring countries where the disease is enzootic to control infection in animals and movement of dogs from known enzootic areas.

II. ECHINOCOCCOSIS DUE TO ICD-9 122.7
ECHINOCOCCUS MULTILOCULARIS
(Alveolar hydatid disease)

1. Identification—This disease is caused by the poorly circumscribed alveolar larval cysts of *Echinococcus multilocularis.* These are usually found in the liver and rarely metastasize to the lungs and brain. Growth of the cysts is not restricted by a thick laminated cyst wall so they continually grow by external proliferation throughout the liver and contiguous organs to produce chronic space-occupying lesions. The clinical effects of the infection depend upon the size and location of the larval masses; the prognosis is grave because of the invasive and metastatic potentials.

Diagnosis is generally based on histopathology: the thin host pericyst and multiple cavities formed by external proliferation. Man is an abnormal host and the cyst rarely produces brood capsules, protoscolices or calcareous corpuscles.

2. Infectious agent—*Echinococcus multilocularis.*

3. Occurrence—Distribution is limited to areas of the Northern Hemisphere: central Europe, USSR, Siberia, northern Japan, Alaska, Canada and northern USA.

4. Reservoir—The adult tapeworms are found in foxes, wolves, dogs, coyotes and cats; the intermediate hosts are voles, lemmings, shrews and mice. *E. multilocularis* is commonly maintained in nature in fox-vole cycles.

5. Mode of transmission—By ingestion of infective eggs passed in the feces of infected Canidae and Felidae. Fecally soiled dog hair, harnesses and environmental fomites serve as vehicles of infection.

6. **Incubation period, 7. Period of communicability, 8. Susceptibility and resistance,** and 9. **Methods of control**—As in Section I., *Echinococcus granulosus,* above, except that surgical removal is less often successful and treatment with mebendazole (Vermox®) may prevent progression of the disease.

ECHINOCOCCOSIS DUE TO *ECHINOCOCCUS VOGELI*

ICD-9 122.9

This disease is caused by the cysts of *Echinococcus vogeli* which have occurred in the liver, lungs and other organs. Symptoms are variable according to cyst size and location. The species is distinguishable on the basis of its rostellar hooks. The polycystic hydatid is unique in that the germinal membrane proliferates externally to form new cysts and internally to form septae that divide the cavity into numerous microcysts. Brood capsules containing many protoscolices develop in the microcysts.

Cases have been reported in Colombia, Ecuador, Panamá and Venezuela. The principal definitive host is the bush dog, *Speothos venaticus;* the main intermediate host is the paca, *Cuniculus paca,* and the spiny rat. Domestic hunting dogs are also definitive hosts, and serve as an important source of human infection.

ENCEPHALOPATHY, SUBACUTE SPONGIFORM*
(Slow virus infections of the central nervous system)

ICD-9 046

A group of subacute and usually noninflammatory degenerative diseases of the brain caused by "unconventional" filterable agents, possibly viruses, with very long incubation periods and no demonstrable immune response. Two such diseases are known to occur in humans (Creutzfeldt-Jakob disease and kuru) and 3 in animals (scrapie of sheep and goats, transmissible mink encephalopathy and wasting disease of American mule deer and elk). Subacute sclerosing panencephalitis (SSPE) and progressive multifocal leukoencephalopathy (PML), caused by measles and papovaviruses respectively, are diseases with similar clinical features following infection with conventional viruses.

CREUTZFELDT-JAKOB DISEASE
(Jakob-Creutzfeldt syndrome, Subacute spongiform encephalopathy)

ICD-9 046.1

1. **Identification**—An insidious onset of confusion, progressive dementia, variable ataxia in patients aged 16 to over 80 years, but almost all

are between 40 and 70. Later, myoclonic jerks appear together with spasticity, wasting and coma. Focal signs sometimes suggest an intracranial mass. No fever. Slight elevation of CSF proteins is common. On occasion mildly abnormal liver function studies. Typical periodic high-voltage complexes are common on an electroencephalogram. Death usually occurs in less than 1 year, with a mean of 7 months (range 1 month to 4.5 years). About 10% of cases have a positive family history of presenile dementia. Pathological changes are limited to the CNS; amorphous amyloid plaques are present in the cerebellum of about 15% of cases.

Creutzfeldt-Jakob disease must be differentiated from other forms of dementia, especially Alzheimer's disease, from toxic and metabolic encephalopathies, and occasionally from tumors or other space-occupying lesions.

Diagnosis is based on clinical signs, EEG, imaging techniques and histopathological findings and can be confirmed by transmission to animals from biopsy specimens.

2. Infectious agent—Caused by a filterable self-replicating agent transmissible to chimpanzees, monkeys, guinea pigs and mice.

3. Occurrence—Creutzfeldt-Jakob disease has been reported from 50 countries. Average annual mortality rates are usually <1/million but vary from 0.25 to >30 cases/million in different population groups. Highest reported incidence is found among Libyan Jews in Israel.

4. Reservoir—Human cases constitute the only known reservoir. There is no documentation of human infection acquired from animals although this has been hypothesized.

5. Mode of transmission—The mode of transmission of most cases is unknown. Three iatrogenic cases have been reported, 1 due to a corneal transplant and 2 to cortical electrodes which had been used on known patients. Several other cases had a history of brain or eye surgery within 2 years of onset.

6. Incubation period—Fifteen months to 2 yrs in the iatrogenic cases (10 months to 8 yrs in animals). Most are unknown; probably as long as in kuru (4 to over 20 years).

7. Period of communicability—CNS tissues are infectious throughout symptomatic illness. Other tissues and CSF are sometimes infectious. Infectivity during incubation period is not known, but studies in animals suggest that lymphoid and other organs are probably infectious before signs of illness appear.

8. Susceptibility and resistance—Genetic differences in susceptibility have been hypothesized to explain patterns of occurrence of the disease in families, resembling those of autosomal dominant traits, and foci of high incidence. Genetic differences in susceptibility to scrapie have been found in animals.

9. **Methods of control—**

A. *Preventive measures:* Great care must be taken to avoid using tissues of infected patients in transplants, or surgical instruments contaminated by tissues from such patients. Instruments must be disinfected before further use.

B. *Control of patient, contacts and the immediate environment:*

1) Report to local health authority: Official case report not ordinarily justifiable. Class 5 (see Preface).
2) Isolation: Blood/body fluid precautions.
3) Concurrent disinfection: Tissues, surgical instruments and all wound drainage should be considered contaminated and must be inactivated. Steam autoclaving is the surest method of disinfection (1 hour at 121°C and 15 psi). 5% sodium hypochlorite and 0.3 N to 1 N sodium hydroxide are effective disinfectants. Aldehydes are ineffective.
4) Quarantine: None.
5) Immunization of contacts: None.
6) Investigation of contacts and source of infections: A complete medical history, including previous surgical or dental procedures, and a family hisotory of dementia or contact with mental illness should be obtained.
7) Specific therapy: None.

C. *Epidemic measures; D. Disaster implication;* and *E. International measures:* None.

KURU   ICD-9 046.0

A disease of the CNS manifested by cerebellar ataxia, incoordination, tremors, rigidity, and progressive wasting in patients ≥4 yrs of age, which occurred in the Fore language group in the Papua New Guinea highlands. Caused by a filterable self-replicating agent transmissible to primates and other animals, similar to that in Creutzfeld-Jakob disease. Kuru was transmitted by traditional burial practices involving intimate contact with infected tissues, including cannibalism. Formerly very common, kuru now occurs in fewer than 50 patients a year.

ENTEROBIASIS
(Pinworm disease, Oxyuriasis)

ICD-9 127.4

1. Identification—A common intestinal infection which often causes no symptoms. There may be anal itching, disturbed sleep, irritability and sometimes secondary infection of the scratched skin. A variety of manifestations including vulvovaginitis, salpingitis and pelvic granuloma have been described and possible associations include appendicitis and enuresis, but these are rare events.

Diagnosis is made by applying transparent adhesive tape to the perianal region and examining the tape microscopically for eggs; the material is best obtained in the morning before bathing or defecation. Examination should be repeated 3 or more times before accepting a negative result. Eggs are sometimes found on microscopic stool and urine examination. Female worms may be found in feces, in the perianal region and during rectal or vaginal examinations.

2. Infectious agent—*Enterobius vermicularis,* an intestinal nematode.

3. Occurrence—Worldwide, affecting all socioeconomic classes, with rates high in some areas. The most common helminth infection in the USA; prevalence is highest in school-age children (in some groups near 50%), next in preschoolers, and lowest in adults except for mothers of infected children. Often occurs in more than one family member. Prevalence is often high in domiciliary institutions.

4. Reservoir—Man. Pinworms of animals are not transmissible to man.

5. Mode of transmission—Direct transfer of infective eggs by hand from anus to mouth of the same or new host, or indirectly through clothing, bedding, food, or other articles contaminated with eggs of the parasite. Dustborne infection is possible in heavily contaminated households and institutions. Eggs become infective within a few hours after being deposited at the anus by migrating gravid females; the eggs survive less than 2 weeks outside the host. Larvae from ingested eggs hatch in the small intestine; young worms mature in the cecum and upper portions of the colon; gravid worms usually migrate actively from the rectum and may enter adjacent orifices.

6. Incubation period—The life cycle requires 4 to 6 weeks to be completed. Symptomatic disease with high worm burden ordinarily builds up from successive reinfections within some months after the initial exposure.

7. Period of communicability—As long as gravid females are discharging eggs on perianal skin and eggs remain infective in an indoor environment—usually about 2 weeks.

8. Susceptibility and resistance—Susceptibility is universal. Differences in frequency and intensity of infection are due primarily to differences in exposure.

9. Methods of control—

A. *Preventive measures:*

1) Remove sources of infection by treatment of cases.
2) Daily morning bathing, with showers (or stand-up baths) preferred to tub baths.
3) Frequent change to clean underclothing, night clothes and bed sheets, preferably after bathing.
4) Clean/vacuum house daily for several days after treatment of cases.
5) Education in personal hygiene, particularly the need to wash hands before eating or preparing food, and to discourage scratching bare anal area and nail-biting. Keep nails short.
6) Reduce overcrowding in living accommodations.
7) Provide adequate toilets; maintain cleanliness in these facilities.

B. *Control of patient, contacts and the immediate environment:*

1) Report to local health authority: Official report not ordinarily justifiable, Class 5 (see Preface).
2) Isolation: None.
3) Concurrent disinfection: Change bed linen and underwear of infected person daily with care to avoid dispersing eggs into the air. Eggs on discarded linen are killed by exposure to temperatures of 55°C (131°F) for a few seconds; either boil or use a properly functioning household washing machine. Clean/vacuum sleeping and living areas daily for several days after treatment.
4) Quarantine: None.
5) Immunization of contacts: None.
6) Investigation of contacts: Examine all members of an affected family or institution.
7) Specific treatment: Pyrantel pamoate (Antiminth®), mebendazole (Vermox®), pyrvinium pamoate (Povan®), or piperazine citrate (Antepar®). In intensive infections, treatment should be repeated after 2 weeks; concurrent treatment of the whole family may be advisable if several are infected.

C. *Epidemic measures:* The occurrence of multiple cases in schools

and institutions can best be controlled by systematic treatment of all infected individuals and their household contacts.

D. *Disaster implications:* None.

E. *International measures:* None.

FASCIOLIASIS   ICD-9 121.3

1. **Identification**—A disease of the liver caused by a large trematode that is a natural parasite of sheep, cattle and related animals throughout the world. Flukes measuring up to about 3 cm live in the bile ducts, and the young stages live in the liver parenchyma, causing tissue damage and enlargement of the liver. During the early period of parenchymal invasion, there may be right upper quadrant pain, liver function abnormalities and eosinophilia. After migration to the biliary ducts, the flukes may cause biliary colic or obstructive jaundice. Ectopic infection, especially by *Fasciola gigantica,* may produce transient or migrating areas of inflammation in the skin over the trunk or other areas of the body.

Diagnosis is based on finding eggs in the feces or in bile aspirated from the duodenum. Serodiagnostic tests, available in some centers, suggest the diagnosis when positive. "Spurious infection" may be diagnosed when eggs appear in the feces after liver from infected animals has been eaten.

2. **Infectious agent**—*Fasciola hepatica* and, less commonly, *F. gigantica.*

3. **Occurrence**—Human infection has been reported in sheep- and cattle-raising areas of S America, the Caribbean, Europe, Australia and the Middle East.

4. **Reservoir**—Sheep and cattle are natural hosts of *F. hepatica;* and cattle, water buffalo, and other large herbivorous mammals harbor *F. gigantica.*

5. **Mode of transmission**—Eggs passed in the feces develop in water and in about 2 weeks a motile ciliated larva (miracidium) hatches; on entering a snail (lymnaeid) it develops to produce large numbers of free-swimming cercaria which attach to aquatic plants and encyst; these encysted forms (metacercariae) are somewhat resistant to drying. Infection is acquired by eating uncooked aquatic plants, such as watercress, bearing metacercariae. On reaching the intestine the larvae migrate through the wall into the peritoneal cavity, enter the liver and, after development, enter the bile ducts and begin laying eggs 3 to 4 months after initial exposure.

6. **Incubation period**—Variable.

7. Period of communicability—Infection is not transmitted directly from person to person.

8. Susceptibility and resistance—People of all ages are susceptible; infection persists indefinitely.

9. Methods of control—

    A. *Preventive measures:* Educate the public in endemic areas on the danger of eating watercress or other aquatic plants from areas where sheep or other animals graze.

    B. *Control of patient, contacts and the immediate environment:*

        1) Report to local health authority: Official report not ordinarily justifiable, Class 5 (see Preface).
        2) Isolation: None.
        3) Concurrent disinfection: None.
        4) Quarantine: None.
        5) Immunization of contacts: None.
        6) Investigation of contacts and source of infection: Determination of source may be useful in preventing additional infection of the patient or exposure of others.
        7) Specific treatment: Praziquantel (Biltricide®) or bithionol (Lorothidol®, Bitin®).

    C. *Epidemic measures:* Determine location and identify plants and snails involved in transmission. Prevent eating of plants from contaminated areas.

    D. *Disaster implications:* None.

    E. *International measures:* None.

FASCIOLOPSIASIS   ICD-9 121.4

1. Identification—A trematode infection of the small intestine, particularly the duodenum. Symptoms result from local inflammation, ulceration of the intestinal wall and systemic toxic effects. Diarrhea usually alternates with constipation; vomiting and anorexia are frequent. Large numbers of flukes may produce acute intestinal obstruction. Patients may show edema of the face, abdominal wall and legs within 20 days after massive infection; ascites is common. Eosinophilia is usual, secondary anemia is occasional. Death is rare; light infections are usually asymptomatic.

Diagnosis is made by finding the large flukes or characteristic eggs in feces; worms are occasionally vomited.

2. Infectious agent—*Fasciolopsis buski,* a large trematode or fluke reaching lengths up to 7 cm.

3. Occurrence—Widely distributed in rural SE Asia, especially Thailand and central and south China. Prevalence is often high.

4. Reservoir—Pig, man and dog are definitive hosts of adult flukes.

5. Mode of transmission—Eggs passed in feces develop in water within 3 to 7 weeks under favorable conditions; miracidia hatch, and penetrate planorbid snails as intermediate hosts; cercariae develop, are liberated and encyst on aquatic plants to become the infective metacercariae. Human infections result from eating these plants uncooked. In China the chief sources of infection are the nuts of the red water caltrop grown in enclosed ponds, and tubers of the so-called "water chestnut"; infection frequently results when the hull or skin is peeled off with teeth and lips.

6. Incubation period—Eggs appear in the feces about 1 month after infection.

7. Period of communicability—As long as viable eggs are discharged in feces; without treatment, probably for years. Not directly transmitted from person to person.

8. Susceptibility and resistance—Susceptibility is universal. In malnourished individuals the ill effects are pronounced; number of worms influences severity of disease.

9. Methods of control—

A. *Preventive measures:*

1) Educate the public in endemic areas on the mode of transmission and life cycle of the parasite.
2) Treat nightsoil to destroy eggs; bar hogs from contaminating areas where water plants are growing.
3) Dry suspected plants, or if eaten fresh, dip into boiling water for a few seconds; both methods kill metacercariae.

B. *Control of patient, contacts and the immediate environment:*

1) Report to local health authority: In selected endemic areas; in most countries not a reportable disease, Class 3C (see Preface).
2) Isolation: None.
3) Concurrent disinfection: Sanitary disposal of feces.
4) Quarantine: None.
5) Immunization of contacts: None.

6) Investigation of contacts and source of infection: In the individual case, of little value. A community problem (see 9C, below).

7) Specific treatment: Praziquantel (Biltricide®) is the drug of choice.

C. *Epidemic measures:* Identify aquatic plants which are eaten fresh and harbor encysted metacercariae; identify infected snail species living in water with such plants; prevent contamination of water with human feces.

D. *Disaster implications:* None.

E. *International measures:* None.

FILARIASIS   ICD-9 125

The term "filariasis" can be used to denote infection with any of the several Filarioidea. However, as commonly used, the term refers only to the lymphatic-dwelling filariae listed below. For others, refer to the specific disease.

FILARIASIS DUE TO *WUCHERERIA*   ICD-9 125.0
BANCROFTI
(Bancroftian filariasis, Wuchereriasis)
FILARIASIS DUE TO *BRUGIA MALAYI*   ICD-9 125.1
(Malayan filariasis, Brugiasis)
TIMOREAN FILARIASIS   ICD-9 125.6

1. Identification—

A. Bancroftian filariasis is an infection with the nematode *Wuchereria bancrofti* which normally develops in the lymphatics of man. Female worms produce microfilariae which reach the bloodstream and circulate. Two forms occur: in one, the microfilariae circulate in the peripheral blood at night (nocturnal periodicity) with greatest concentrations between 10 pm and 2 am; in the other form, microfilariae circulate continuously in the peripheral blood but occur in greater concentration in the daytime (diurnal subperiodicity). The latter form is endemic in the S Pacific, and in small rural foci in SE Asia where the principal vectors are day-biting mosquitoes. The spectrum of clinical manifestations in regions of endemic filariasis include: people who are exposed but remain asymptomatic and parasitologically negative; people who are asymptomatic with microfilaremia; people with acute recurrent filarial fever, lymphadenitis and retrograde lymphangitis who may or may not have microfilaremia; people with chronic signs including hydrocele, chyluria and elephantiasis of the limbs, breast and genitalia who have low level or undetectable microfilaremia; and people with tropical eosinophilia manifested by paroxysmal, nocturnal asthma, chronic interstitial lung disease and degenerating microfilariae in tissues but not in blood (occult filariasis).

B. Malayan filariasis is caused by the nematode *Brugia malayi*. The nocturnally periodic form occurs in rural populations living in open rice-growing areas throughout much of Asia. The subperiodic form infects man, monkeys and wild and domestic carnivores in the forests of Malaya, Sumatra, and Borneo. Clinical manifestations are similar to those of Bancroftian filariasis except that the recurrent acute attacks of filarial fever, adenitis and descending lymphangitis are more severe while chyluria is uncommon and elephantiasis is usually confined to below the knee.

C. Timorean filariasis results from infection with *Brugia timori* and has been described on Timor (Indonesia). Clinical manifestations are comparable to those seen in *B. malayi* infections.

Clinical manifestations of filariasis often occur with no demonstrable circulating microfilariae (occult filariasis). In several thousand cases seen in American military personnel during World War II, microfilariae were found in only 10–15 patients despite repeated blood examinations. In some of these cases, infection was manifested by marked eosinophilia associated with pulmonary infiltrates (tropical eosinophilia or tropical pulmonary eosinophilia).

Microfilariae are best detected during periods of maximal microfilaremia. Live microfilariae can be seen under low power in a drop of peripheral blood on a slide or in hemolyzed blood in a counting chamber. Microfilariae may be concentrated by filtration through a Nuclepore filter (5 micron pore size) and the Knott technique (centrifugal sedimentation of blood laked with 2% formalin). During periods of minimal microfilaremia the provocative test with diethylcarbamazine may be used except in areas where onchocerciasis or loiasis are also endemic. Species identification is made with Giemsa-stained blood smears.

2. Infectious agents—*Wuchereria bancrofti, Brugia malayi* and *B. timori*.

3. Occurrence—*W. bancrofti* is endemic in most of the warm humid regions of the world, including Latin America, Africa, Asia, and the Pacific Islands; it is common in urban areas with inadequate sanitation favoring breeding of vector mosquitoes. *B. malayi* is endemic in rural southwest India, Sri Lanka, SE Asia, central China, and S Korea. *B. timori* occurs on the rural eastern islands of Indonesia. High prevalence depends upon a large reservoir of infection and abundant vectors.

4. Reservoir—Man with microfilariae in the blood for *W. bancrofti,*

periodic *B. malayi* and *B. timori;* in Malaya, Borneo and probably Sumatra, cats and nonhuman primates serve as reservoirs for subperiodic *B. malayi.*

5. Mode of transmission—By bite of a mosquito harboring infective larvae. *W. bancrofti* is transmitted by many species, the most important being *Culex quinquefasciatus, Anopheles gambiae, An. funestus, Aedes polynesiensis,* and *Ae. pseudoscutellaris. B. malayi* is transmitted by various species of *Mansonia, Anopheles,* and *Aedes. B. timori* is transmitted by *An. barbirostris.* In the mosquito, ingested microfilariae penetrate the stomach wall and develop in the thoracic muscles to infective larvae which migrate to the proboscis and finally into the punctured skin following the mosquito bite.

6. Incubation period—While allergic inflammatory manifestations may appear as early as a month after infection, microfilariae may not appear in the blood until 2–3 months in *B. malayi* or 8–12 months in *W. bancrofti* infections.

7. Period of communicability—Not directly transmitted from person to person. Man may infect mosquitoes if microfilariae are present in the peripheral blood; microfilaremia may persist for 5 yrs or longer after initial infection. The mosquito becomes infective about 10 days after an infective blood meal.

8. Susceptibility and resistance—Universal susceptibility to infection but considerable geographic differences in the type and severity of disease. Repeated infections occur in endemic regions and lead to the severe manifestations such as elephantiasis.

9. Methods of control—

  A. Preventive measures:

  1) Identify the vectors by detecting infective larvae in mosquitoes caught on human bait; identify times and places of mosquito biting and locate breeding places; if indoor night-biters are responsible, spray inside walls with a residual insecticide, screen houses or use bed nets and insect repellents. Eliminate breeding places such as open latrines, old tires, coconut husks, etc., and treat others with larvicides. Where *Mansonia* species are vectors, clear ponds of vegetation *(Pistia)* or apply herbicides to plants which serve as sources of air for the larvae.

  2) Public education on the mode of transmission and methods of mosquito control.

  3) Long-term control may involve changes in housing construction to include screening and environmental control to eliminate mosquito breeding sites.

B. *Control of patient, contacts and the immediate environment:*

1) Report to local health authority: In selected endemic regions; in most countries, not a reportable disease, Class 3C (see Preface). Reporting of cases with demonstrated microfilariae provides information on potential areas of transmission.

2) Isolation: Not practicable. So far as possible, patients with microfilaremia should be protected from mosquitoes to reduce transmission.

3) Concurrent disinfection: None.

4) Quarantine: None.

5) Immunization of contacts: None.

6) Investigation of contacts and source of infection: Only as part of a general community effort (see 9A and 9C).

7) Specific treatment: Diethylcarbamazine (DEC, Hetrazan®, Banocide®) results in rapid disappearance of most or all microfilariae from the blood but may not destroy the adult worms. Low level microfilariae may reappear after treatment. Therefore, treatment must usually be repeated at specified intervals. Low level microfilaremia can be detected only by concentration techniques. DEC may cause acute generalized reactions during the first 24 days of treatment due to death and degeneration of microfilariae; these are often controlled by aspirin and corticosteroids. Localized lymphadenitis and lymphangitis may follow the death of the adult worms.

C. *Epidemic measures:* Vector control is the fundamental measure. In areas of high endemicity it is essential to appraise correctly the bionomics of mosquito vectors, prevalence and incidence of disease, and environmental factors responsible for transmission in each locality. Even partial control by anti-mosquito measures may reduce incidence and restrict the endemic focus. Measurable results are slow because of the long incubation period. Mass treatment with DEC often is an effective measure although in some instances adverse reactions have discouraged community participation, particularly where onchocerciasis is endemic. (See Mazzotti reaction).

D. *Disaster implications:* None.

E. *International measures:* None.

DIROFILARIASIS
ICD-9 125.6
(Zoonotic filariasis)

Certain species of filaria, commonly seen in wild or domestic animals, occasionally infect man but microfilaremia rarely occurs. The genus *Dirofilaria* causes pulmonary and cutaneous disease in man. *D. immitis*, the dog heartworm, has caused pulmonary disease in the USA (about 50 cases), with a few infections in Japan and Australia. Transmission to man is by mosquito bite. The worm lodges in a pulmonary artery where it forms the nidus of a thrombus which leads to vascular occlusion, coagulation, necrosis and fibrosis. Common symptoms are chest pain, cough and hemoptysis. Eosinophilia is infrequent. The fibrotic nodule, 1–3 cm in diameter is recognizable by x-ray as a "coin lesion." Cutaneous disease is caused by various species including *D. tenuis*, a parasite of the raccoon in the USA, and adult *D. repens*, a parasite of dogs and cats in Europe, Africa and Asia; the worms develop in or migrate to the conjunctivae and the subcutaneous tissues of the scrotum, breast, arms and legs, but there is rarely microfilaremia. Others *(Brugia)* localize in lymph nodes. Diagnosis is usually by the finding of worms in tissue sections of surgically excised lesions.

OTHER NEMATODES PRODUCING MICROFILARIAE IN MAN

Several other nematodes may infect man and produce microfilariae. These include *Onchocerca volvulus* and *Loa loa* causing onchocerciasis and loiasis, respectively. (See under each disease listing). Other infections are forms of mansonellosis (ICD-9 125.4); *Mansonella (Dipetalonema, Tetrapetalonema, Acanthocheilonema) perstans* is widely distributed in west Africa and northeastern S America; the adult is found in the body cavities and the unsheathed microfilariae circulate with nocturnal subperiodicity. Infection is usually asymptomatic. In some countries of west and central Africa infection with·*M. streptocerca* (ICD-9 125.6) is common and is suspected of causing cutaneous edema and thickening of the skin, hypopigmented macules, pruritis and papules. The adults and unsheathed microfilariae occur in the skin as in onchocerciasis. *M. ozzardi* (ICD-9 125.5) occurs from the Yucatan to northern Argentina and in the West Indies; diagnosis is based on the demonstration of the circulating unsheathed nonperiodic microfilaria; infection is generally asymptomatic but may be associated with allergic manifestations such as articular pain, pruritis, headaches and lymphadenopathy. *Culicoides* midges are the main vectors for the last three parasites. *M. ozzardi* is transmitted by blackflies. Diethylcarbamazine is effective against *M. streptocerca*, and possibly is occasionally effective against *M. perstans* and *M. ozzardi*.

FOODBORNE INTOXICATION   ICD-9 005
(Food poisoning; Foodborne disease)

Foodborne intoxication or food poisoning are generic terms applied to illnesses acquired through consumption of contaminated food or water. The terms apply to intoxications caused by chemical contaminants (heavy metals and others), toxins elaborated by bacterial growth *(Staphylococcus aureus, Clostridium botulinum)*, and a variety of organic substances that may be present in natural foods such as certain mushrooms, mussels, eels, scombroid fish, and other seafood. This definition also includes acute foodborne infections such as salmonellosis, discussed elsewhere (see Salmonellosis).

This chapter will present those conditions with short incubation periods which could be considered to be intoxications, i.e., caused by toxins produced by infectious agents which are present in the ingested food. Included are botulism and food poisonings caused by *S. aureus, Clostridium perfringens, Vibrio parahaemolyticus* and *Bacillus cereus*.

Food poisoning outbreaks are usually recognized by the occurrence of illness within a short period of time among individuals who had eaten foods in common. Prompt and thorough laboratory evaluation of cases and implicated foods is essential. Single cases of food poisoning are difficult to identify unless, as in botulism, there is a distinctive clinical syndrome. Food poisoning may be one of the most common causes of acute illness, yet cases and outbreaks are underrecognized and underreported.

Prevention and control of these diseases are based on the same technical principles—to avoid or minimize contamination, to destroy or denature the contaminant, and to prevent further spread or multiplication of the contaminant. Specific problems and appropriate modes of intervention will vary from one country to another depending on environmental, economic, political, technological and sociocultural factors. Ultimately, prevention will depend on education of foodhandlers in proper practices in cooking and storage of food, and in personal hygiene.

I. STAPHYLOCOCCAL FOOD POISONING   ICD-9 005.0

1. **Identification**—An intoxication (not an infection) of abrupt and sometimes violent onset, with severe nausea, cramps, vomiting, and prostration; often accompanied by diarrhea; sometimes with subnormal temperature and lowered blood pressure. Deaths are rare; duration of

illness is commonly not more than a day or two but the intensity of symptoms may require hospitalization and may result in surgical exploration in sporadic cases. Diagnosis is easier when a group of cases is recognized with the characteristic acute, predominantly upper gastrointestinal symptoms and the short interval between eating a common food item and the onset of symptoms.

Differential diagnosis includes other recognized forms of food poisoning as well as chemical poisons.

Recovery of large numbers of enterotoxin-producing staphylococci ($\geqq 10^5$ organisms/g) on routine culture media from vomitus, feces or a suspected food item supports the diagnosis. Absence of staphylococci on culture of a heated food does not rule out the diagnosis. It may be possible to identify enterotoxin or thermonuclease in the food in the absence of viable organisms. Phage typing and enterotoxin tests may help epidemiologic investigations but are not routinely available or indicated.

2. **Toxic agent**—Several enterotoxins of *Staphylococcus aureus*, stable at boiling temperature. Staphylococci multiply in food and produce the toxins.

3. **Occurrence**—Widespread and relatively frequent; one of the principal acute food poisonings in the USA.

4. **Reservoir**—Man in most instances; occasionally cows with infected udders.

5. **Mode of transmission**—By ingestion of a food product containing staphylococcal enterotoxin. Foods involved are particularly those which are contacted by foodhandlers' hands either without subsequent cooking or with inadequate heating or refrigeration, such as pastries, custards, salad dressings, sandwiches, sliced meats and meat products. Toxin has also developed in inadequately cured hams and salami, and in nonprocessed and inadequately processed cheese. When these foods remain at room temperature for several hours before being eaten, toxin-producing staphylococci multiply and elaborate the toxin. The organisms may be of human origin from purulent discharges of an infected finger, infected eyes, abscesses, acneiform facial eruptions, nasopharyngeal secretions, or apparently normal skin; or of bovine origin such as contaminated milk or milk products.

6. **Incubation period**—Interval between eating food and onset of symptoms is 30 minutes to 7 hours, usually 2–4 hours.

7. **Period of communicability**—Not applicable.

8. **Susceptibility and resistance**—Most persons are susceptible.

9. **Methods of control**—

A. *Preventive measures:*

1) Food handling time (initial preparation to service) should be reduced to an absolute minimum unless the temperature can be controlled. Perishable foods should be kept **hot** ($>60°C/140°F$) or **cold** ($\leqq4°C/39°F$) in shallow containers and covered, if they are to be stored for more than 2 hours.

2) Temporary exclusion from food handling of persons with boils, abscesses and other purulent lesions of hands, face or nose.

3) Educate foodhandlers in strict food hygiene, sanitation and cleanliness of kitchens, proper temperature control, handwashing, cleaning of fingernails; and to the danger of working with skin, nose or eye infections.

B. *Control of patient, contacts and the immediate environment:*

1) Report to local health authority: Report promptly. Obligatory report of outbreaks of suspected or confirmed cases, Class 4 (see Preface).

2), 3), 4), 5), 6): Not pertinent. Control is of outbreaks; single cases are rarely identified.

7) Specific treatment: Fluid replacement when indicated.

C. *Epidemic measures:*

1) By quick review of reported cases, determine time and place of exposure and the population at risk; obtain a complete listing of the foods served and embargo under refrigeration all foods still available. The prominent clinical features, coupled with an estimate of the incubation period, provides useful leads to the most probable etiological agent. Collect specimens of feces and vomitus for laboratory examination. Alert laboratory to suspected etiologic agents. Interview a random sample of those who were exposed. Compare the attack rates for specific food items eaten and not eaten; the implicated food item(s) will have the greatest difference in attack rates. Most of the sick will have eaten the contaminated food.

2) Inquire about the origin of the incriminated food and the manner of its preparation and storage before serving. Look for possible sources of contamination and periods of inadequate refrigeration and heating that would permit growth of staphylococci. Submit any leftover suspected foods promptly for laboratory examination; failure to

isolate staphylococci does not exclude the presence of the heat-resistant enterotoxin if the food had been heated.

3) Search for foodhandlers with skin infections, particularly of the hands. Culture all purulent lesions and collect nasal swabs from all foodhandlers. Antibiograms and/or phage-typing of representative strains of enterotoxin-producing staphylococci isolated from foods and foodhandlers and from vomitus or feces of patients may be helpful.

D. *Disaster implications:* A potential hazard in situations involving mass feeding and lack of refrigeration facilities. A particular problem of air travel.

E. *International measure:* WHO Collaborating Centres (see Preface).

II. BOTULISM ICD-9 005.1

1. Identification—A severe intoxication resulting from ingestion of toxin preformed in contaminated food and not from toxin produced in the gut as occurs in infant botulism (see Botulism, Infant). The illness is characterized by clinical manifestations relating primarily to the nervous system. Ptosis, visual difficulty (blurred or double vision), dry mouth and sore throat are often the first complaints. These symptoms may be followed by descending symmetrical flaccid paralysis in an alert person. Vomiting and diarrhea may be present initially. Fever is absent unless a complicating infection occurs. Unless adequately treated, about one-third of patients may die within 3 to 7 days after onset, usually from respiratory failure or from superimposed infection; with good respiratory care and specific antitoxin, the case fatality rate in the USA during the last decade has generally been under 15%. Recovery may be slow (months and rarely years).

The same clinical picture has been seen rarely after the causal organism contaminated a wound in which anaerobic conditions develop; this is known as wound botulism.

Diagnosis is established by demonstration of the specific toxin in serum or stool, or by culture of *Clostridium botulinum* from a wound in a clinical case. Identification of organisms in a suspected food is helpful but not diagnostic since botulinum spores are so often present in the environment; the presence of toxin is more significant.

2. Toxic agent—Toxins produced by *Clostridium botulinum*. Most human outbreaks are due to types A, B and E with rare cases due to type F and type G toxins of *C. botulinum*. Type E outbreaks are usually related to fish, seafood and meat from marine mammals. Toxin is produced in improperly processed canned low-acid or alkaline foods or in pasteurized or lightly cured foods held without refrigeration, especially in airtight packaging. Toxin is destroyed by boiling; inactivation of spores requires much higher temperatures. Type E toxin can be produced slowly at temperatures as low as 3°C (37.4°F), which is lower than that of ordinary refrigeration.

3. Occurrence—Worldwide; sporadic cases, family and general outbreaks occur where food products are prepared or preserved by methods which do not destroy the spores and which permit toxin formation. Cases rarely result from contaminated commercially processed products; outbreaks have occurred from contamination after processsing through damaged cans.

4. Reservoir—Soil, marine sediment and the intestinal tract of animals, including fish.

5. Mode of transmission—By ingestion of food in which toxin had been formed, predominantly after inadequate heating during canning, and eaten without subsequent adequate cooking. Most poisonings in the USA are due to home-canned vegetables and fruits; meats are infrequent vehicles. Cases associated with baked potatoes and improperly handled commercial potpies have been reported. A recent outbreak was attributed to sautéed onions. In Canada outbreaks have been associated with seal meat, smoked salmon and fermented salmon eggs. In Europe, most cases are due to sausages and to smoked or preserved meats; in Japan, to fish. These differences have been attributed in part to the greater use in the USA of sodium nitrite for preserving meats. Rare cases of botulism secondary to wound infection have been reported.

6. Incubation period—Neurologic symptoms usually appear within 12-36 hours, sometimes several days, after eating contaminated food. In general, the shorter the incubation period, the more severe the disease and the higher the fatality rate.

7. Period of communicability—Not applicable.

8. Susceptibility and resistance—Susceptibility is general.

9. Methods of control—

    A. Preventive Measures:

        1) Ensure effective control of processing and preparation of commercially canned and preserved foods.

        2) Educate housewives and others concerned with home canning and other food preservation techniques regarding the proper time, pressure and temperature required to destroy spores, the need for adequately refrigerated storage of incompletely processed foods and the effective-

ness in destroying botulism toxins by boiling, with stirring, home-canned vegetables for at least 3 minutes.

3) *C. botulinum* may or may not cause container lids to bulge and the contents to have "off-odors." Other contaminants can also cause cans or bottle lids to bulge. Bulging containers should not be opened and foods with "off-odors" should not be eaten or "taste tested." Commercial cans with bulging lids should be returned unopened to the vendor.

B. *Control of patient, contacts and the immediate environment:*

1) Report to local health authority: Case report of suspected and confirmed cases obligatory in most states and countries, Class 2A (see Preface); immediate telephone report indicated.

2) Isolation: None.

3) Concurrent disinfection: The contaminated food(s) should be detoxified by boiling before discarding or else the containers broken and buried deeply in soil to prevent ingestion by animals. Contaminated utensils should be sterilized by boiling or by chlorine disinfection to inactivate any remaining toxin.

4) Quarantine: None.

5) Management of contacts: None for simple direct contacts. Those who are known to have eaten the incriminated food should be purged with cathartics, given gastric lavage and high enemas and kept under close medical observation. The decision to provide presumptive treatment with polyvalent antitoxin to asymptomatic individuals should be weighed carefully, balancing the potential protection when antitoxin is administered early (within 1–2 days after eating the implicated meal) against the risk of adverse reactions and sensitization to horse serum.

6) Investigation of contacts and source of toxin: Study recent food history of those ill and recover all suspected foods for appropriate testing and disposal.

7) Specific treatment: Intravenous and i.m. administration of trivalent botulinal antitoxin (types A, B and E), available from CDC, Atlanta (see Preface), as soon as possible is considered a part of routine treatment. Serum should be collected to identify the specific toxin before antitoxin is administered, but antitoxin should not be withheld pending test results. Most important is immediate access to an intensive care unit so that respiratory failure, the usual cause of death, can be anticipated and managed promptly.

C. *Epidemic measures:* Suspicion of a single case of botulism should immediately raise the question of a group outbreak involving a family or others who have shared a common food. Home- preserved foods should be the prime suspect until ruled out, although widely distributed commercially preserved foods are occasionally identified as the source of intoxication and pose a far greater threat to the public health. In addition, since recent outbreaks have implicated unusual food items, even theoretically unlikely foods should be considered. When any food is implicated by epidemiologic or laboratory findings, immediate recall of the product is necessary, as is immediate search for persons who shared the suspected food and a search for any remaining food from the same source that may be similarly contaminated; such food, if found, should be submitted for laboratory examination. Sera and stools from patients and, when indicated, from others exposed but not ill should be collected before administration of antitoxin and forwarded immediately to a reference laboratory.

D. *Disaster implications:* None.

E. *International measures:* Commercial products may have been distributed widely; international efforts may be required to recover or test implicated foods.

III. *CLOSTRIDIUM PERFRINGENS* FOOD POISONING   ICD-9 005.2
(*C. welchii* food poisoning, Enteritis necroticans, Pigbel)

1. **Identification**—An intestinal disorder characterized by sudden onset of colic followed by diarrhea; nausea is common but vomiting and fever are usually absent. Generally a mild disease of short duration, one day or less, and rarely fatal in healthy persons. Outbreaks of severe disease with a high case fatality rate associated with a necrotizing enteritis have been documented in post-war Germany and in New Guinea.

Diagnosis is supported by demonstration of *C. perfringens* in semiquantitative anaerobic cultures of food ($\geqq 10^5/g$) and patients' stools ($\geqq 10^6/g$) in addition to clinical and epidemiologic evidence. When serotyping can be performed, the same serotype is usually demonstrated in different specimens; serotyping is done routinely only in Japan and the UK.

2. **Infectious agent**—Type A strains of *C. perfringens (C. welchii)* cause typical food poisoning outbreaks; type C strains cause necrotizing enteritis. Disease is produced by toxins elaborated by these organisms.

3. Occurrence—Widespread and relatively frequent in countries with cooking practices that favor multiplication of *Clostridia* to high levels.

4. Reservoir—Soil; also the gastrointestinal tract of healthy persons and animals (cattle, pigs, poultry and fish).

5. Mode of transmission—Ingestion of food contaminated by soil or feces, held under conditions which permit multiplication of the organism. Almost all outbreaks are associated with inadequately heated or reheated meats, usually stews, meat pies, or gravies made of beef, turkey or chicken. Spores survive normal cooking temperatures, germinate and multiply during slow cooling, storage at ambient temperature, and/or inadequate rewarming. Outbreaks are usually traced to food catering firms, restaurants, cafeterias and schools which have inadequate cooking and refrigeration facilities for large-scale service. Heavy bacterial contamination ($>10^5$ organisms/g of food) is usually required for clinical disease.

6. Incubation period—From 6–24 hours, usually 10–12 hours.

7. Period of communicability—Not applicable.

8. Susceptibility and resistance—Most persons are probably susceptible. In volunteer studies, no resistance was observed after repeated exposures.

9. Methods of control—

    A. Preventive measures:

        1)   Serve meat dishes hot, as soon as they are cooked, or cool them rapidly in a properly designed chiller and refrigerate until serving time; reheating, if necessary, should be thorough (internal temperature of $\geqq75°C/167°F$) and rapid. Do not partially cook meat and poultry one day and reheat the next, unless it can be stored at a safe temperature. Large cuts of meat should be thoroughly cooked; for more rapid cooling of cooked foods, divide stews and similar dishes prepared in bulk into many shallow containers to place in a rapid chiller.

        2)   Educate foodhandlers on the risks inherent in large-scale cooking, especially of meat dishes. Where possible, encourage serving hot dishes while still hot from initial cooking.

    B. Control of patient, contacts and the immediate environment; C. Epidemic measures; and D. Disaster implications: See Staphylococcal Food Poisoning, (19, above).

    E. International measures: None.

IV. *VIBRIO PARAHAEMOLYTICUS*   ICD-9 005.4
FOOD POISONING
(*Vibrio parahaemolyticus* infection)

1. **Identification**—An intestinal disorder characterized by watery diarrhea and abdominal cramps in the majority of cases, and sometimes with nausea, vomiting, fever and headache. Occasionally a dysentery-like illness is observed with bloody or mucoid stools, high fever, and high WBC count. A disease of moderate severity with duration generally 1–7 days; systemic infection and death rarely occur.

Diagnosis is confirmed by isolating the organism from the patient's stool on appropriate media.

2. **Infectious agent**—*Vibrio parahaemolyticus,* a halophilic vibrio. Twelve different "O" antigen groups and approximately 60 different "K" antigen types have been identified. Pathogenic strains are generally capable of producing a characteristic hemolytic reaction (the "Kanagawa phenomenon").

3. **Occurrence**—Sporadic cases and common source outbreaks have been reported from many parts of the world, particularly Japan, SE Asia, and the USA. Occurs primarily in warm months of the year.

4. **Reservoir**—Marine coastal environs are the natural habitat. During the cold season, organisms are found in marine silt; during the warm season, they are found free in coastal waters and in fish and shellfish.

5. **Mode of transmission**—Ingestion of raw or inadequately cooked seafood, or any food cross-contaminated by handling raw seafood in the same environment, or by rinsing with contaminated seawater. A period of time at room temperature is generally necessary to allow multiplication of organisms to the usual infectious level ($\geq 10^6$).

6. **Incubation period**—Usually between 12–24 hours, but can range from 4–96 hours.

7. **Period of communicability**—Noncommunicable from person to person.

8. **Susceptibility and resistance**—Most persons are probably susceptible.

9. **Methods of control**—

    A. Preventive measures:

        1) Assure that cooked seafood reaches temperatures adequate to kill the organism (may survive at 60°C (140°F) for up to 15 minutes and at 80°C (176°F) for several minutes).

        2) Handle cooked seafood in a manner that precludes con-

tamination from raw seafood, or from contaminated seawater.

3) Keep all seafood, raw or cooked, adequately refrigerated prior to eating.

4) Educate seafood handlers and processors on these preventive measures.

5) Avoid use of seawater in foodhandling areas, e.g., on cruise ships.

6) Education regarding risks associated with eating raw seafood.

B. Control of patient, contacts and immediate environment; C. Epidemic measures; and D. Disaster implications: See Staphylococcal Food Poisoning (I9, above) except for 9B2, Isolation: Enteric precautions.

E. International measures: None.

V. BACILLUS CEREUS FOOD POISONING   ICD-9 005.8

1. Identification—A gastrointestinal disorder characterized in some cases by sudden onset of nausea and vomiting and in others by colic and diarrhea. Generally persists no longer than 24 hours and is rarely fatal.

Diagnosis is supported by identifying the causative organism in the suspect food and in feces of patients, and by performing quantitative cultures with selective media to estimate the number of organisms present (generally $>10^5$ organisms/g of food are required). Enterotoxin testing is valuable but may not be widely available.

2. Infectious agent—*Bacillus cereus*, an aerobic spore former. Two enterotoxins have been identified—one heat stable causing vomiting and one heat labile causing diarrhea.

3. Occurrence—A well-recognized cause of foodborne disease in Europe; rarely reported in the USA.

4. Reservoir—A ubiquitous organism of soil and commonly found in raw, dried and processed foods.

5. Mode of transmission—Ingestion of food that has been kept at ambient temperatures after cooking, permitting multiplication of the organisms. Outbreaks associated with vomiting have been most commonly associated with rice (such as fried rice served in Asian restaurants). Vegetables and meat dishes mishandled after cooking are also often responsible.

6. **Incubation period**—From 1–6 hours in cases where vomiting is the predominant symptom; from 6–16 hours where diarrhea is predominant.

7. **Period of communicability**—Not communicable from person to person.

8. **Susceptibility and resistance**—Unknown.

9. **Methods of control**—

A. *Preventive measures:* Foods should not remain at ambient temperature after cooking since the ubiquitous *B. cereus* spores can survive boiling, germinate, and multiply rapidly at room temperature. Leftover food should be refrigerated promptly; thorough reheating should be performed rapidly to avoid multiplication of microorganisms.

B. *Control of patient, contacts and the immediate environment; C. Epidemic measures;* and D. *Disaster implications:* See Staphylcoccal Food Poisoning (I9, above).

E. *International measures:* None.

GASTROENTERITIS, ACUTE VIRAL   ICD-9 078

Viral gastroenteritis is comprised of at least two entities with distinct epidemiological differences. "Sporadic viral gastroenteritis," or more properly rotaviral enteritis, affects mainly infants and young children as a diarrheal illness which may be severe enough to require hospitalization. "Epidemic viral gastroenteropathy," a self-limited mild illness, tends to occur in family, school or community outbreaks affecting both adults and children.

I. ROTAVIRAL ENTERITIS   ICD-9 008.8
(Sporadic viral gastroenteritis, Severe viral gastroenteritis of infants and children)

1. **Identification**—A sporadic severe gastroenteritis of infants and young children characterized by diarrhea and vomiting, often with severe dehydration and occasional deaths in the young age group. Milder forms of gastroenteritis also occur. Secondary cases among family contacts are relatively rare, while subclinical infections occur frequently. Rotaviral infection has occasionally been found in pediatric patients with a variety of clinical manifestations including intussusception, gastrointestinal bleeding, fatal Reye syndrome, encephalitis, upper and lower respiratory illness,

exanthem subitum, neonatal necrotizing enterocolitis, Kawasaki syndrome and others; further studies are needed to establish whether the virus is coincidental or etiological. It is a major cause of nosocomial diarrhea.

The virus is identified in stool or rectal swab by EM, or immunological techniques for which commercial kits are available. Evidence of infection can be demonstrated by ELISA, CF, IF, neutralization in cell culture, and other serological techniques. Adenoviruses 40 and 41 have been implicated in some cases of acute infantile gastroenteritis, detected by genus-specific ELISA.

2. Infectious agent—The 70 nm rotavirus (formerly designated orbivirus, reovirus-like, duovirus) belongs to the reoviridae family. There are at least 4 serotypes of human rotaviruses. They also share subgroup specificity which further defines the serotypes into 1 of 2 subgroups. The human rotaviruses are related by a common antigen to some animal rotaviruses.

3. Occurrence—Worldwide; sporadically and in outbreaks. Rotavirus is associated with up to 50% of the hospitalized cases of diarrheal illness in infants and young children (6–24 month age group) and up to 25% of all diarrheal illness in this age group. Outbreaks are being detected in geriatric units. In temperate climates, almost exclusively in the cooler months; in tropical climates, throughout the year and with less pronounced peaks. Infection of adults is usually subclinical; subclinical infections occur commonly in neonates in certain settings.

4. Reservoir—Probably man. The pathogenicity of animal viruses for man is not defined.

5. Mode of transmission—Probably fecal-oral and possibly fecal-respiratory.

6. Incubation period—Approximately 48 hours.

7. Period of communicability—During acute stage of disease and later while virus shedding continues. Virus is not usually detectable after about the 8th day of illness, although individuals excreting virus for up to 23 days have been reported.

8. Susceptibility and resistance—Susceptibility is universal but by 3 years of age most individuals have acquired rotavirus antibody.

9. Methods of control—

    A. Preventive measures:

        1)   Undetermined. Hygienic measures applicable to diseases transmitted via fecal-oral route (see Typhoid Fever, 9A), or possibly fecal-respiratory route.

    2) Prevent exposure of infants and young children to individuals with acute gastroenteritis.

    3) Passive immunization by oral administration of IG has been shown to protect low-birth-weight neonates. Studies are underway on the efficacy of a live attenuated bovine rotavirus as an orally administered vaccine.

B. *Control of patient, contacts and the immediate environment:*

    1) Report to local health authority: Obligatory report of epidemics; no individual case report, Class 4 (see Preface).

    2) Isolation: Enteric precautions.

    3) Concurrent disinfection: None.

    4) Quarantine: None.

    5) Immunization of contacts: None.

    6) Investigation of contacts and source of infection: Sources of infection should be sought, especially in family and home.

    7) Specific treatment: Fluid and electrolyte replacement; oral glucose-electrolyte solution is adequate in most cases. Parenteral fluids are needed in cases with vascular collapse (see Cholera, 9B7).

C. *Epidemic measures:* Search for vehicles of transmission and source on epidemiologic bases.

D. *Disaster implications:* A potential problem.

E. *International measures:* WHO Collaborating Centres (see Preface).

II. EPIDEMIC VIRAL GASTROENTEROPATHY   ICD-9 078.8

(Epidemic viral gastroenteritis, Norwalk type disease, Acute infectious nonbacterial gastroenteritis, Viral diarrhea, Epidemic diarrhea and vomiting, Winter vomiting disease, Epidemic nausea and vomiting)

1. Identification—Usually a self-limited mild disease that often occurs in outbreaks with clinical symptoms of nausea, vomiting, diarrhea, abdominal pain, myalgia, headache, malaise, low-grade fever or a combination thereof. Gastrointestinal symptoms characteristically last 24–48 hours.

The viruses may be identified in stools of ill individuals by IEM or, for the Norwalk virus, also by RIA. Serologic evidence of infection may be demonstrated by IEM, or, for the Norwalk virus, by the blocking RIA test.

2. Infectious agent—The small 27 nm Norwalk virus (unclassified but with some characteristics of caliciviruses) has been implicated as the etiologic agent of about one-third of the nonbacterial gastroenteritis outbreaks. Other agents which are morphologically similar but antigenically distinct have been associated with gastroenteritis outbreaks. These include Hawaii, Ditchling or W, Cockle, Parramatta, Snow Mountain (Colorado) and Marin County agents. Outbreaks have been associated with adenoviruses, astroviruses, caliciviruses, the 33–39 nm Sapporo agent, the similar Otofuke agent and coronaviruses; with the exception of the enteric adenoviruses, the role of these agents as a cause of severe diarrhea of infants and young children is inconclusive.

3. Occurrence—Worldwide and common; most often in outbreaks but also sporadically affecting all age groups. In a study in the USA, antibody to Norwalk agent was acquired slowly; by the 5th decade of life, >60% of the population had antibody. In most developing countries studied, antibody is acquired much earlier. Seroresponses to Norwalk virus were detected in infants and young children in Bangladesh and this agent was associated with 1–2% of diarrhea episodes.

4. Reservoir—Man is the only known reservoir.

5. Mode of transmission—Unknown; probably by fecal-oral route. Several recent outbreaks have strongly suggested foodborne and waterborne transmission.

6. Incubation period—24–48 hours; in volunteer studies with Norwalk agent, the range was 10–51 hours.

7. Period of communicability—During acute stage of disease.

8. Susceptibility and resistance—Susceptibility is widespread. Short-term immunity lasting up to 14 wks after induced Norwalk illness in volunteers has been demonstrated but long-term immunity was variable; some individuals became ill on rechallenge 27–42 months later. Levels of preexisting serum antibody to Norwalk virus did not correlate with susceptibility or resistance.

9. Methods of control—

    A. *Preventive measures:* Undetermined. Use hygienic measures applicable to diseases transmitted via fecal-oral route (see Typhoid Fever, 9A).

    B. *Control of patient, contacts and the immediate environment:*

        1) Report to local health authority: Obligatory report of epidemics; no individual case report, Class 4 (see Preface).

        2) Isolation: Enteric precautions.

        3) Concurrent disinfection: None.

        4) Quarantine: None.

     5)   Immunization of contacts: None.
     6)   Investigation of contacts and source of infection: Search for means of spread of infection in outbreak situations.
     7)   Specific treatment: Electrolyte and fluid replacement in severe cases.

C.   *Epidemic measures:* Search for vehicles of transmission and source; determine course of outbreak to define the epidemiology.

D.   *Disaster implications:* A potential problem.

E.   *International measures:* None.

GIARDIASIS   ICD-9 007.1
(Giardia enteritis, Lambliasis)

1. Identification—A protozoan infection principally of the upper small intestine; while often asymptomatic, it may also be associated with a variety of intestinal symptoms such as chronic diarrhea, steatorrhea, abdominal cramps, bloating, frequent loose and pale greasy stools, fatigue and weight loss. Malabsorption of fats or of fat-soluble vitamins may occur. There is no extra-intestinal invasion; damage to duodenal and jejunal mucosal cells may occur in severe giardiasis.

Diagnosis is made by the identification of cysts or trophozoites in feces (repeated at least 3 times before considered negative) or of trophozoites in duodenal fluid (by aspiration or string test) or in mucosa obtained by small intestine biopsy; the latter may be more reliable when results of stool examination are questionable, but is rarely necessary. Because *Giardia* infection can be asymptomatic, the presence of *G. lamblia* (in either stools or duodenum) does not necessarily indicate that *Giardia* is the cause of illness.

2. Infectious agent—*Giardia lamblia,* a flagellate protozoan.

3. Occurrence—Worldwide. Children are infected more frequently than adults. Prevalence is higher in areas of poor sanitation and in institutions including day-care centers. The prevalence of stool positivity in different areas may range between 1% and 30%, depending on the community and age group surveyed. Waterborne outbreaks in the USA are common in mountain communities that derive drinking water from streams or rivers without a water filtration system. Prevalent in temperate as well as in tropical countries with frequent infection of tour groups related epidemiologically to drinking tap water.

4. Reservoir—Man; possibly beaver and other wild or domestic animals.

5. Mode of transmission—Localized outbreaks occur from ingestion of cysts in fecally contaminated water and less often from fecally contaminated food. Person-to-person transmission occurs by hand-to-mouth transfer of cysts from the feces of an infected individual in institutions or day-care centers. Asymptomatic individuals are probably more important in transmission than those with diarrhea. Concentrations of chlorine used in routine water treatment do not kill *Giardia* cysts; unfiltered stream or lake waters that are open to contamination by human and animal feces are a frequent source of infection.

6. Incubation period—5–25 days or longer; median 7–10 days.

7. Period of communicability—Entire period of infection.

8. Susceptibility and resistance—Asymptomatic carrier rate is high; infection is frequently self-limited. Pathogenicity of *G. lamblia* for humans has been established by clinical studies. Host factors associated with resistance have not been defined.

9. Methods of control—

   A.   Preventive measures:

   1)   Filter public water supplies that are at risk of human or animal fecal contamination.
   2)   Protect public water supplies against contamination with human or animal feces.
   3)   Educate families, personnel and inmates of institutions in personal hygiene; especially adult personnel of day-care centers.
   4)   Sanitary disposal of feces.
   5)   Emergency water supplies are best boiled, or treated with hypochlorite or iodine, using 0.1 to 0.2 ml (2 to 4 drops) of household bleach or 0.5 ml of 2% tincture of iodine per liter for 20 minutes (longer if the water is cold).

   B.   Control of patient, contacts and the immediate environment:

   1)   Report to local health authority: Case report in selected areas, Class 3B (see Preface).
   2)   Isolation: Enteric precautions.
   3)   Concurrent disinfection: Of feces and articles soiled therewith. In communities with a modern and adequate sewage disposal system, feces can be discharged directly into sewers without preliminary disinfection. Terminal cleaning.
   4)   Quarantine: None.

5) Immunization of contacts: None.
6) Investigation of contacts and source of infection: Microscopic examination of feces of household members and other suspected contacts, especially those who are symptomatic, supplemented by search for environmental contamination.
7) Specific treatment: Quinacrine hydrochloride (Atabrine®) is the drug of choice; metronidazole (Flagyl®) is also effective. Furazolidone is available in pediatric suspension for young children and infants. Relapses may occur with any drug.

C. *Epidemic measures:* Epidemiological investigation of clustered cases in an area or institution to determine source of infection and mode of transmission; a common vehicle, such as water or association with a day-care center, should be sought; institute applicable preventive or control measures. Control of person-to-person transmission requires special emphasis on personal cleanliness and sanitary disposal of feces.

D. *Disaster implications:* None.

E. *International measures:* None.

GONOCOCCAL INFECTIONS   ICD-9 098

Urethritis, epididymitis, proctitis, cervicitis, Bartholinitis, salpingitis (pelvic inflammatory disease), and pharyngitis of adults; vulvovaginitis of children and conjunctivitis of the newborn and adults are localized inflammatory conditions which are caused by *Neisseria gonorrhoeae.* Gonococcal bacteremia results in the arthritis-dermatitis syndrome, occasionally associated with endocarditis or meningitis. Other complications include perihepatitis and the neonatal amniotic infection syndrome.

Clinically indistinguishable infections of the same genital structures may be caused by *Chlamydia trachomatis* and other infectious agents.

I. GONOCOCCAL INFECTION OF   ICD-9 098.0-098.3
GENITOURINARY TRACT
(Gonorrhea, Gonococcal urethritis, Gonococcal vulvovaginitis, Gonococcal cervicitis, Gonococcal bartholinitis, Clap, Strain, Gleet, Dose)

1. **Identification**—A sexually transmitted bacterial disease limited to columnar and transitional epithelium which differs in males and females in

course, severity and ease of recognition.

In males, a purulent discharge from the anterior urethra with dysuria appears 2–7 days after an infecting exposure. The infection may be self-limited, or may extend to the posterior urethra to produce epididymitis and may result in a chronic carrier state. Asymptomatic anterior urethral carriage also may occur. Rectal infection, common among homosexual males, is at times asymptomatic but may cause pruritis, tenesmus and discharge.

In females, a few days after exposure an initial urethritis or cervicitis occurs, frequently so mild as to pass unnoticed. In about 20% there is uterine invasion at the 1st, 2nd, or later menstrual period, with symptoms of endometritis, salpingitis or pelvic peritonitis with subsequent risk of infertility. Chronic endocervical infection is common. Prepubescent girls may develop gonococcal vulvovaginitis subsequent to direct genital contact with exudate from infected adults.

In both sexes, pharyngeal and anal infections are common. Conjunctivitis occurs rarely in adults. Septicemia may occur, with arthritis, skin lesions, endocarditis, and meningitis. Death is rare except among cases with endocarditis. Arthritis can produce permanent joint damage if appropriate antibiotic treatment is delayed.

Nongonococcal urethritis (NGU) and nongonococcal mucopurulent cervicitis may also be of sexual origin and seriously complicate the clinical diagnosis of gonorrhea; frequently these coexist with gonococcal infections. In many countries the incidence of NGU exceeds that of gonorrhea. About 40% of NGU in the USA and the UK is caused by *Chlamydia trachomatis* (see Chlamydial Infections).

Bacteriologic culture on special media (e.g., modified Thayer-Martin medium) confirms the diagnosis of gonococcal infection. Typical gram-negative intracellular diplococci can be considered diagnostic in male urethral smears; they are highly suggestive when seen in smears from the cervix. In females, repeated cervical and rectal cultures may be necessary to detect infection. Presently available serological tests lack specificity and are not recommended.

2. Infectious agent—*Neisseria gonorrhoeae,* the gonococcus. The presence in some strains of plasmids coding for β-lactamases render these resistant to penicillin (Penicillinase-Producing *Neisseria Gonorrhoeae* or PPNG strains). Chromosomally mediated (β-lactamase-negative) penicillin-resistant strains are seen with increasing frequency.

3. Occurrence—Common worldwide, affects both sexes and practically all ages, especially younger adult groups among whom sexual activity is greatest; it is grossly underreported. Common in the USA among male homosexuals with multiple partners. In the last two decades, incidence has increased worldwide; in the USA, the number of reported cases has decreased since 1975. Both PPNG and chromosomally mediated gonococcal resistance to penicillin are apparently increasing worldwide.

4. **Reservoir**—Strictly a human disease.

5. **Mode of transmission**—By contact with exudates from mucous membranes of infected persons, almost always as a result of sexual activity. Even in children older than 1 yr, it is most frequently a result of sexual contact or molestation.

6. **Incubation period**—Usually 2–7 days, sometimes longer.

7. **Period of communicability**—May extend for months if untreated, especially in asymptomatic individuals. Effective therapy usually ends communicability within hours.

8. **Susceptibility and resistance**—Susceptibility is general. Humoral and secretory antibodies have been demonstrated, but gonococcal strains are antigenically heterogeneous and reinfection is common. Women using an intrauterine contraceptive device have higher risks of salpingitis; some persons deficient in complement are uniquely susceptible to bacteremia. Since only columnar and transitional epithelium can be infected by the gonococcus, the vaginal epithelium of adult women, which is covered by stratified squamous epithelium, is resistant to infection whereas the prepubertal columnar or transitional vaginal epithelium is susceptible.

9. **Methods of Control**—

  A. *Preventive measures:* Same as for syphilis (see Syphilis, 9A), except for measures applying specifically to gonorrhea, i.e., primarily the use of prophylactic agents in the eyes of the newborn (II, 9A1, below) and special attention (prophylactic treatment) to contacts of infectious patients (I, 9B6, below).

  B. *Control of patient, contacts and the immediate environment:*

   1) Report to local health authority: Case report is required in many states and countries, Class 2B (see Preface).
   2) Isolation: None. Effective antibiotics in adequate dosage promptly render discharges noninfectious. Patients should refrain from sexual intercourse until post-treatment cultures are free of gonococci, and with untreated previous sexual partners to avoid reinfection.
   3) Concurrent disinfection: Care in disposal of discharges from lesions and articles soiled therewith.
   4) Quarantine: None.
   5) Immunization of contacts: Not available.
   6) Investigation of contacts: Interview patients and trace contacts as fundamental elements of a control program.

Trained interviewers obtain the best results with uncooperative patients, but clinicians can motivate most patients to help arrange for treatment of their partners. Locate, examine and treat at once (prophylactic treatment) all sexual contacts of male cases of acute urethritis within 14 days, all contacts of women with acute salpingitis within 60 days of onset of symptoms, and all recent contacts of asymptomatic cases. Orogastric and rectal cultures should be made on all infants born to infected mothers. Examine serologically for syphilis initially and 6 wks after starting treatment of gonorrhea.

7) Specific treatment: On clinical, laboratory or epidemiological grounds (contacts of a diagnosed case), adequate treatment must be given as follows:

a) For uncomplicated gonorrhea in adults (if less than 5% of strains are resistant to penicillin or tetracycline): Aqueous procaine penicillin G, 4.8 million units, half i.m. in each buttock (2.4 m.u. each) at one visit, together with 1 g of oral probenecid; *Or* Ampicillin 3.5 g or amoxicillin 3.0 g as a single oral dose with 1 g oral probenecid; *Or* Tetracycline hydrochloride 500 mg orally 4 times/d for 7 days for a total dose of 14.0 g or doxycycline hyclate 100 mg by mouth twice/d for 7 days. Cultures should be taken 4–7 days after completion of treatment to detect any treatment failures. Because of the frequency of coexisting chlamydial infection, which has been documented in up to 45% of gonorrhea patients for whom adequate chlamydial cultures were done, a single-dose regimen of ampicillin or amoxicillin could be administered, immediately followed by the tetracycline/doxycycline or, in pregnant women, erythromycin.

b) For treatment failures or infection known to be caused by PPNG or for infections acquired in areas with a high prevalence of these organisms: spectinomycin (2 g as a single i.m. dose) is indicated; *Or* alternate treatments include cefoxitin 2.0 g i.m., in a single injection plus probenecid 1.0 g by mouth; *Or* cefotaxime 1.0 g i.m., in a single injection without probenecid; or Kanamycin A, 2 g i.m.; *Or* thiamphenicol, 2.5 g by mouth; *Or* TMP-SMX, 10 tablets orally daily for 3 days. Rule out concurrent syphilis (9B6, above).

c) For patients allergic to penicillin, use spectinomycin or tetracyclines. Concurrent syphilis must be ruled out (see 9B6, above).

C. *Epidemic measures:* Intensification of routine procedures, especially therapy of contacts on epidemiologic grounds.

D. *Disaster implications:* None.

E. *International measures:* See Syphilis, 9E.

II. GONOCOCCAL CONJUNCTIVITIS (NEONATORUM)   ICD-9 098.40
(Gonorrheal ophthalmia neonatorum)

1. Identification—Acute redness and swelling of the conjunctiva of one or both eyes, with mucopurulent or purulent discharge in which gonococci are identifiable by microscopic and culture methods. Corneal ulcer, perforation and blindness may occur if specific treatment is not given promptly.

Gonococcal ophthalmia neonatorum is only one of a number of acute inflammatory conditions of the eye or the conjunctiva occurring within the first 3 wks of life and collectively known as ophthalmia neonatorum. The gonococcus is the most serious, but not the most frequent, infectious agent. The most common cause is *Chlamydia trachomatis,* producing chlamydial conjunctivitis which tends to be less acute than gonococcal conjunctivitis and usually appears 5–14 days after birth (see Conjunctivitis, Chlamydial). All purulent neonatal conjunctivitides should be considered gonococcal until proven otherwise.

2. Infectious agent—*Neisseria gonorrhoeae,* the gonococcus.

3. Occurrence—Varies widely according to the prevalence of maternal infection and the measures for prevention of infection of eyes of the newborn at delivery. Infrequent where infant eye prophylaxis is adequate. Globally, the disease continues to be an important cause of blindness.

4. Reservoir—Infection of the cervix.

5. Mode of transmission—Contact with the infected birth canal during childbirth.

6. Incubation period—Usually 1–5 days.

7. Period of communicability—While discharge persists if untreated; for 24 hours following initiation of specific treatment.

8. Susceptibility and resistance—Susceptibility is general.

9. Methods of control—

A. *Preventive measures:*

1) Use of an established effective preparation for protection

of babies' eyes at birth; instillation of 1% silver nitrate solution stored in individual wax capsules remains the prophylactic agent most widely used. Erythromycin and tetracycline ophthalmic ointments are also effective; they may be effective in preventing neonatal chlamydial conjunctivitis.

2) Depends fundamentally on control of sexually transmitted disease (see Syphilis, 9A). Routine cervical and rectal culturing for gonococci during prenatal period, especially in third trimester, should be considered in high-risk populations.

B. *Control of patient, contacts and the immediate environment:*

1) Report to local health authority: Case report is required in most states and countries, Class 2B (see Preface).

2) Isolation: Contact isolation for the first 24 hours after administration of effective therapy. Cases should be hospitalized if possible. Where β-lactamase-producing gonococci are prevalent, bacterial cure after penicillin therapy should be confirmed by culture.

3) Concurrent disinfection: Care in disposal of conjunctival discharges and articles soiled therewith.

4) Quarantine: None.

5) Immunization of contacts: Not applicable; prompt treatment on diagnosis or clinical suspicion of infection.

6) Investigation of contacts: Examination and treatment of mothers and their sexual partners.

7) Specific treatment: Aqueous crystalline penicillin G, 50,000 units/kg/d, in 2 daily doses given i.v. for 7 days. Topical penicillin in addition is not essential but may be used. If response to treatment is poor, the involvement of PPNG organisms must be ruled out; if present, cefotaxime, 25 mg/kg/d i.m. in 4 doses for 3 days.

C. *Epidemic measures:* None.

D. *Disaster implications:* None.

E. *International measures:* None.

GRANULOMA INGUINALE   ICD-9 099.2
(Donovanosis)

1. Identification—A nonfatal, chronic and progressive bacterial disease of the skin and mucous membranes of the external genitalia, inguinal and anal region with low communicability. A small nodule, vesicle or papule becomes a slowly spreading, exuberant, granulomatous, ulcerative, or cicatricial process which is frequently painless and extends peripherally with characteristic rolled edges and formation of fibrous tissue. In many cases the lesion is predominantly granulomatous. Lesions have a predilection for warm and moist surfaces such as the folds between scrotum and thighs or labia and vagina. If neglected, the process may result in extensive destruction of genital organs and spread to other parts of the body. Occasionally, this infection is associated with squamous cell carcinoma of the penis. Clinically similar lesions have been proven to be a variant of chancroid (q.v.).

Laboratory diagnosis is based on demonstrating intracytoplasmic Donovan bodies in Giemsa-stained smears of granulation tissue or by histologic examination of biopsy specimens. *Haemophilus ducreyi* should be excluded by culture on appropriate selective media.

2. Infectious agent—*Calymmatobacterium granulomatis (Donovania granulomatis)* is the presumed etiologic agent; this is not certain.

3. Occurrence—An infrequent disease of tropical and subtropical areas; endemic in southern India, Papua New Guinea, central, west and southern Africa, West Indies and S America. Apparently more frequent among males than females and among persons of lower socioeconomic status; predominantly at ages 20–40. In USA, more common among homosexuals; relatively rare in heterosexual partners of cases.

4. Reservoir—Infected persons.

5. Mode of transmission—Presumably by direct contact with lesions during sexual activity.

6. Incubation period—Unknown; probably between 8–80 days.

7. Period of communicability—Unknown; probably for the duration of open lesions on the skin or mucous membranes.

8. Susceptibility and resistance—Susceptibility is variable; immunity apparently does not follow attack.

9. Methods of control—

    A.   *Preventive measures:* Except for those measures applicable only to syphilis, preventive measures are those described in syphilis, 9A.

B. *Control of patient, contacts and the immediate environment:*

1) Report to local health authority: A reportable disease in most states and countries, Class 3B (see Preface).

2) Isolation: None; avoid close personal contact until lesions are healed.

3) Concurrent disinfection: Care in disposal of discharges from lesions and articles soiled therewith.

4) Quarantine: None.

5) Immunization of contacts: Not applicable; prompt treatment upon recognition or clinical suspicion of infection.

6) Investigation of contacts: Examination of sexual contacts.

7) Specific treatment: Tetracyclines, TMP-SMX, and chloramphenicol have been reported to be effective; recurrence is not rare but usually responds to a 2nd course of therapy unless malignancy is present.

C. *Epidemic measures:* Not applicable.

D. *Disaster implications:* None.

E. *International measures:* See Syphilis, 9E.

HEMORRHAGIC FEVER WITH RENAL SYNDROME   ICD-9 078.6
(Hemorrhagic nephrosonephritis, Epidemic hemorrhagic fever, Korean hemorrhagic fever, Nephropathia epidemica)

1. **Identification**—An acute zoonotic infectious disease characterized by an abrupt onset of fever of 3–8 days duration, conjunctival injection, prostration, backache, headache, abdominal pain, anorexia and vomiting. Hemorrhagic manifestations are uncommon but may appear about the 3rd day, followed by proteinuria, hypotension and sometimes shock. Renal abnormalities may be mild or progress to acute renal failure and continue for several weeks. The majority of deaths (case fatality rate is about 7% in Korea, 0.5% in Scandinavia) occur during the anuric phase from renal shutdown. Convalescence is usually rapid and complete during the 3rd week.

Diagnosis is made by IFA or ELISA, available from highly specialized laboratories. Presence of proteinuria, leukocytosis, thrombocytopenia and elevated blood urea nitrogen assist in supporting the diagnosis.

2. **Infectious agent**—Hantaan virus, a 3-segmented RNA virus, is an ungrouped member of the Bunyaviridae, with spherical to oval particles,

95–110 nm in diameter. Several antigenic subtypes exist. Laboratory-adapted strains can be propagated in tissue cultures and laboratory rats and mice. A closely related agent thought to cause nephropathia epidemica in Scandinavia has been isolated from voles.

3. **Occurrence**—Recognized in Korea in the vicinity of the 38th parallel among United Nations troops in 1951 and among military personnel and civilians since then. Earlier, Japanese and Soviets reported its presence in Manchuria along the Amur River. Also recognized in Japan and central and southern China. A few cases occur throughout the year, but in Korea there are two peaks of seasonal incidence, one in May-June and one in October-November. The majority of cases are isolated events but outbreaks have involved 5–20 persons within a small area, apparently acquired at the same time and place. In rural areas of Korea, 100–800 cases are hospitalized per year. Disease in medical research personnel in Japan was traced to naturally infected laboratory rats. Occurs as a milder disease in European USSR, Scandinavia and other countries of eastern Europe. Serological mapping indicates that Hantaan or related viruses have infected large numbers of people in the region from Japan across central and north Asia to the Scandinavian peninsula. Recently agents similar or identical to Hantaan virus have been identified in urban rats captured in major Asian and Western cities, including the USA; associated human illness has occurred in several European countries, including France, Belgium and Greece.

4. **Reservoir**—Field rodents (*Apodemus* spp. in Korea, *Clethrionomys* voles in Scandinavia and USSR, *Peromyscus* and *Microtus* rodents in USA), perhaps urban rats, with man only an accidental host.

5. **Mode of transmission**—Unknown; virus is present in urine, feces and saliva of persistently infected asymptomatic rodents; highest virus concentration is found in the lungs. Aerosol transmission from rodent excreta is presumed.

6. **Incubation period**—Usually 12–16 days, but varying from 9 to 35.

7. **Period of communicability**—Not transmitted directly from person to person.

8. **Susceptibility and resistance**—Newcomers to endemic areas are uniformly susceptible; indigenous populations may have acquired resistance. Inapparent infections occur; second attacks have not been observed.

9. **Methods of control**—

   A. Preventive measures:

   1) While details of transmission are unknown, specific rodent control is indicated where the reservoir host has been

    identified; in endemic areas, minimize personal and environmental exposure to wild rodents.

    2)   Laboratory rat and mouse colonies should be checked to assure freedom from asymptomatic Hantaan infection.

B.   *Control of patient, contacts and the immediate environment:*

    1)   Report to local health authority: In selected endemic areas; in most countries not a reportable disease, Class 3A (see Preface).

    2)   Isolation: None.

    3)   Concurrent disinfection: None.

    4)   Quarantine: None.

    5)   Immunization of contacts: None.

    6)   Investigation of contacts: None.

    7)   Specific treatment: None. Appropriate treatment for shock or for renal failure.

C.   *Epidemic measures:* Rodent control. Laboratory-associated outbreaks call for evaluation of the associated rodents and, if positive, elimination of the rodents and careful thorough cleaning with sodium hypochlorite or phenolics.

D.   *Disaster implications:* None.

E.   *International measurés:* None.

HEPATITIS, VIRAL   ICD-9 070

    Several distinct infections are grouped as the viral hepatitides; they are similar in many ways but differ in etiology and in some epidemiological, immunological, clinical and pathological characteristics. Their prevention and control vary greatly. Therefore, each will be presented in a separate section.

I. VIRAL HEPATITIS A   ICD-9 070.1
(Infectious hepatitis, Epidemic hepatitis, Epidemic jaundice, Catarrhal jaundice, Type A hepatitis, HA).

    1. Identification—Onset is usually abrupt with fever, malaise, anorexia, nausea and abdominal discomfort, followed within a few days by jaundice. Varies from a mild illness lasting 1–2 wks, rarely to a severely disabling disease lasting several months. Convalescence usually is prolonged. In general, severity increases with age but complete recovery without sequelae or recurrences is the rule. Many infections are asymptomatic; many are mild and without jaundice, especially in children, and recognizable only by liver function tests. The case fatality rate is <0.1%; the rare death usually occurs in an older patient in whom the disease has a fulminant course.

Differential diagnosis usually depends on epidemiologic evidence (which will not differentiate this from fecal-oral non-A non-B hepatitis) and clinical laboratory results for the exclusion of other causes of febrile jaundice.

Diagnosis is usually established by the demonstration of IgM antibodies against hepatitis A virus in the serum of acutely or recently ill patients; IgM may remain detectable for 6 wks to 4–6 months after onset. In research facilities, diagnosis may also be made by a fourfold or greater rise in specific antibodies in paired sera. Virus and antibody can be detected by RIA or ELISA tests. Assay kits for the detection of IgM and total antibodies to the virus are available commercially.

2. Infectious agent—Hepatitis A virus, a 27 nm picornavirus with the characteristics of an enterovirus.

3. Occurrence—Worldwide, sporadic and epidemic, with a tendency to cyclic recurrences in the past. Outbreaks commonly occur in institutions, day-care centers, low-cost housing projects, rural areas, and military forces particularly during wars. Where environmental sanitation is poor, infection is common and occurs at an early age. Thus, in developing countries, adults are usually immune and epidemics of HA are rare. In developed countries, epidemics often evolve slowly, involve wide geographic areas and last many months, but common source epidemics may evolve explosively. Most common among school-age children and young adults; a major problem in day-care centers. Seroepidemiologic studies suggest diminishing frequency in the USA and other developed areas.

4. Reservoir—Man, and rarely captive chimpanzees; less frequently, certain other nonhuman primates. An enzootic focus has been identified in Malaysia but there is no suggestion of transmission to man.

5. Mode of transmission—Person-to-person by the fecal-oral route. The infectious agent is found in feces, reaching peak levels the week or two before onset of symptoms and diminishing rapidly after liver dysfunction or symptoms appear, which is concurrent with the appearance of circulating antibodies. Common vehicle outbreaks have been related to contaminated water and food, including milk, sliced meats, salads, and raw or undercooked molluscs. Although rare, instances of transmission by transfusion of blood from a donor in the incubation period have been reported.

6. Incubation period—From 15–50 days, depending on dose; average 28–30 days.

7. Period of communicability—Studies of transmission in humans and epidemiological evidence indicate maximum infectivity during the latter half of the incubation period, continuing for a few days after onset of jaundice (or during peak aminotransferase activity in anicteric cases). Most cases are probably noninfectious after the first week of jaundice.

8. Susceptibility and resistance—Susceptibility is general. Low incidence of manifest disease in infants and preschool children suggests that mild and anicteric infections are common. Homologous immunity after attack probably lasts for life.

9. Methods of control—

   A.   *Preventive measures:*

   1)   Educate the public about good sanitation and personal hygiene, with special emphasis on sanitary disposal of feces and careful handwashing.

   2)   Management of day-care centers should stress measures to minimize the possibility of fecal-oral transmission, including thorough handwashing after **every** diaper change and before eating. If one or more HA cases are associated with a center, IG should be administered to the staff and attendees and should be considered for family contacts of attending children age 2 years or less.

   3)   Travelers to highly endemic areas, including north and tropical Africa, the Middle East, Asia, and parts of Central and S America, may be given prophylactic doses of IG. For expected exposures up to 2 months, a single dose of 0.02–0.04 ml/kg or 2 ml for adults is recommended; for more prolonged exposures, 0.06 ml/kg (5 ml for adults) should be given and repeated every 4–6 months if exposure continues.

   4)   Proper sterilization of syringes and needles and other equipment used for parenteral injections or use of disposable units, although the virus is rarely transmitted by this route.

   5)   Vaccines for active immunization, both killed and attenuated, are being developed but are not yet available for general use.

   B.   *Control of patient, contacts and the immediate environment:*

   1)   Report to local health authority: Obligatory in all states of

the USA and in Canada, although not now required in many countries; Class 2A (see Preface).

2) Isolation: For proven hepatitis A, enteric precautions during the first 2 wks of illness, but no more than 1 wk after onset of jaundice; until a specific diagnosis of HA is made, the maintenance of blood and body fluid precautions may be considered advisable.

3) Concurrent disinfection: Sanitary disposal of feces, urine, and blood.

4) Quarantine: None.

5) Immunization of contacts: Passive immunization with IG, 0.02–0.04 ml/kg of body weight, should be given i.m. as soon as possible after exposure, but within 2 wks, to all household and sexual contacts. In a day-care center, IG should be given to all classroom contacts. If the center admits children in diapers, IG should be given to all children and staff in the center. It is not indicated for contacts in the usual office, school or factory situation.

6) Investigation of contacts: Search for missed cases and maintain surveillance of contacts in the patient's household or, in a common source outbreak, persons exposed to the same risk.

7) Specific treatment: None.

C. *Epidemic measures:*

1) Epidemiologic investigation to determine mode of transmission, whether from person to person or by common vehicle, and to identify the population exposed to increased risk of infection. Eliminate any common sources of infection. If HA occurs in a foodhandler, IG should be given to other foodhandlers in the establishment. IG is usually not offered to patrons, but may be considered if the foodhandlers were involved in the preparation of foods which were not heated and deficiencies in personal hygiene are noted and if the IG can be given within 2 wks after last exposure.

2) Special efforts to improve sanitary and hygienic practices to eliminate fecal contamination of foods and water.

3) Focal outbreaks in institutions may warrant mass prophylaxis with IG.

D. *Disaster implications:* A potential problem in a large collection of people with crowding, inadequate sanitation and water supplies; if cases occur, increased efforts should be exerted to improve sanitation and safety of water supplies. Mass administration of IG is not a substitute for environmental measures.

E. *International measures:* None.

II. VIRAL HEPATITIS B   ICD-9 070.3
(Type B hepatitis, Serum hepatitis, Homologous serum jaundice,
Australia antigen hepatitis, HB).

1. **Identification**—Onset is usually insidious with anorexia, vague abdominal discomfort, nausea and vomiting, sometimes arthralgias and rash, often progressing to jaundice. Fever may be absent or mild. Severity ranges from inapparent cases detectable only by liver function tests to fulminating, fatal cases of acute hepatic necrosis. The case fatality rate in hospitalized patients is <1%. Prolonged hepatitis B antigenemia (the HBV carrier state), without overt signs of disease, is found in 0.1–0.5% of adults in N America and in 0.1–20% of persons from other parts of the world. HBV carriers may or may not have a history of clinical hepatitis. About one-third have an elevated aminotransferase; biopsy findings range from normal to chronic active hepatitis, with or without cirrhosis. The prognosis of the liver disease in such individuals is variable. About one-third of patients with histological findings of chronic hepatitis or cryptogenic cirrhosis have hepatitis B surface antigen detectable in their sera. HBV is the cause of up to 80% of all cases of hepatocellular carcinoma worldwide, second only to tobacco among known human carcinogens. Perinatal infection has a high likelihood of chronic antigenemia culminating in chronic hepatitis, cirrhosis, or primary hepatocellular carcinoma.

Diagnosis is confirmed by demonstration of hepatitis B surface antigen (HBsAg) or recent development of antibody to core and/or surface antigens (anti-HBc, anti-HBs, respectively). Three antigen-antibody systems have been identified for HB: HBsAg and anti-HBs, core antigen and antibody (HBcAg and anti-HBc), and e antigen and antibody (HBeAg and anti-HBe). Commercial kits (RIA or EIA) are available for all markers except HBcAg. HBsAg can be detected in the serum for up to several weeks before onset of symptoms to days, weeks or months after onset; it persists in chronic infections. Anti-HBc appears at the onset of illness and persists indefinitely. IgM anti-HBc is present in high titer during acute infection and usually disappears within 6 months; this test may reliably diagnose acute HBV infection.

2. **Infectious agent**—The hepatitis B virus (HBV), a 42 nm double stranded DNA virus, is composed of a 27 nm nucleocapsid core (HBcAg), surrounded by an outer lipoprotein coat containing the surface antigen (HBsAg). HBsAg is antigenically heterogeneous, with a common antigen designated *a,* and two pairs of mutually exclusive antigens, *d* and *y,* and *w* (including several subdeterminants) and *r,* resulting in 4 major subtypes: *adw, ayw, adr,* and *ayr.* The distribution of subtypes varies geographically;

protection against one subtype appears to confer protection against the other subtypes.

A third hepatitis B antigen, the e antigen (HBeAg) has been identified as a soluble antigen, probably a component of the nucleocapsid. The hepatitis B virion also contains a DNA-dependent DNA polymerase. In common usage, antigens are identified as indicated, and the respective antibodies as anti-HBc, anti-HBs, and anti-HBe. The detection of e antigen (HBeAg) is associated with relatively high infectivity; conversely, presence of anti-HBe correlates with a relative (but not absolute) lack of infectivity.

3. Occurrence—Worldwide; endemic with little seasonal variation. In areas of Africa and Asia, widespread infection may occur in infancy and childhood; in N America infection is most common in young adults. In the USA and Canada serologic evidence of previous infection varies depending on age and socioeconomic class. Overall, 5% of the adult USA population has anti-HBs, and 0.3% are HBsAg positive; among those from some areas of Asia, overall antigen carrier rates may be 10–15%. In developed countries, HBV infection is common in certain high-risk groups. These include parenteral drug abusers, homosexual men, clients and staff in institutions for the retarded, patients and employees in hemodialysis centers and certain persons in health occupations. Frequent and routine exposure to blood or serous fluids is the common denominator of health occupation exposure; surgeons, oral surgeons, pathologists, operating room and emergency room staff, and clinical laboratory workers who handle blood are at highest risk. In the past, recipients of blood products were at high risk. In the many countries in which pretransfusion screening of blood for HBsAg has been required, this risk has been virtually eliminated except for recipients of pooled blood-clotting factors (especially anti-hemophilic factor). In the past, contaminated and inadequately sterilized syringes and needles have resulted in outbreaks of hepatitis B among patients in clinics and physician's offices. Occasionally, outbreaks have been traced to tattoo parlors and acupuncturists.

4. Reservoir—Man. Chimpanzees are susceptible but an animal reservoir in nature has not been recognized.

5. Mode of transmission—HBsAg has been found in virtually all body secretions and excretions; however, only blood (and serum-derived fluids), saliva, semen and vaginal fluids have been shown to be infectious. The presence of e antigen greatly enhances the infectivity of these fluids. Transmission occurs by percutaneous (i.v., i.m., s.c. or intradermal) or permucosal exposure to infective body fluids as may occur in needle stick accidents or sexual exposure. Human blood, plasma, serum, thrombin, fibrinogen, packed RBCs, cryoprecipitate, and other blood products may transmit infection if not screened for HBsAg. IG, heat-treated plasma protein fraction, albumin and fibrinolysin are generally considered safe. Contaminated needles, syringes and other i.v. equipment are important vehicles of spread, especially among drug addicts. The infection may be spread through contamination of wounds or lacerations, or by exposure of mucous membranes to infective blood; this route is probably an important source of transmission in health occupations, institutions for the retarded, and in less developed countries where HBV is endemic. Perinatal transmission is common in hyperendemic areas of SE Asia and the Far East, especially when HBsAg carrier mothers are also HBeAg positive. Infection may also be transmitted in the course of close personal contact, especially between sexual partners, most frequently between male homosexuals. Accidental percutaneous inoculations by communally used razors or toothbrushes have been implicated as occasional transmitters of HB. Fecal-oral transmission has not been demonstrated.

6. Incubation period—Usually 45–180 days, average 60–90 days. As short as 2 wks to the appearance of HBsAg, and rarely as long as 6–9 months; the variation is related in part to the amount of virus in the inoculum and the mode of transmission as well as to host factors.

7. Period of communicability—Blood from experimentally inoculated volunteers has been shown to be infective many weeks before the onset of first symptoms and remains infective through the acute clinical course of the disease and during the chronic carrier state, which may persist for years. Most, if not all, carriers have demonstrable HBsAg and anti-HBc. Chronic antigenemia may follow asymptomatic infections and is common in individuals infected in infancy and in those with immunodeficiency, such as patients with Down's syndrome or lymphoproliferative disease and patients on hemodialysis. The infectivity of chronically infected individuals varies from highly infectious (HBeAg positive) to sparingly infectious (anti-HBe positive). The former may progress to the latter but rarely does the reverse occur.

8. Susceptibility and resistance—Susceptibility is general. Usually, the disease is milder and often anicteric in children; in infants it is predominantly asymptomatic. Solid immunity follows infection if antibody to HBsAg (anti-HBs) develops and HBsAg is negative.

9. Methods of control—

    A. Preventive measures:

        1)   Inactivated vaccines against HB have been licensed and are commercially available. Studies have shown that they are safe and highly protective against all subtypes of HBV. Laboratory studies confirm that each of the 3 inactivating processes used in the production of the plasma-derived vaccine licensed in the USA is sufficient to inactivate all

human retroviruses including HTLV-III (see AIDS). Combined passive-active immunoprophylaxis with HBIG and vaccine has been shown to stimulate anti-HBs comparable to vaccine alone.

a) In hyperendemic areas of the world, only widescale immunization of infants and children can be expected to produce signficant disease control; strategies for control differ from those in areas of low endemicity. Currently, the high cost of HB vaccine precludes its widespread use, but many countries are exploring the feasibility of local production of vaccines with lower cost. In addition, newer technologies hold the promise of significantly less costly vaccines in the future.

b) For areas with overall low endemicity of infection, where risk is limited to a few high-risk groups, vaccination is recommended for those who are at increased and continuing risk of infection with hepatitis B virus. These include health care personnel (especially those who come into contact with blood and secretions), patients who require repeated blood transfusions or clotting factor concentrates, household contacts of carriers, the sexually promiscuous (especially male homosexuals), staff and clients in institutions for the retarded, hemodialysis patients and users of illicit injectable drugs.

c) Tests to exclude preexisting anti-HBs or HBsAg are not required prior to vaccination but may be desirable as a cost-saving method where there is a high level of preexisting immunity. Vaccines licensed in different parts of the world may have varying dosages and schedules; the vaccine licensed in the USA should be administered in 3 i.m. doses: initially and 1 and 6 months later. Recommended doses are 0.5 ml (10 μg) for newborns and children under 10 yrs; 1.0 ml (20 μg) for adults and older children; and 2.0 ml (40 μg) (two-1.0 ml doses at different sites) for dialysis and immunocompromised patients. Pregnancy is not a definitive contraindication for receiving this inactivated vaccine.

2) All pregnant women belonging to groups at high risk of hepatitis B infection should be tested for the presence of HBsAg; if positive, their infants should be managed as outlined in 9B5, below. These groups include, but are not limited to, women from hepatitis B hyperendemic areas such as parts of Asia and Africa, parenteral drug abusers,

and women who work in health care occupations that involve routine contact with human blood or in institutions for the retarded (see section 3, above).

3) Enforce strict discipline in blood banks. All donated blood should be tested for HBsAg by sensitive tests (RIA or EIA); reject as donors all individuals who have a history of viral hepatitis, show evidence of drug addiction, or have received a blood transfusion or tattoo within the preceding 6 months. Use paid donors only in emergencies.

4) Limit administration of unscreened whole blood or potentially hazardous blood products to those patients in clear and immediate need of such therapeutic measures.

5) Maintain surveillance for all cases of post-transfusion hepatitis, including a register of all persons who donated blood for each case. Notify blood banks of these potential carriers so that future donations may be promptly identified.

6) Adequately sterilize all syringes and needles (including acupuncture needles) and stylets for finger puncture or preferably use disposable equipment whenever possible. A fresh sterile syringe and needle are essential for each individual receiving skin tests, other parenteral inoculations, or venipuncture. Discourage tattooing; enforce aseptic sanitary practices in tattoo parlors.

7) Persons with e antigen should exert great care to avoid opportunities for transmission, especially medical and dental personnel who routinely perform invasive procedures, sexually active persons, and children in day-care centers or special education classes.

B. Control of patient, contacts and the immediate environment:

1) Report to local health authority: Official report is obligatory in the USA, although not now required in many countries; Class 2A (see Preface).

2) Isolation: Blood and body fluid precautions until disappearance of HBsAg and appearance of anti-HBs.

3) Concurrent disinfection: Of equipment contaminated with blood, saliva, or semen.

4) Quarantine: None.

5) Immunization of contacts: Products available for postexposure prophylaxis include hepatitis B immunoglobulin (HBIG) and IG, in addition to hepatitis B vaccine. Most lots of IG in the USA since the mid 1970s have moderate amounts of anti-HBs; HBIG has high titers of anti-HBs (>1:100,000). HBIG is preferable when

specific immunoprophylaxis is indicated but is much more expensive. When indicated, it is important to administer the globulin as soon after exposure as possible.

a) Studies of various regimens to prevent or modify mother-to-infant transmission of HBV have shown that 3 doses of HBIG or 3 doses of hepatitis B vaccine alone were about 75% effective and that combinations of the 2 were about 90% effective. Thus, infants born to HBsAg-positive mothers should be given a single dose of HBIG (0.5 ml, i.m.) within a few hours of birth (at least within the first 24 hours) to provide immediate passive protection. In addition, a complete series of 3 doses of vaccine should be given to provide long lasting active immunity; the 1st dose (0.5 ml; 10 µg) is given within the first 7 days of life and can be given concurrently with HBIG at birth but in a separate site. The 2nd and 3rd doses of vaccine (without HBIG) are given 1 and 6 months later. If vaccine is delayed until 3 months of age, a 2nd dose of HBIG is needed at that time.

After percutaneous (e.g., needle-stick) or mucous membrane exposures to HBsAg-positive material (unless a rapid test indicates the presence of anti-HBs in the exposed person) a single dose of HBIG (0.06 ml/kg or 5 ml for adults) should be given as soon as possible, but at least within 24 hours after high-risk needle-stick exposure and the HBV vaccine series should be started. If HBIG is unavailable, a similar dosage of IG may be given (5 ml for adults). If active immunization is not accepted, a second dose of HBIG should be given 1 month after the first. HBIG is not usually given for needle-stick exposure to blood which is not known or highly suspected to be positive for HBsAg since the risk of infection in these instances is small.

After sexual exposure to an HBsAg-positive contact, a similar dose of HBIG (or IG if HBIG is unavailable) is recommended if it can be given within 14 days of the last sexual contact. In exposures among heterosexuals, a 2nd dose of HBIG should be given if the index case remains antigen-positive 3 months after detection and if ongoing sexual contact has been occurring; if the index case is a known HBsAg carrier or remains HBsAg-positive for 6 months, active immunization with hepatitis B vaccine should be offered to regular sexual contacts. Among homosexual men, the vaccine

series should be started at the time HBIG is given, since vaccine is recommended for all such men.
6) Investigation of contacts: See 9C, below.
7) Specific treatment: None. Anti-inflammatory drugs such as steroids are not indicated in acute or chronic hepatitis B. Studies with antiviral agents such as adenine arabinoside are under way.

C. *Epidemic measures:* When two or more cases occur in association with some common exposure, conduct a search for additional cases. Institute strict aseptic techniques. If a plasma derivative such as antihemophilic factor, fibrinogen, pooled plasma or thrombin is implicated, withdraw the lot from use and trace all recipients of the same lot in a search for additional cases.

D. *Disaster implications:* Relaxation of sterilization precautions and emergency use of unscreened blood for transfusions may result in an increased number of cases.

E. *International measures:* None.

III. DELTA HEPATITIS   ICD-9 070.5
(Δ hepatitis, Delta agent hepatitis, Delta-associated hepatitis)

1. Identification—Onset is usually abrupt, with signs and symptoms resembling those of hepatitis B. Hepatitis may be severe and is always associated with a coexistent hepatitis B virus infection. Delta hepatitis may be self-limiting or it may progress to chronic hepatitis. The delta agent and hepatitis B virus may coinfect, or delta infection may be superimposed upon the inapparent HBV carrier state. In the latter case, delta hepatitis can be misdiagnosed as an exacerbation of chronic hepatitis B. In several studies throughout Europe and the USA, 25–50% of fulminant hepatitis thought to be caused by hepatitis B virus was associated with concurrent infection with the delta agent.

Diagnosis is made by demonstration of the viral antigen in the serum or liver or, more commonly, by detection of seroconversion or IgM antibody to the viral antigen. RIA or ELISA are the methods of choice.

2. Infectious agent—The delta agent is a 35–37 nm virus-like particle consisting of a coat of hepatitis B surface antigen and a unique internal antigen, delta antigen. Encapsulated with the delta antigen is a linear single-stranded RNA that is thought to be the genome of the delta agent. The RNA does not hybridize with hepatitis B viral DNA. The delta agent is defective and requires coinfection with the hepatitis B virus for its synthesis. Synthesis of the delta agent, in turn, results in temporary suppression of synthesis of hepatitis B viral components.

3. Occurrence—Worldwide, but its prevalence varies widely. Occurs epidemically or endemically in populations at high risk of acquiring hepatitis B virus infection, including populations among which HB is endemic in southern Italy, Africa and S America, and hemophiliacs, drug addicts, others who come in frequent contact with blood and, to a lesser extent, male homosexuals. Severe epidemic outbreaks have been observed in Venezuela in an Indian community, and among drug addicts in Worcester, Massachusetts.

4. Reservoir—Man. Can be transmitted experimentally to chimpanzees that are infected with hepatitis B virus.

5. Mode of transmission—Thought to be similar to that of hepatitis B virus, including blood and serous body fluids, contaminated needles and syringes, plasma derivatives such as antihemophilic factor and mother-to-infant transmission.

6. Incubation period—Approximately 2–10 wks for experimental infections in chimpanzees; not firmly established in man.

7. Period of communicability—Blood is potentially infectious during all phases of active delta infection. Peak infectivity probably occurs just prior to onset of illness, when particles containing the delta antigen are readily detected in the blood. Following onset, viremia probably falls rapidly to low or undetectable levels. The delta agent has been transmitted to chimpanzees from the blood of chronically infected patients in which delta antigen-containing particles could not be detected.

8. Susceptibility and resistance—All persons susceptible to HB or who are HBV carriers can be infected with delta. Severe disease can occur even in children.

9. Methods of control—

    A. *Preventive measures:* For persons susceptible to HB, as for hepatitis B, above. Prevention of hepatitis B virus infection will prevent infection with the delta agent. Among HBV carriers, avoidance of exposure to any potential source of delta agent is the only effective measure. Neither HBIG, IG or HBV vaccine is useful in protecting HBV carriers after exposure to delta agent.

    B. *Control of patient, contacts and the immediate environment: C. Epidemic measures: D. Disaster implications:* and *E. International measures:* Same as for Hepatitis B, above.

IV. NON-A NON-B HEPATITIS   ICD-9 070.9

There is epidemiologic evidence for viral hepatitis caused by at least two yet unidentified agents that are serologically distinct from hepatitis A and hepatitis B virus. Epidemiologically, one of these resembles hepatitis A and the other resembles hepatitis B. Each will be presented separately.

IV.A. EPIDEMIC NON-A NON-B   ICD-9 070.5
HEPATITIS
(Fecal-oral non-A non-B hepatitis, A-like non-A non-B hepatitis)

1. Identification—Onset and severity are similar to that of hepatitis A. No evidence for a chronic form. The case fatality rate is similar to that of hepatitis A except in pregnant women where the rate may reach 10% during the 3rd trimester of pregnancy. Differential diagnosis depends on exclusion of other etiologies of hepatitis, especially hepatitis A, by serologic means. At present there is no serologic test available for the agent or agents of epidemic non-A non-B hepatitis.

2. Infectious agent—At present not characterized. There is preliminary evidence for a 27 nm virus-like particle resembling hepatitis A virus and found in the stool during early acute phase of infection.

3. Occurrence—Epidemics consistent with an epidemic non-A non-B virus etiology have been identified principally in India but also in Burma, Nepal, USSR, Algeria, and probably Libya. Often occur as waterborne epidemics but sporadic cases and epidemics not clearly related to water have been reported. Attack rate highest in young adults, often with male predominance. Uncommon in children and the elderly.

4. Reservoir—Man; possibly transmissible to marmosets and chimpanzees.

5. Mode of transmission—Contaminated water and probably person-to-person by the fecal-oral route.

6. Incubation period—From 15–64 days; mean incubation period has varied from 26–42 days in different epidemics.

7. Period of communicability—Not known but may be similar to HA.

8. Susceptibility and resistance—Susceptibility unknown. Estimates of secondary transmission in households are low. The occurrence of major epidemics among young adults in geographic regions in which other enteric viruses are highly endemic, and infect most of the population in infancy, is unexplained.

9. Methods of control—

A. *Preventive measures:* Educational programs to stress sanitary disposal of feces and careful postdefecatory and prefoodhandling handwashing. Basic measures to prevent fecal-oral transmission, as listed under Typhoid Fever, 9A. It is not known whether IG prepared from the serum of donors in the USA or Europe will protect against epidemic non-A non-B hepatitis.

B. *Control of patient, contacts and the immediate environment:*

1) Report to local health authority; 2) Isolation; and 3) Concurrent disinfection: Same as for hepatitis A, above.
4) Quarantine: None.
5) Immunization of contacts: None. The efficacy of IG other than locally prepared lots has not been established.
6) Investigation of contacts: Same as for hepatitis A, above.
7) Specific treatment: None.

C. *Epidemic measures:* Same as for hepatitis A, except that administration of IG is not indicated. Administration of IG to prevent possible concurrent hepatitis A should be considered, however.

D. *Disaster implications:* Same as for hepatitis A, above.

E. *International measures:* None.

IV.B. NON-A NON-B, B-LIKE HEPATITIS   ICD-9 070.5
(Non-B transfusion-associated hepatitis, Post-transfusion non-A non-B hepatitis, Hepatitis C)

1. **Identification**—Onset is usually insidious with anorexia, vague abdominal discomfort, nausea and vomiting, progressing to jaundice less frequently than hepatitis B. Severity ranges from inapparent cases to, rarely, fulminating, fatal cases. It is usually less severe in the acute stage, but chronicity is common, occurring possibly more frequently than with hepatitis B. Chronic infection may be symptomatic or asymptomatic. Chronic non-A non-B hepatitis may progress to cirrhosis but more often improves clinically after 2–3 yrs. Differential diagnosis depends on the exclusion of hepatitis types A and B and on epidemiology.

2. **Infectious agent**—There is some evidence for more than one type of non-A non-B hepatitis agent from epidemiologic studies and transmission studies in primates. To date these agents have not been unequivocally visualized or characterized. A suspect retrovirus is under investigation. Despite intensive efforts, serologic tests suitable for a diagnosis of non-A non-B hepatitis have not been developed.

3. Occurrence—Non-A non-B hepatitis has been found in every part of the world where it has been sought. It is the most common post-transfusion hepatitis in the USA, accounting for approximately 90% of such disease, and is more common when paid donors are used. It also causes sporadic community-acquired hepatitis, accounting for 15–40% of cases. The epidemiology of this type of non-A non-B hepatitis resembles that of hepatitis B except that sexual transmission has not been well documented. Recipients of blood transfusions and parenteral drug abusers are at highest risk.

4. Reservoir—Man; has been transmitted experimentally to chimpanzees.

5. Mode of transmission—Percutaneous transmission via contaminated blood or plasma derivatives or by use of an improperly sterilized needle and syringe has been well documented; other means of transmission similar to those of hepatitis B virus are suspected but have not been confirmed. There is no evidence of fecal-oral transmission.

6. Incubation period—Range from 2 wks to 6 months but most fall within 6–9 wks.

7. Period of communicability—From one or more weeks before onset of first symptoms through the acute clinical course of the disease and indefinitely in the chronic carrier stages. Based upon infectivity studies in chimpanzees, the titer of non-A non-B hepatitis in the blood appears to be relatively low.

8. Susceptibility and resistance—Susceptibility is general. The degree of immunity following infection is not known; repeated bouts of acute non-A non-B hepatitis have been reported but it is not known whether these represent infection by different agents or recrudescence of the original infection.

9. Methods of control—

    A.   Preventive measures: General control measures against HBV infection apply. (See Hepatitis B, above). The value of prophylactic IG is not clear.

    B.   Control of patient, contacts and the immediate environment: Control measures against HBV infection apply. The value of prophylactic IG has not been established for contacts.

    C.   Epidemic measures: Same as for hepatitis B, above.

    D.   Disaster measures: Same as for hepatitis B, above.

E.   International measures: None.

HERPES SIMPLEX   ICD-9 054
(Alphaherpesviral disease*, Herpesvirus hominis, Human
herpesviruses 1 and 2)

1. **Identification**—Herpes simplex is a viral infection characterized by a localized primary lesion, latency and a tendency to localized recurrence. The two etiological agents, designated herpes simplex virus (HSV) types 1 and 2, generally produce distinct clinical syndromes, depending on the portal of entry.

The primary infection with HSV type 1 may be mild and inapparent and occur in early childhood. In approximately 10% of primary infections, overt disease may appear as an illness of varying severity, marked by fever and malaise lasting a week or more; it may be associated with gingivostomatitis accompanied by vesicular lesions in the oropharynx, severe keratoconjunctivitis, a generalized cutaneous eruption complicating chronic eczema, meningoencephalitis, or some of the fatal generalized infections in newborn infants (congenital herpes simplex, ICD-9 771.2). It causes about 10% of acute pharyngotonsillitis, usually as a primary infection. Reactivation of latent infection commonly results in herpes labialis (fever blisters or cold sores) manifested by superficial clear vesicles on an erythematous base, usually on the face and lips, which crust and heal within a few days. Reactivation is precipitated by various forms of trauma, fever, physiological changes, or intercurrent disease, and may also involve other body tissues; it occurs in the presence of circulating antibodies which are not elevated by reactivation. Severe and extensive disease may occur in immunosuppressed individuals.

CNS involvement usually occurs in association with a primary infection but may appear following a recrudescence. HSV type 1 is a common cause of meningoencephalitis. Fever, headache, leukocytosis, meningeal irritation, drowsiness, confusion, stupor, coma and focal neurological signs frequently referable to one or the other temporal region, may occur. The condition may be confused with a variety of other intracranial lesions including brain abscess and tuberculous meningitis.

HSV type 2 usually produces genital herpes. This occurs principally in adults and is sexually transmitted. Primary and recurrent infections occur, with or without symptoms. In women, the principal site of primary disease is the cervix as well as the vulva; recurrent disease generally involves the vulva, perineal skin, legs, and buttocks. In men, lesions appear on the glans penis or prepuce, and in the anus and rectum of homosexuals. Other genital or perineal sites, as well as the mouth, may be involved in either sex, depending on sexual practices. This virus has been associated with aseptic meningitis and radiculitis rather than meningoencephalitis. Vaginal delivery of pregnant women with active genital infections, particularly if primary, carries a high risk of infection to the fetus or newborn, causing disseminated visceral infection, encephalitis and death. Genital infection with HSV type 2 in adult women may be a risk factor in cancer of the cervix.

Diagnosis is suggested by characteristic cytologic changes (multinucleated giant cells with intranuclear inclusions in tissue scrapings or biopsy), but is confirmed by direct FA tests or isolation of the virus from oral or genital lesions or from a brain biopsy in cases of encephalitis. Diagnosis of primary infection can be confirmed by testing paired sera by neutralization or other serological tests; demonstration of herpes-specific IgM is suggestive but not conclusive evidence of primary infection. Reliable techniques to differentiate type 1 antibody from type 2 antibody are not yet available; virus isolates can be readily distinguished.

2. Infectious agent—Herpes simplex virus (HSV). HSV types 1 and 2 can be differentiated immunologically (especially when highly specific or monoclonal antibodies are used) and differ somewhat in tissue culture, embryonated eggs and experimental animals.

3. Occurrence—Worldwide. Seventy to 90% of adults possess circulating antibodies against HSV type 1. Initial infection with HSV type 1 usually occurs before the fifth year of life, but more primary infections in adults are now being reported. HSV type 2 infection begins with sexual activity and is rare before adolescence; type 2 antibody is found in about 20% of adults. The prevalence is greater (to 60%) in lower socioeconomic groups and in sexually promiscuous individuals.

4. Reservoir—Man.

5. Mode of transmission—Contact with type 1 virus in saliva of carriers is probably the most important mode of spread. Infection of the hands of health personnel, e.g., dentists, from patients shedding HSV results in herpetic whitlow; preexisting lesions in the recipient may play a significant rôle. Transmission of HSV type 2 to nonimmune adults usually is by means of sexual contact. Both types 1 and 2 may be transmitted to various sites during homosexual activity or by oral-genital or oral-anal contact.

6. Incubation period—Two to 12 days.

7. Period of communicability—Secretion of virus in the saliva has been reported for as long as 7 weeks after recovery from stomatitis. Patients with primary genital lesions are infective for about 7–12 days, with recurrent disease for 4 days to a week. Asymptomatic oral as well as genital infections, with transient viral shedding, are probably common. Reactivation of genital herpes may occur repeatedly in up to 50% or more of women following either symptomatic or asymptomatic primary infection; reactivation may be asymptomatic with viral shedding only.

8. Susceptibility and resistance—Humans are probably universally susceptible.

9. Methods of control—

A. *Preventive measures:*

1) Personal hygiene and health education directed toward minimizing the transfer of infectious material.
2) Avoid contaminating the skin of eczematous patients with infectious material.
3) Health personnel should wear gloves when in direct contact with potentially infected lesions.
4) Cesarean section is advised before membranes rupture when primary or recurrent genital herpes infections occur in late pregnancy because of the risk of highly fatal neonatal infection.
5) Using a condom in sexual practice may decrease the risk of infection; no anti-viral agent has yet been proved to be practical in prophylaxis although acyclovir may reduce the incidence of recurrences and of herpes infection in immunodeficient patients.

B. *Control of patient, contacts and the immediate environment:*

1) Report to local health authority: Official case report not ordinarily justifiable, Class 5 (see Preface).
2) Isolation: For neonatal and for disseminated or primary severe lesions, contact isolation; for recurrent lesions, drainage/secretion precautions. Patients with herpetic lesions should be kept away from newborns, children with eczema or burns, and immunosuppressed patients.
3) Concurrent disinfection: None.
4) Quarantine: None.
5) Immunization of contacts: None.
6) Investigation of contacts: Seldom of practical value.
7) Specific treatment: Topical 5-iodo-2'deoxyuridine (Idoxuridine®) may modify the acute manifestations of herpetic keratitis and early dendritic ulcers. Corticosteroids should never be used for ocular involvement unless administered by an ophthalmologist. Adenine arabinoside (vidarabine, Vira-A® or Ara-A®) is effective as an ophthalmic ointment and is of value in herpes simplex encephalitis but may not prevent residual neurological problems. Acyclovir, used orally, i.v. or topically, has been shown to reduce

shedding of virus, diminish pain and accelerate healing time in primary genital herpes. The oral preparation is most convenient to use and may benefit patients with extensive recurrent infections as well.

C. *Epidemic measures:* Not applicable.

D. *Disaster implications:* None.

E. *International measures:* None.

MENINGOENCEPHALITIS DUE TO *CERCOPITHECID HERPESVIRUS 1*
(B-virus, Simian B disease)

ICD-9 054.3

While HSV type 1, or rarely type 2, can cause meningoencephalitis, it is distinctly different from B-virus infection, or encephalomyelitis caused by *Herpesvirus simiae,* a virus closely related to HSV. This is an ascending encephalomyelitis occurring in veterinarians, laboratory workers and other individuals having close contact with Old World monkeys or monkey cell cultures. After an incubation period of up to 3 weeks, there is an acute febrile onset with headache, lymphocytic pleocytosis and variable neurological patterns, usually ending in death 1 day to 3 weeks after onset of symptoms in over 70% of cases. The occasional recoveries have been associated with considerable residual disability.

The virus causes a natural infection of monkeys analogous to HSV infection in man. Human disease is acquired by the bite of apparently normal monkeys, or by exposure of naked skin to infected saliva or to monkey tissue cultures. There is no known effective treatment. Prevention depends on use of proper protective gauntlets and care to minimize exposure to monkeys. If there has been exposure to bites by a monkey with known or suspicious lesions of B-virus, wash thoroughly with soap and water; specific immune serum globulin, if available, may be given in large doses.

HISTOPLASMOSIS

ICD-9 115

Two clinically different mycoses have been designated as histoplasmosis because the pathogens that cause them cannot be distinguished morphologically when growing on culture media as molds. Detailed information will be given for the infection caused by *Histoplasma capsulatum* var. *capsulatum,* followed by a brief resumé of histoplasmosis caused by *H. capsulatum* var. *duboisii.*

INFECTION BY *HISTOPLASMA CAPSULATUM*

ICD-9 115.0

(Histoplasmosis capsulati*, Histoplasmosis due to *H. capsulatum* var. *capsulatum**, American histoplasmosis)

1. **Identification**—A systemic mycosis of varying severity, with the primary lesion usually in the lungs. While infection is common, overt clinical disease is not. Five clinical forms are recognized: (1) asymptomatic with only hypersensitivity to histoplasmin; (2) acute benign respiratory, which varies from mild respiratory illness to temporary incapacity with general malaise, weakness, fever, chest pains, and dry or productive cough, occasional erythema multiforme and erythema nodosum, and sometimes multiple, small scattered calcifications in the lung, hilar lymph nodes and spleen; (3) acute disseminated with hepatosplenomegaly, accompanied by septic-type fever, prostration, and a rapid course often resembling miliary tuberculosis, most frequent in infants and young children and, without therapy, usually fatal;(4) chronic disseminated with variable symptoms, such as unexplained fever, anemia, patchy pneumonia, hepatitis, endocarditis, meningitis, mucosal ulcers of mouth, larynx, stomach or bowel, adrenal infection common but usually asymptomatic, more common in the adult male and may follow cytotoxic or corticosteroid therapy, subacute course with progression over weeks up to a few years and usually fatal unless treated; and (5) chronic pulmonary which clinically and radiologically resembles chronic pulmonary tuberculosis, is more common in males over 40 years old and progresses over months or years, with periods of quiescence and sometimes spontaneous cure.

Clinical diagnosis is confirmed by culture or by visualizing the fungus in Giemsa- or Wright-stained smears of ulcer exudates, bone marrow, sputum or blood; special stains are necessary to demonstrate the fungus in biopsies of ulcers, liver, lymph nodes, or lung. Among the available serologic tests, the immunodiffusion test is the most specific and reliable. A rise in CF titers in paired sera is strong evidence for active disease, but recent positive skin tests with histoplasmin can raise the titer and the serological tests can cross-react with other mycoses. False negative tests are common enough that negative serological tests do not exclude the diagnosis.

2. **Infectious agent**—*Histoplasma capsulatum* var. *capsulatum (Ajellomyces capsulatus)*, a dimorphic fungus growing as a mold in soil and as a yeast in animal and human hosts.

3. **Occurrence**—Focal infections are common over wide areas of the Americas, Europe, Africa, eastern Asia and Australia; clinical disease is far less frequent and severe progressive disease is rare. Histoplasmin hypersensitivity, sometimes in as much as 80% of a population and indicating antecedent infection, is prevalent in parts of eastern and central USA. Prevalence increases from childhood to 30 years of age; differences

by sex are usually not observed except that the chronic pulmonary form is more common in males. Outbreaks have occurred in families or in groups of workmen with common exposure to bird or bat droppings or recently disturbed contaminated soil. Histoplasmosis also occurs in dogs, cats, rats, skunks, opossums, foxes and other animals.

4. **Reservoir**—Soil around old chicken houses, in caves harboring bats and around starling roosts; also around houses sheltering the common brown bat, in other soils with high organic content and in decaying trees.

5. **Mode of transmission**—Inhalation of airborne conidia.

6. **Incubation period**—Symptoms appear within 5–18 days after exposure, commonly 10 days.

7. **Period of communicability**—Not transmitted from person to person.

8. **Susceptibility and resistance**—Susceptibility is general. Inapparent infections are extremely common in endemic areas and usually result in increased resistance to infection.

9. **Methods of control**—

    A. *Preventive measures:* Minimize exposure to dust in a contaminated and enclosed environment such as chicken coops and their surrounding soil, spray with water to reduce dust; use protective masks. Infectious foci can be decontaminated with 3% formalin.

    B. *Control of patient, contacts and the immediate environment:*

        1) Report to local health authority: In selected endemic areas (USA); in many countries not a reportable disease, Class 3B (see Preface).
        2) Isolation: None.
        3) Concurrent disinfection: Of sputum and articles soiled therewith. Terminal cleaning.
        4) Quarantine: None.
        5) Immunization of contacts: None.
        6) Investigation of contacts: Household and occupational contacts for evidence of infection from a common environmental source.
        7) Specific treatment: For disseminated or chronic pulmonary cases, amphotericin B (Fungizone®) is the drug of choice. There is evidence that ketoconazole may be effective.

    C. *Epidemic measures:* Occurrence of grouped cases of acute pulmonary disease in or outside of an endemic area, particularly with history of exposure to dust within a closed space as within caves or construction sites, should arouse suspicion of histoplasmosis. Suspected sites such as chicken houses, barns, silos, caves, starling roosts, attics or basements should be investigated.

D. *Disaster implications:* None. Possible hazard if large groups, especially from nonendemic areas, are forced to move through or to live in areas where the mold is prevalent.

E. *International measures:* None.

HISTOPLASMOSIS DUBOISII ICD-9 115.1
(Histoplasmosis due to *H. capsulatum* var. *duboisii,* African histoplasmosis)

This usually presents as a subacute granuloma of the skin or bone. Infection, though usually localized, may be disseminated in the skin, subcutaneous tissue, lymph nodes, bones and joints, lungs and abdominal viscera. Disease is more common in males and may occur at any age, but especially in the second decade of life. Thus far, the disease has been recognized only in Africa and Madagascar. Diagnosis is made by culture and by demonstrating the yeast cells of *H. capsulatum* var. *duboisii* from tissue by smear or biopsy. These cells are much larger than the yeast cells of *H. capsulatum* var. *capsulatum.* The true prevalence of African histoplasmosis, its reservoir, mode of transmission, and incubation period are unknown. It is not communicable from person to person. Amphotericin B (Fungizone®) is an effective therapeutic agent.

HOOKWORM DISEASE ICD-9 126
(Ancylostomiasis, Uncinariasis, Necatoriasis)

1. Identification—A common chronic parasitic infection with a variety of symptoms, usually in proportion to the degree of anemia. The bloodletting activity of the nematode leads to iron deficiency and hypochromic microcytic anemia, the major cause of disability. Children with heavy, long-term infection may have hypoproteinemia and may be retarded in mental and physical development. Occasionally severe acute pulmonary and gastrointestinal reactions follow the exposure to infective larvae. Death is infrequent and then usually can be attributed to other infections. Light hookworm infections generally produce few or no clinical effects.

Infection is confirmed by finding hookworm eggs in feces; stool examination may be negative early in the course of the infection until the worms mature. Species differentiation requires microscopic examination of larvae cultured from the feces, or examination of adult worms expelled by purgation following a vermifuge.

2. Infectious agents—*Necator americanus, Ancylostoma duodenale* and *A. ceylanicum.*

3. Occurrence—Widely endemic in those tropical and subtropical countries where disposal of human feces is inadequate, and the soil, moisture, and temperature conditions favor development of infective larvae. May also occur in temperate climates in similar environmental conditions (e.g., mines). Both *Necator* and *Ancylostoma* occur in many parts of Asia (particularly in SE Asia), the S Pacific and in east Africa. *N. americanus* is the prevailing species throughout most of tropical Africa and America; *A. duodenale* prevails in north Africa, including the Nile Valley, in northern India, northern parts of the Far East and in the Andean areas of S America. *A. ceylanicum* occurs in SE Asia but is less common than either *N. americanus* or *A. duodenale.*

4. Reservoir—Man for *N. americanus* and *A. duodenale;* cats and dogs for *A. ceylanicum.*

5. Mode of transmission—Eggs in feces are deposited on the ground and hatch; under favorable conditions of moisture, temperature and type of soil, larvae develop to the third stage, becoming infective in 7 to 10 days. Infection of man occurs when the infective larvae penetrate the skin, usually of the foot; in so doing they characteristically produce a dermatitis (ground itch). The larvae normally enter the skin and pass via lymphatics and bloodstream to the lungs, enter the alveoli, migrate up the trachea to the pharynx, are swallowed, and reach the small intestine where they attach to the intestinal wall, develop to maturity and produce eggs in 6 to 7 weeks; earlier (3–4 weeks) in *A. ceylanicum.* Infection with *Ancylostoma* may also be acquired by the oral route by ingesting infective larvae.

6. Incubation period—Symptoms may develop after a few weeks to many months, depending on intensity of infection and iron intake of the host. Pulmonary infiltration, cough, and tracheitis may occur during the lung migration phase of infection, particularly in *Necator* infections.

7. Period of communicability—Not transmitted from person to person, but infected persons can contaminate soil for several years in the absence of treatment. Under favorable conditions, larvae remain infective in soil for several weeks.

8. Susceptibility and resistance—Universal; some immunity is thought to develop with infection.

9. Methods of control—

A. *Preventive measures:*

1) Prevent soil contamination by installation of sanitary disposal systems for human feces, especially sanitary privies in rural areas. Nightsoil and sewage effluents are hazardous, especially where they are used as fertilizer.

2) Educate the public as to dangers of soil contamination and in preventive measures, including wearing shoes in endemic areas.

3) Examine and treat people migrating from endemic to receptive nonendemic areas, especially those who will work in mines, constructing dams or in the horticultural sector.

B. *Control of patient, contacts and the immediate environment:*

1) Report to local health authority: Official report not ordinarily justifiable, Class 5 (see Preface).

2) Isolation: None.

3) Concurrent disinfection: Sanitary disposal of feces to prevent contamination of soil.

4) Quarantine: None.

5) Immunization of contacts: None.

6) Investigation of contacts: Each infected contact and carrier is a potential or actual indirect spreader of infection.

7) Specific treatment: Mebendazole (Vermox®) or pyrantel pamoate (Antiminth®); adverse reactions are infrequent. Bephenium hydroxynaphthoate (Alcopar®) and tetrachloroethylene are effective alternatives. Follow-up stool examination is indicated after 2 weeks and therapy repeated if a heavy worm burden persists. Iron supplementation will correct the anemia without worm eradication.

C. *Epidemic measures:* Surveys for prevalence in highly endemic areas, periodic mass treatment, health education in sanitation of the environment and in personal hygiene, and provision of facilities for excreta disposal.

D. *Disaster implications:* None.

E. *International measures:* None.

HYMENOLEPIASIS
(Hymenolepidosis, Dwarf tapeworm infection)

ICD-9 123.6

1. **Identification**—An intestinal infection with tapeworms that usually are too small to be seen in feces. Usually asymptomatic when infection is light. Massive numbers of the worms may cause enteritis with or without diarrhea, abdominal pain, or other vague symptoms such as pallor, loss of weight, and weakness.

Diagnosis is made by microscopic identification of eggs in feces.

2. **Infectious agent**—*Hymenolepis nana* (dwarf tapeworm).

3. **Occurrence**—Cosmopolitan, more common in warm than in cold, and especially common in dry more than in wet, climates. Dwarf tapeworm is the most common human tapeworm in southeastern USA, Latin America, Australia, Mediterranean countries, the Near East and India.

4. **Reservoir**—Infected humans; possibly also mice.

5. **Mode of transmission**—Eggs of *H. nana* are infective when passed in the feces; infection in man is acquired either by ingestion of eggs in contaminated food or water, directly from fecally contaminated fingers, or ingestion of an insect-bearing larva that developed from eggs ingested by the insect. When *H. nana* eggs are ingested, they hatch in the intestine, liberating an oncosphere that enters a mucosal villus and develops into a cysticercoid which ruptures into the lumen; this in turn produces the adult tapeworm. Some *H. nana* eggs are immediately infective when released from the proglottids in the human gut, so autoinfections can occur. If *H. nana* eggs are ingested by meal worms, larval fleas or other insects, they hatch in the insect's intestine liberating an oncosphere that penetrates into the insect's body cavity and develops into a cysticercoid that is infective to man as well as to rodents when ingested.

6. **Incubation period**—Onset of symptoms variable, the development of mature worms requires about 2 wks.

7. **Period of communicability**—As long as eggs are passed in the feces. *H. nana* infections may persist for several years.

8. **Susceptibility and resistance**—Universal; children are more susceptible than adults; infection produces resistance to reinfection. Intensive infection occurs in immunodeficient and malnourished children.

9. **Methods of control**—

    A. *Preventive measures:*

        1)   Education in personal hygiene and sanitary disposal of feces.

        2)   Provide and maintain clean toilet facilities.

3) Protect food and water from contamination with human and rodent feces.
4) Treatment to remove sources of infection.
5) Eliminate rodents from the home environment.

B. *Control of patient, contacts and the immediate environment:*

1) Report to local health authority: Official report not ordinarily justifiable, Class 5 (see Preface).
2) Isolation: None.
3) Concurrent disinfection: Sanitary disposal of feces.
4) Quarantine: None.
5) Immunization of contacts: Not applicable.
6) Investigation of contacts and source of infection: Fecal examination of family or institution members.
7) Specific treatment: Praziquantel (Biltricide®) and niclosamide (Yomesan®, Niclocide®) are effective.

C. *Epidemic measures:* Outbreaks in schools and institutions can be controlled best by treatment of infected individuals and by special attention to personal and group hygiene.

D. *Disaster implications:* None.

E. *International measures:* None.

HYMENOLEPIASIS DUE TO
HYMENOLEPIS DIMINUTA
ICD-9 123.6
(Rat tapeworm infection, Hymenolepiasis diminuta)

Rat tapeworm, caused by *H. diminuta,* occurs accidentally in man, most usually in young children. The eggs passed in rodent feces are ingested by insects such as flea larvae, grain beetles and cockroaches in which cysticercoids develop in the hemocele of the insect. The mature tapeworm develops in rats, mice or other rodents when the insect is ingested. Man is a rare accidental host, usually of a single or few tapeworms, rarely symptomatic. Definitive diagnosis is based on the characteristic egg in the feces; treatment as for *H. nana.*

DIPYLIDIASIS
ICD-9 123.8
(Dog tapeworm infection)

Toddler-age children are occasionally infected with dog tapeworm *(Dipylidium caninum),* the adult of which is found worldwide in dogs and cats. It rarely if ever produces symptoms in the child but is distressful to the parent who sees motile, seed-like proglottids (tapeworm segments) at the anus or on the surface of the stool. Infection is acquired when the child ingests fleas which had, in their larval stage, eaten eggs from proglottids which had migrated from the anus of the animal or had been passed in the feces. In 3–4 weeks the tapeworm becomes mature. Infection is prevented by keeping dogs and cats free of fleas and of worms; niclosamide and praziquantel are effective for treatment.

INFLUENZA   ICD-9 487

1. **Identification**—An acute viral disease of the respiratory tract characterized by fever, chilliness, headache, myalgia, prostration, coryza and mild sore throat. Cough is often severe and protracted. Usually self-limited, with recovery in 2–7 days. Recognition is commonly by epidemiologic characteristics; sporadic cases can be identified only by laboratory procedures. Influenza in children may be indistinguishable from disease caused by other respiratory viruses. The common cold, croup and viral pneumonia, and undifferentiated acute respiratory disease are often caused by influenza virus in children. Gastrointestinal tract manifestations (nausea, vomiting, diarrhea) are rare, but have been reported in up to 25% of children in school outbreaks of influenza A (H1N1).

Influenza derives its importance from the rapidity with which epidemics evolve, the widespread morbidity, and the seriousness of complications, notably viral and bacterial pneumonias. During major epidemics, severe disease and deaths occur primarily among the elderly and those debilitated by chronic cardiac, pulmonary, renal or metabolic disease. However, in the 1918 epidemic the highest fatality rates were among young adults. While fatality generally is low, most epidemics are associated with a general mortality much in excess of nonepidemic expectancy. Reye syndrome involving the CNS and liver is a rare complication in children; cases have been associated with influenza B disease and more rarely with influenza A. It has been suggested by several studies that salicylates play a rôle in this syndrome.

During the early febrile stage of disease, laboratory confirmation is made by recovery of influenza viruses from pharyngeal or nasal secretions in tissue culture, by direct identification of the virus in nasopharyngeal cells by FA or ELISA tests, or by demonstration of a specific serologic response in acute and convalescent sera.

2. **Infectious agent**—Three types of influenza virus are recognized: A, B and C. Type A has been associated with widespread epidemics and pandemics; type B has usually been associated with localized epidemics; type C thus far has appeared only in sporadic cases and in minor localized outbreaks. Identification of the broad types of influenza virus is deter-

mined by serological tests with type-specific antisera. Strains of influenza A are described by geographic origin, strain number and year of isolation as well as by an index identifying the character of the hemagglutinin (H) and the neuraminidase (N) antigens. For the subtypes of influenza A isolated from man, prototype strains by this nomenclature are A/PR/8/34 (H0N1), A/FM/1/47 (H1N1), A/Japan/305/57 (H2N2) and A/Hong Kong/1/68 (H3N2). Completely new subtypes (antigenic shift) appear at irregular intervals; they are responsible for pandemics. Continuous minor antigenic changes (antigenic drift) in the strains are responsible for the interpandemic epidemics. Influenza B (and to a lesser extent influenza C) also undergoes antigenic drift.

3. Occurrence—In pandemics, epidemics, localized outbreaks, and as sporadic cases. During the past 90 years, pandemics began in 1889, 1918, 1947, 1957, and 1968. Attack rates during epidemics range from <15%–25% in large communities to ≧40% in closed populations. Epidemics of influenza A have appeared in the USA at intervals of roughly 1–3 yrs, influenza B usually every 3–4 years. Mixed epidemics also occur. In temperate zones, epidemics tend to occur in winter; in the tropics often without seasonal preference.

Influenza viral infections also occur in swine, horses, and many domestic and wild avian species in many parts of the world. Transmission from animals to man has been demonstrated only on very rare occasions.

4. Reservoir—Of human infections, man; although animal reservoirs are suspected as sources of new human subtypes, perhaps by recombination with human strains.

5. Mode of transmission—By direct contact through droplet infection; airborne spread among crowded populations in enclosed spaces. Influenza virus may persist for hours in dried mucus and be transmitted by direct contact.

6. Incubation périod—Short, usually 24–72 hours.

7. Period of communicability—Probably limited to 3 days from clinical onset.

8. Susceptibility and resistance—With a new subtype, susceptibility is universal. Infection produces immunity to the specific infecting virus, but the duration and breadth of immunity depends on the degree of antigenic drift. Vaccines produce serologic responses specific for the viruses used and elicit booster responses to related strains with which the individual has had prior experience.

Age-specific attack rates during an epidemic reflect existing immunity from past experience with strains related to the epidemic subtype and the amount of exposure, so that incidence of infection is often highest in school-age children. Thus, with the recent H1N1 influenza epidemics, incidence of disease was greatest among those born after 1947, the date of the last pandemic of H1N1 disease.

9. Methods of control—

A. *Preventive measures:*

1) Active immunization gives effective protection against infection or reduces the severity of disease when a sufficient mass of antigen closely matching the prevailing wild strain of virus is administered. A single dose may suffice for those with prior exposure to the antigens; two doses of vaccine are required for persons with no previous exposure to one or more of the vaccine strains. Because of the uncertainty that epidemic influenza will occur in any given year and that available vaccines will be effective, routine immunization programs should be directed primarily at persons with greatest risk of serious complication or death (see section 1, above) or of infection (health care personnel, military recruits). However, any adult may benefit from routine immunization. When a widespread epidemic of influenza A is anticipated, immunization may be considered for those engaged in essential community services. Immunization should be accomplished before influenza is expected. Yearly recommendations for vaccine components are based on the viral strains currently circulating, as determined by international surveillance. (During the swine influenza vaccine program in 1976, an increased risk of developing Guillain-Barré Syndrome (GBS) within 9–10 weeks following receipt of the vaccine was reported in the USA. Continuing surveillance since then has shown no such association with subsequent influenza vaccinations; there are data suggesting that the association may be spurious and the study continues).

2) Amantadine hydrochloride or rimantadine, 100 mg twice daily for those 9 yrs of age or older (for younger children, daily dose is 4–8 mg/kg in 2–3 divided doses, to a maximum of 150 mg/d), is effective in the chemoprophylaxis of influenza A, but not type B. The degree of protection approximates that of the vaccine. Amantidine is associated with CNS side effects in 5–10% of uses; these may be more severe in the elderly or those with impaired kidney function. Rimantidine (which is not licensed in the USA) has fewer CNS side effects; protection is comparable in those with some prior immunity to the prevalent virus strains. The use of these drugs should be considered in

persons or groups at high risk of complications who are not immunized or when an appropriate vaccine is not available.

3) Educate the public in basic personal hygiene, especially the danger of unprotected coughs and sneezes.

B. *Control of patient, contacts and the immediate environment:*

1) Report to local health authority: Obligatory report of outbreaks or laboratory-confirmed cases as a Disease under Surveillance by WHO. Report identity of the infectious agent as determined by laboratory examination, if possible. Class 1A (see Preface).

2) Isolation: Generally impractical under most circumstances because of the delay in diagnosis, unless rapid direct viral tests are available. In epidemics, due to increased patient load, it may be necessary to isolate patients, especially infants and young children, believed to have influenza by placing them in the same room (cohorting).

3) Concurrent disinfection: None.

4) Quarantine: None.

5) Protection of contacts: A specific rôle has been shown for antiviral chemoprophylaxis against type A strains with amantadine (see 9A2).

6) Investigation of contacts: Of no practical value.

7) Specific treatment: Amantadine given early in the course of influenza A reduces symptoms. Antibiotics should be administered only for bacterial complications. Because of possible association with Reye syndrome, salicylates should be avoided.

C. *Epidemic measures:*

1) The severe and often disrupting effects of epidemic influenza on community activities may be reduced in part by effective health planning and education, particularly at the local level. Surveillance by health authorities of the extent and progress of outbreaks is important.

2) Closing of schools has not proven to be an effective control measure but may be necessary due to high absenteeism of students or staff.

3) Hospital administrators should anticipate the increased demand for medical care during epidemic periods; there may also be excessive absenteeism of health care personnel as a result of influenza. Health care personnel should be immunized annually or use amantidine while influenza A epidemics are in progress.

D. *Disaster implications:* Aggregations of people in emergency shelters will favor outbreaks of disease if the virus is introduced.

E. *International measures:* A Disease under Surveillance by WHO. The following is recommended:

1) Report epidemics within a country to WHO.

2) Identify the causative virus with report and submit prototype strains to one of the two WHO Centres for Reference and Research on Influenza in Atlanta and London. Throat washings, nasopharyngeal aspirates and paired blood samples may be sent to any WHO recognized national influenza center in the country.

3) Continuing epidemiologic studies and prompt identification of viruses by national health agencies.

4) Continuing effort to ensure enough commercial and/or governmental facilities to provide for rapid production of sufficient quantities of vaccine, and existence of programs for its administration to high-risk and essential personnel.

5) Maintain adequate supplies of amantidine for use by selected high-risk people and essential personnel in the event of a new pandemic strain for which no suitable vaccine is available.

KAWASAKI SYNDROME ICD-9 446.1
(Kawasaki disease, Mucocutaneous lymph node syndrome, Acute febrile mucocutaneous lymph node syndrome)

1.Identification—An acute febrile syndrome of childhood with a high, spiking fever unresponsive to antibiotics, and usually more than 5 days in duration, associated with pronounced irritability and mood change, nonsuppurative cervical adenopathy, bilateral conjunctival injection; an enanthem consisting of a "strawberry" tongue, an injected oropharynx or dry fissured or erythematous lips; limb changes consisting of edema, erythema, or periungual or generalized desquamation; and a polymorphous erythematous exanthem which is usually truncal. Typically there are 3 phases: (1) an acute febrile phase for about 10 days characterized by high spiking fever, rash, adenopathy, peripheral erythema or edema, conjunctivitis, and enanthem; (2) a subacute phase lasting about 2 wks characterized by thrombocytosis, desquamation, and resolution of fever; and (3) a lengthy convalescent phase during which clinical signs fade.

Coronary artery aneurysms due to coronary arteritis occur in 15–30% of patients; the case fatality rate is between 1–2% with the majority of deaths occuring between the 3rd and 6th weeks of illness. Complications can involve any organ of the body. Long-term prognosis is unknown.

There is no pathognomonic laboratory test for Kawasaki syndrome; diagnosis is based on the presence of fever lasting more than 5 days, exclusion of other causes, and at least 4 of the following: (1) bilateral conjunctival injection; (2) injected or fissured lips, or injected pharynx, or "strawberry tongue"; (3) erythema of palms or soles, or edema of the hands or feet, or generalized or periungual desquamation; (4) rash; and (5) cervical lymphadenopathy (at least 1 node $\geqq 1.5$ cm). The ESR is elevated during the acute phase; the platelet count rises above 500,000/mm^3 during the 2nd and 3rd weeks of the illness and remains elevated approximately 3 weeks.

2. Infectious agent—Unknown. Antecedent viral respiratory illnesses and exposure to mites in association with specific bacterial species have been suggested as causal or possible predisposing risk factors.

3. Occurrence—Worldwide, although most cases (>20,000) are reported in Japan. Most cases are diagnosed in infants and children less than 5 yrs old; more in boys than in girls. In the USA, attack rates are highest in children of Asian ancestry and in black children; cases are more frequent in the winter and spring. Outbreaks of Kawasaki syndrome have been reported in New York City as well as upstate New York, Los Angeles, Denver, Massachusetts, Hawaii, Wisconsin, Illinois and Michigan.

4. Reservoir—Unknown.

5. Mode of transmission—Unknown; little evidence of person-to-person transmission. Outbreak occurrence in communities is consistent with infectious etiology.

6. Incubation period—Unknown.

7. Period of communicability—Unknown.

8. Susceptibility and resistance—Children under 5 yrs, especially those of Asian ancestry, are most likely to develop Kawasaki syndrome. Recurrences are very infrequently reported.

9. Methods of control—

A. *Preventive measures:* Unknown.

B. *Control of patient, contacts and the immediate environment:*

   1) Report to local health authority: Voluntary in the USA. Clusters and epidemics should be reported immediately, Class 5 (see Preface).
   2) Isolation: None.
   3) Concurrent disinfection: None.

4) Quarantine: None.
5) Immunization of contacts: Not applicable.
6) Investigation of contacts: Not profitable.
7) Specific therapy: None. High-dose IG may reduce fever and aneurysm formation. High-dose aspirin is recommended during the acute phase, followed by low doses for several weeks.

C. *Epidemic measures:* Outbreaks and clusters should be investigated to elucidate etiology and risk factors.

D. *Disaster implications:* None.

E. *International measures:* None.

KERATOCONJUNCTIVITIS, ADENOVIRAL

ICD-9 077.1

(Epidemic keratoconjunctivitis, Shipyard conjunctivitis, Shipyard eye, Infectious punctate keratitis)

1. **Identification**—An acute viral disease of the eye with unilateral or bilateral inflammation of conjunctivae and edema of the lids and periorbital tissues. Onset is sudden, with pain, photophobia, blurred vision, and occasionally low-grade fever, headache, malaise and tender preauricular lymphadenopathy. Approximately 7 days after onset in about half of the cases, the cornea exhibits several small round subepithelial infiltrates, which may eventually form punctate erosions that stain with fluorescein. Duration of acute conjunctivitis is about 2 wks although the keratitis may continue to evolve, leaving discrete subepithelial opacities which may interfere with vision for a few weeks. In severe cases conjunctival membranes develop which may be followed by conjunctival scarring.

Diagnosis is confirmed by recovery of virus from appropriate cell cultures inoculated with eye swabs or conjunctival scrapings and by titer rises in serum neutralization or HAI tests. Virus may be visualized by FA staining of scrapings or by IEM.

2. **Infectious agent**—Type 3, 7, 8, 19 and 37 adenovirus and rarely other types, e.g., 4, 10, 11 and 14.

3. **Occurrence**—Presumably worldwide. Both sporadic cases and large outbreaks have occurred in Asia, Hawaii, N America and Europe.

4. **Reservoir**—Man.

5. **Mode of transmission**—Direct contact with eye secretions of an

infected person or indirectly through contaminated instruments or solutions. In industrial plants epidemics are centered in first aid stations or dispensaries where treatment is frequently administered for minor trauma to the eye; transmission then occurs through fingers, instruments or other contaminated items. Similar outbreaks have originated in eye clinics and medical offices. When dispensary and clinic personnel acquire the disease they may act as sources of infection. Family spread is common, with children introducing the infection.

6. **Incubation period**—Probably 5–12 days.

7. **Period of communicability**—From late in the incubation period to 14 days after onset. Prolonged viral shedding has been reported.

8. **Susceptibility and resistance**—There is usually complete immunity after adenovirus 8 infection. Similar conjunctivitis with minor keratitis may occur with other adenoviruses. Trauma and eye manipulation increase the risk of infection.

9. **Methods of control**—

A. *Preventive measures:*

1) Avoid communal eye droppers, medicines, instruments, towels, etc.
2) In ophthalmologic procedures in dispensaries, clinics and offices, asepsis should include vigorous handwashing before examining each patient and systematic sterilization of instruments after use. Medical personnel with overt conjunctivitis should be kept out of contact with patients.
3) Use safety measures such as goggles in industrial plants.
4) Education about personal cleanliness and the danger in using common towels and toilet articles.

B. *Control of patient, contacts and the immediate environment:*

1) Report to local health authority: Obligatory report of epidemics; no individual case report, Class 4 (see Preface).
2) Isolation: Drainage/secretion precautions; patients should use separate towels and linen during the acute stage. Infected medical personnel should not come in contact with patients.
3) Concurrent disinfection: Of conjunctival and nasal discharges and articles soiled therewith. Terminal cleaning.
4) Quarantine: None.
5) Immunization of contacts: None.
6) Investigation of contacts and source of infection: In outbreaks the source of infection should be identified and precautions taken to prevent further transmission.

7) Specific treatment: None during the acute phase. If the residual opacities interfere with the patient's ability to work, topical corticosteroids may be tried.

C. *Epidemic measures:*

1) Educate medical personnel to wash hands and sterilize instruments carefully before and after eye examinations.
2) Organize convenient facilities for prompt diagnosis and treatment.

D. *Disaster implications:* None.

E. *International measures:* WHO Collaborating Centres (see Preface).

LASSA FEVER   ICD-9 078.89

1. **Identification**—An acute viral illness with a duration of 1 to 4 weeks. Onset is gradual with malaise, fever, headache, sore throat, cough, nausea, vomiting, diarrhea, myalgia, chest and abdominal pain; fever is persistent or intermittent-spiking. Inflammation and enanthem of pharynx, hypotension, conjunctivitis and swelling of the face or neck are commonly observed. In severe cases shock, pleural effusion, hemorrhagic manifestations, and encephalopathy are often noted. Leukopenia, albuminuria, and hemoconcentration are common, but leukocytosis has been noted in some cases. Transient alopecia may occur in convalescence and deafness is a recognized sequela. Case fatality rate is about 15% among hospitalized cases, varying widely in different areas; inapparent infections, diagnosed serologically, are common.

Diagnosis is made by isolation of virus from blood, urine or throat washings and serologically by IFA; half of the patients have specific IgM at the time of admission. Neutralizing antibodies may not appear until several months later and then in low titer. Laboratory specimens may be hazardous and must be handled under maximal biosafety conditions (P4 containment). A mobile laboratory is available on request to CDC for this purpose. (See 9B3, below).

2. **Infectious agent**—An arenavirus, serologically related to lymphocytic choriomeningitis, Machupo, and Junin viruses.

3. **Occurrence**—Widely distributed over west and central Africa. Serologically related viruses from Central African Republic, Mozambique, and Zimbabwe of lesser virulence for laboratory hosts have not yet been associated with human infection or disease.

4. **Reservoir**—Wild rodents; in west and central Africa, the multimammate mouse, *Mastomys natalensis*, is implicated.

5. **Mode of transmission**—Primarily through direct or indirect contact with urine of infected rodents in dust or on food. Person-to-person and laboratory infections occur, especially in the hospital environment, by direct contact with blood, pharyngeal secretions or urine of a patient, including inoculation with contaminated needles. Transmission by droplet or aerosol exposure has been implicated in one situation.

6. **Incubation period**—Commonly 6 to 21 days.

7. **Period of communicability**—Person-to-person infections may occur during the acute febrile phase when virus is present in the throat. Virus may be excreted in urine of patients for 3 to 9 weeks from onset of illness.

8. **Susceptibility and resistance**—All ages are susceptible; the duration of immunity following infection is unknown.

9. **Methods of control**—

A. *Preventive measures:* Specific rodent control.

B. *Control of patient, contacts and the immediate environment:*

1) Report to local health authority: Individual cases should be reported, Class 2A (Preface).

2) Isolation: Strict isolation in a hospital room away from traffic patterns should be instituted immediately. Transfer to special isolation units is no longer considered essential because of the absence of nosocomial infections in hospitals with high aseptic standards; however, if such facilities are available (plastic isolator or room with laminar flow air, high efficiency particulate air (HEPA) filters on exhaust air and at negative pressure to an anteroom) may be considered. Advice on management of a possible patient is available from CDC.

3) Concurrent disinfection: Patients' excreta, sputum, blood and all objects with which the patients had contact, including laboratory equipment used to carry out tests on blood, etc., with 0.5% sodium hypochlorite solution disinfection and, so far as possible, appropriate heating methods such as autoclaving, incineration or sterilization. For safety in carrying out necessary laboratory tests, in the USA, a Vickers Mobile Laboratory, together with a qualified laboratory technician, can be obtained from CDC. Thorough terminal disinfection with 0.5% sodium

hypochlorite solution or a phenolic compound; formaldehyde fumigation can be considered.

4) Quarantine: Three weeks from the time of exposure for face-to-face contacts who are not expected to cooperate fully in surveillance. (See 9B6, below.)

5) Immunization of contacts: None.

6) Investigation of contacts and source of infection: Identify all face-to-face contacts from time of onset of fever; establish close surveillance with body temperature checks at least 2 times daily for at least 3 weeks after last exposure. In case of any temperature elevation, immediate hospitalization in strict isolation facilities. Determine place of residence of patient during two weeks prior to onset and search for unreported or undiagnosed cases. To minimize contacts, laboratory tests should be carried out in special containment facilities; if there is no such facility, tests should be kept to a minimum and handled with extreme care.

7) Specific treatment: If the patient is seen within the first six days of clinical illness, administer ribavirin i.v., 1.0 g every 6 hours; after 6 days of illness, use ribavirin and 1 or 2 units of convalescent plasma, tested and found free of Lassa virus and containing neutralizing antibodies.

C. *Epidemic measures:* Not determined.

D. *Disaster implications:* None.

E. *International measures:* Notification to receiving countries of possible exposures by infected travelers.

LEGIONELLOSIS   ICD-9 482.8
(Legionnaires' disease; Legionnaires' pneumonia; Pontiac fever)

1. **Identification**—An acute bacterial disease with two currently recognized distinct clinicoepidemiologic manifestations: "Legionnaires' disease" and "Pontiac fever." Both are characterized initially by anorexia, malaise, myalgia, and headache. Within a day, there is usually a rapidly rising fever associated with chills. A nonproductive cough is common; abdominal pain and diarrhea occur in many patients. Temperatures commonly reach 39°–40.5°C (102°–105°F). In Legionnaires' disease, chest x-ray may show patchy areas of consolidation which may progress to bilateral involvement and ultimately to respiratory failure; the overall case

fatality rate has been as high as 15% in hospitalized cases of legionnaires' disease; it is generally higher in those with compromised immunity. Pontiac fever is not associated with pneumonia or death; patients recover spontaneously in 2–5 days without treatment.

Diagnosis depends on isolation of the causative organism or its demonstration by direct IF stain of involved tissue or respiratory secretions, either an expectorated sputum sample or a transtracheal aspirate. A diagnostic rise in IFA titer (more than fourfold) between an acute phase serum and one drawn ≧3 weeks later is diagnostic.

2. **Infectious agent**—*Legionella pneumophila*, a poorly staining gram-negative rod that is difficult to grow in vitro. Serogroups 1–9 are currently recognized. Related organisms have been isolated from pneumonia cases predominantly in immunosuppressed patients, including *L. micdadei, L. bozemanii, L. longbeachae,* and *L. dumoffii;* additional species are currently being described.

3. **Occurrence**—Legionellosis is neither new nor localized. The earliest documented case occurred in 1947 and the earliest documented outbreak in 1957 in Minnesota. Since then the disease has been identified in most states as well as in Australia, Africa, Canada, S America and Europe. Although cases occur throughout the year, both sporadic cases and outbreaks are recognized more commonly in summer and autumn. Serologic surveys suggest a prevalence of antibodies to *L. pneumophila* serogroup 1 at a titer of ≧1:128 in 1–5% of the general population in the few locations studied. The proportion of cases with sporadic, otherwise undiagnosed, pneumonias that are legionnaires' disease, appears to range from 0.5 to 4%.

Outbreaks of legionellosis usually occur with low attack rates (0.1–5%) in the population at risk. Epidemic Pontiac fever has had a high attack rate (about 95%) in several outbreaks.

4. **Reservoir**—Probably aqueous; soil has been suspected. Hot water systems and air-conditioning cooling towers or evaporative condensers have been implicated epidemiologically; the organism has been isolated from water in these as well as from hot and cold water taps and showers, and from creeks and ponds and the soil from their banks. The organism survives for months in tap or distilled water.

5. **Mode of transmission**—Epidemiologic evidence supports airborne transmission; other modes are possible but none has been proven conclusively.

6. **Incubation period**—Legionnaires' disease, 2–10 days, most often 5–6 days; Pontiac fever, 5–66 hours, most often 24–48 hours.

7. **Period of communicability**—Person-to-person transmission has not been documented.

8. Susceptibility and resistance—Susceptibility is general but the disease is rare in those under 20 yrs of age; several outbreaks have occurred among hospitalized patients. Unrecognized infections may be common but prospective studies indicate that at least half of *Legionella* infections are associated with pneumonia. More serious illness tends to occur with increasing age, especially in smokers and the immunocompromised. The male/female ratio is about 2.5:1; and the average age of cases is in the 50s.

9. Methods of control—

   A. *Preventive measures:* Unknown, other than appropriate disinfection of cooling tower waters and adequate treatment of water supplies where these sources have been implicated.

   B. *Control of patient, contacts and the immediate environment:*

   1) Report to local health authorities: In selected endemic areas (USA); in many countries not a reportable disease, Class 3B (see Preface).

   2) Isolation: None.

   3) Concurrent disinfection: None.

   4) Quarantine: None.

   5) Immunization of contacts: None.

   6) Investigation of contacts: Search for additional cases (households, business, etc.) due to infection from a common environmental source.

   7) Specific treatment: Erythromycin appears to be the agent of choice. Rifampin may be a valuable adjunct but should not be used alone. Penicillin, the cephalosporins, and the aminoglycosides are ineffective.

   C. *Epidemic measures:* Search for possible environmental sources of infection. Chlorination of cooling tower water, super-chlorination of the water supply and/or periodic superheating of the water supply have been used.

   D. *Disaster implications:* None known.

   E. *International measures:* None.

LEISHMANIASIS
I. LEISHMANIASIS, CUTANEOUS   ICD-9 085.1-085.5
(Aleppo, Baghdad or Delhi boil, Oriental sore; in the Americas—
Espundia, Uta, Chiclero ulcer)

1. **Identification**—A polymorphic disease of skin and mucous membranes caused by tissue flagellates. The disease starts with a nodular lesion which may remain indolent or become painful and ulcerate. Lesions may be single, multiple or diffuse; and may be self-limiting or chronic. With some strains mainly from the New World, even years after the primary lesion has healed, or with no recognized initial lesion, mucocutaneous lesions (espundia) may develop that involve the nasopharyngeal tissues. This form can be fatal.

Diagnosis is made by culture of the flagellates on suitable media from biopsies or aspirates, or by microscopic identification of the non-flagellated form (amastigotes) in stained smears of scrapings or aspirates from the edges of lesions. An intradermal test (Montenegro's test) with material derived from the flagellated forms (promastigotes) generally becomes positive early in the disease and remains so thereafter; not helpful in very early lesions or anergic disease. Serology (IFA or ELISA) testing usually shows antibodies in those in the New World with active lesions but is mostly negative in Old World cutaneous leishmaniasis. Species identification is difficult; isozyme analysis and other research techniques are required.

2. **Infectious agents**—Old World, *Leishmania tropica, L. major, L. aethiopica;* New World, *L. braziliensis* and *L. mexicana* complexes of species and probably others. *L. braziliensis* strains produce more severe infections with mucocutaneous lesions; *L. mexicana* produces self-limiting cutaneous lesions. *L. donovani,* in the Old World, may cause single cutaneous lesions as well as post-kala-azar dermal leishmaniasis.

3. **Occurrence**—Northwest India and Pakistan, the Middle East including Iran and Afghanistan, southern USSR, the Mediterranean littoral; the sub-Sahara African savanna and Sudan, the highlands of Ethiopia, Kenya and Namibia; southcentral Texas, Mexico (especially Yucatan), most of Central America and every country of S America except Chile. In some areas, such as the Old World, large population groups, including children, may be at risk; in the New World, disease is restricted usually to occupational groups such as those involved in work in forested areas or to those whose homes are in or next to a forest. Generally more common in rural than urban areas.

4. **Reservoir**—Man, wild rodents, sloths, marsupials, and Canidae, often including domestic dogs; unknown hosts in many areas.

5. **Mode of transmission**—From the zoonotic reservoir host through

the bite of infective female phlebotomines (sandflies). After feeding on an infected host, flagellate forms develop in the gut and in 8–20 days infective forms are present which are either injected during biting or contaminate the bite wound. In man, or other mammal, the organisms lose their flagella and the amastigote forms multiply in histiocytes until the cells rupture, enabling spread to other histiocytes.

6. **Incubation period**—At least a week to many months.

7. **Period of communicability**—As long as parasites remain in lesions; in untreated cases usually 5 months to 2 years. Spontaneous healing is the rule with *L. tropica, L. major* and *L. mexicana* infections except when the ear (pinna) is involved. Most infections with *L. aethiopica* and *L. m. amazonensis* also heal spontaneously, but a proportion of patients develop diffuse cutaneous lesions which are rich in parasites and do not heal spontaneously. Infections with parasites of the *L. braziliensis* complex also heal, but up to 80% of infections with *L. b. braziliensis* are followed, months or years later, by metastatic mucocutaneous lesions.

8. **Susceptibility and resistance**—Susceptibility is probably general. Immunity is usual after lesions heal. Factors responsible for late mutilating disease such as espundia are unknown; occult infections may be activated years after the primary infection.

9. **Methods of control**—

    A. Preventive measures:

        1) Control measures vary from area to area, depending on the habits of the vector phlebotomines and vertebrate hosts. Where their habits are known, applicable control measures may be carried out. These include:

            a) Systematic case detection and rapid treatment applies to all forms as one of the important preventive measures, particularly in those situations where the reservoir is largely or solely in man.

            b) Periodic application of insecticides with residual action. Phlebotomine flies have a short flight range and are highly susceptible to control by systematic spraying with residual insecticides. Spraying should cover exterior and interior of doorways and other openings if infection takes place in dwellings, as well as possible breeding places of Old World sandflies such as stone walls, animal houses and rubbish heaps.

            c) Eliminate rubbish heaps and other breeding places for Old World phlebotomines.

            d) Destroy animals implicated locally as reservoirs.

            e) In the New World, avoid sandfly-infested or thickly

forested areas, particularly after sundown; use insect repellents and protective clothing if exposure to sandflies is unavoidable.

2) Educate the public concerning modes of transmission and methods of controlling phlebotomines.

B. *Control of patient, contacts and the immediate environment:*

1) Report to local health authority: Official report not ordinarily justifiable, Class 5 (see Preface).

2) Isolation: None. If transmission occurs locally, protect patient from phlebotomines by fine mesh screen (10–12 holes to the linear cm or 25–30 to the linear inch, aperture size not more than 0.89 mm or 0.035 inches); by spraying quarters with residual-action insecticide; and by use of repellents.

3) Concurrent disinfection: None.

4) Quarantine: None.

5) Immunization of contacts: None.

6) Investigation of contacts and source of infection: Determine local transmission cycle and interrupt it in most practical fashion.

7) Specific treatment: Mainly pentavalent antimonials. Sodium antimony gluconate (Pentostam®), the recommended drug, is available in the USA from CDC, Atlanta (see Preface). Other compounds, including meglumine antimonate (Glucantime®) are in use in S America and elsewhere. Cycloguanil pamoate (Camolar®) may be effective. Amphotericin B (Fungizone®) may be required in South American mucocutaneous disease when disease does not respond to antimonial therapy. While spontaneous healing of simple cutaneous lesions occurs with certain strains, infections with *L. braziliensis* should always be treated with drugs.

C. *Epidemic measures:* In areas of high incidence, intensive efforts to control the disease by provision of diagnostic facilities, by mass treatment campaigns and by appropriate measures against phlebotomine flies and the mammalian reservoir hosts.

D. *Disaster implications:* None.

E. *International measures:* WHO Collaborating Centres (see Preface).

II. LEISHMANIASIS, VISCERAL
(Kala-azar)

ICD-9 085.0

1. **Identification**—A chronic systemic disease caused by a tissue flagellate. The disease is characterized by fever, hepatosplenomegaly, lymphadenopathy, anemia with leukopenia, and progressive emaciation and weakness. Untreated, usually a fatal disease. Fever is of gradual or sudden onset, continued and irregular, often with 2 daily peaks; alternating periods of apyrexia and low-grade fever follow. Post-kala-azar leishmanoid dermal lesions may occur after apparent cure.

Diagnosis is made preferably by culture of the organism from biopsy or aspirated material, or by demonstration of intracellular amastigotes (Leishman-Donovan bodies) in stained smears from bone marrow, spleen, liver, lymph node or blood. (See Leishmaniasis, Cutaneous, above).

2. **Infectious agents**—*Leishmania donovani, L. infantum* and *L. chagasi.*

3. **Occurrence**—A rural disease of some tropical and subtropical areas, occurring in discrete foci in India, the Middle East including Turkey, the Mediterranean basin, Mexico and Central and S America, and in Sudan and Kenya. In many affected areas, common as scattered cases among infants, children and adolescents, but occasionally occurs in epidemic waves. Incidence is modified by the use of antimalarial insecticides. Where dog populations have been drastically reduced, disease in man has been reduced.

4. **Reservoir**—Known or presumed reservoirs include man, wild Canidae and domestic dogs, and rodents. Man is the only known reservoir in India.

5. **Mode of transmission**—Through bite of infective phlebotomine sandflies. (See Leishmaniasis, Cutaneous, above).

6. **Incubation period**—Generally 2–4 months; range is 10 days to 2 yrs.

7. **Period of communicability**—As long as parasites persist in the circulating blood or skin of the mammalian reservoir host. If man is the reservoir host, infectivity for phlebotomines may persist even after clinical recovery. Transmission from person to person, and by blood transfusion and sexual contact have been reported.

8. **Susceptibility and resistance**—Susceptibility is general. Kala-azar induces apparent lasting homologous immunity; recovery from cutaneous leishmaniasis does not confer immunity against kala-azar.

9. **Methods of control**—

   A. *Preventive measures:* See Leishmaniasis, Cutaneous 9A, above. Eliminate domestic canine reservoir.

B. *Control of patient, contacts and the immediate environment:*

1) Report to local health authority: In selected endemic areas, Class 3B (see Preface).

2) Isolation: None; (see Leishmaniasis, Cutaneous, 9B2, above).

3) Concurrent disinfection: None.

4) Quarantine: None.

5) Immunization of contacts: None.

6) Investigation of contacts and source of infection: Ordinarily none.

7) Specific treatment: Sodium antimony gluconate (Pentostam®), available from CDC, Atlanta (see Preface) or meglumine antimonate (Glucantime®) is effective. Antimony-resistant cases may be treated by diamidine compounds such as pentamidine; these are not used routinely because of toxicity. In some regions, such as Kenya, the parasite is more resistant than in India, requiring much longer antimonial therapy.

C. *Epidemic measures:* Effective control must include an understanding of the local ecology and transmission cycle, followed by adoption of practical measures to stop transmission.

D. *Disaster implications:* None.

E. *International measures:* Coordinated programs of control among neighboring countries where the disease is endemic. WHO Collaborating Centres (see Preface).

LEPROSY
(Hansen's disease)

ICD-9 030

1. **Identification**—A chronic bacterial disease of the skin, peripheral nerves and (in lepromatous patients) the nasal mucosa. The manifestations of the disease vary from patient to patient in a continuous spectrum from lepromatous to tuberculoid leprosy. In lepromatous leprosy, nodules, papules, macules and diffuse infiltrations are bilaterally symmetrical and usually numerous and extensive. In lepromatous leprosy, involvement of the nasal mucosa may lead to crusting, obstructed breathing and epistaxis; iritis and keratitis are common. In tuberculoid leprosy, skin lesions are single or few, sharply demarcated, anesthetic or hypesthetic, and bilaterally asymmetrical; peripheral nerve involvement tends to be relatively severe. Borderline leprosy has features of both polar forms, and the disease form

is more labile with a tendency to shift toward lepromatous in the untreated and toward the tuberculoid form in the treated patient. An early form of the disease manifested by a hypopigmented macule with ill-defined borders is known as indeterminate and, if untreated, may progress to tuberculoid, borderline, or lepromatous disease. The clinical manifestations include the "reactions" of leprosy, acute adverse episodes: erythema nodosum leprosum (ENL) in lepromatous patients and reversal reactions in borderline leprosy; reactions are more frequent in treated patients.

Clinical diagnosis is based on complete skin examination; search for signs of peripheral nerve involvement (hypesthesia, anesthesia, paralysis, muscle wasting, trophic ulcers), palpation of peripheral nerves (ulnar nerve at the elbow, peroneal nerve at the head of the fibula and the greater auricular nerves) for enlargement and tenderness. Skin lesions are tested for sensation (light touch, pin-prick, temperature discrimination).

Differential diagnosis includes many skin diseases, none of which has anesthesia. Diffuse cutaneous leishmaniasis may resemble lepromatous leprosy, but acid-fast bacilli and nerve involvement are not present.

The diagnosis is strongly supported by the demonstration of acid-fast bacilli in skin smears made by the scraped-incision method; in tuberculoid disease the bacilli may be so few they are not demonstrable. Whenever possible, a skin biopsy confined to the affected area should be sent to a pathologist experienced in leprosy diagnosis. Nerve involvement with acid-fast bacilli is pathognomonic of leprosy.

2. Infectious agent—*Mycobacterium leprae.* The organism has not been grown in bacteriologic media or tissue cultures. It can be grown in mouse foot pads to 10^6/g of tissue; in the nine-banded armadillo it grows to 10^9–10^{10}/g.

3. Occurrence—The world prevalence is estimated at about 12 million. Prevalence rates of $\geq 10{:}1000$ are common in the rural tropics and subtropics; socioeconomic conditions may be more important than climate itself. The chief endemic areas are SE Asia, Philippines, Papua New Guinea, India, Korea, China, tropical Africa, some Pacific islands and some areas of Latin America. Reported rates in the Americas range from <0.1–$5{:}1000$. Newly recognized cases in the USA are diagnosed principally in California, Hawaii, Texas, Florida, Louisiana, Puerto Rico and New York City. Most of these cases represent infections acquired in endemic areas elsewhere; the disease remains endemic in Hawaii, Puerto Rico, Texas and Louisiana.

4. Reservoir—Man is the only reservoir of proven significance. Feral armadillos in Louisiana and Texas have been found naturally afflicted with a disease identical to experimental leprosy in this animal, and there have been reports suggesting that disease in armadillos has been naturally transmitted to humans. Naturally acquired leprosy has been observed in a mangabey monkey and in a chimpanzee, captured in Nigeria and Sierra Leone, respectively.

5. Mode of transmission—Not clearly established, but household and prolonged close contact are important. Millions of bacilli are liberated daily in the nasal discharges of untreated lepromatous patients. Bacilli have been shown to remain viable for at least 7 days in dried nasal secretions. The organisms probably gain entrance through the upper respiratory tract and possibly through broken skin.

6. Incubation period—The average is probably 4 yrs for tuberculoid leprosy and twice that for lepromatous leprosy, although many years may elapse before the disease is recognized. The disease is rarely seen in children under age 3.

7. Period of communicability—Clinical and laboratory evidence suggests that infectiousness is lost in most instances within 3 months of continuous and regular treatment with dapsone (4,4'-diamino-diphenylsulfone, DDS) or clofazimine, or with 3 days of rifampicin.

8. Susceptibility and resistance—No proven racial immunity. The persistence and form of leprosy depend upon the ability to develop effective cell-mediated immunity. The lepromin test is the intradermal injection of autoclaved *M. leprae*. The Mitsuda reaction, which is read at 28 days, is negative in lepromatous leprosy and positive in tuberculoid disease and in a proportion of normal adults; thus, the test gives prognostic information but is of no diagnostic value. The rate of positive tests in the general population increases with age. In addition, a high prevalence of specific lymphocyte transformations and specific *M. leprae* antibodies among close contacts of leprosy patients suggests that infection is frequent but disease eventuates in only a small proportion.

9. Methods of control—The availability of drugs effective in treatment and in suppressing infectiousness has changed the management of the patient with leprosy from isolation from society with attendant despair, to one of ambulatory treatment with hospitalization only for managing reactions, surgical correction of deformities and the treatment of ulcers resulting from the anesthesia of the disease.

A. Preventive measures:

    1) Early detection of infectious cases and regularly adminis-tered therapy, on an outpatient basis whenever possible.

    2) Health education stressing the availability of effective multidrug therapy, the absence of infectivity of patients under continuous treatment and the prevention of physical and social disabilities.

    3) In field trials in Uganda and Papua New Guinea, prophylac-

tic BCG apparently effected a considerable reduction in the incidence of tuberculoid leprosy among contacts. A study in Burma showed less protection. Chemoprophylactic studies suggest that approximately 50% protection against disease can be achieved with dapsone or acedapsone.

B. Control of patient, contacts and the immediate environment:

1) Report to local health authority: Case reporting obligatory in many states and countries and desirable in all, Class 2B (see Preface).

2) Isolation: None for cases of tuberculoid leprosy; contact isolation for cases of lepromatous leprosy. Hospitalization is often indicated during the treatment of reactions. No special procedures are required when cases are hospitalized but in a general hospital a separate room may be desirable. No restrictions in employment or attendance at school are indicated for patients whose disease is regarded as noninfectious.

3) Concurrent disinfection: Of nasal discharges of infectious patients. Terminal cleaning.

4) Quarantine: None.

5) Protection of contacts: None, but initial leprosy examination of all household and family contacts deserves high priority. (See 9A3, above).

6) Control of contacts: The initial examination is most productive, but periodic examination of household and other close contacts at 12-month intervals for at least 5 yrs after last contact with an infectious case is recommended.

7) Specific treatment: With the widespread prevalence of dapsone resistance and the emergence of resistance to rifampicin, combined chemotherapy regimens are essential. The minimal regimen recommended by WHO for multibacillary leprosy is rifampicin 600 mg once monthly, dapsone (DDS) 100 mg/d and clofazimine 300 mg once monthly along with 50 mg/d. The monthly rifampicin and clofazimine are administered under supervision. The treatment should be continued until skin smears become negative but for at least 2 yrs. For paucibacillary (tuberculoid) leprosy the recommended regimen is rifampicin 600 mg once a month (supervised) and dapsone 100 mg/d, both for a period of 6 months. Patients under treatment should be monitored for side effects of drugs, for leprosy reactions, and for the development of trophic ulcers. Some complications may need to be treated in a referral center.

C. *Epidemic measures:* Not applicable.

D. *Disaster implications:* Any interruption of therapy schedules is serious. During wars the diagnosis and treatment of leprosy patients has often been neglected.

E. *International measures:* International controls should be limited to untreated infectious cases only. WHO Collaborating Centres (see Preface).

LEPTOSPIROSIS   ICD-9 100
(Weil's disease, Canicola fever, Hemorrhagic jaundice, Mud fever, Swineherd's disease)

1. **Identification**—A group of zoonotic diseases with protean manifestations including fever, headache, chills, severe malaise, vomiting, myalgia and conjunctival suffusion; occasionally meningitis, rash and uveitis. Sometimes jaundice, renal insufficiency, hemolytic anemia and hemorrhage in skin and mucous membranes occur. Clinical illness lasts from a few days to 3 weeks; often a biphasic illness. Infections may be asymptomatic; severity varies with the infecting serovar. Case fatality rate is low, but increases with advancing age and may reach $\geq 20\%$ in patients with jaundice and kidney damage who have not been treated with renal dialysis; deaths are predominantly due to hepatorenal failure or from myocardial involvement.

Diagnosis is confirmed by rising titers in serological tests and by isolation of leptospires from blood or CSF during the acute illness or from urine after the first week in special media or by inoculation of young guinea pigs, hamsters or gerbils. IF methods and ELISA techniques are also used for identification of the isolates.

2. **Infectious agent**—Leptospires, members of the order Spirochaetales. Pathogenic leptospires belong to the species *Leptospira interrogans,* which is subdivided into serovars. More than 170 serovars have been identified and these fall into about 20 serogroups based on antigenic overlap. Commonly identified serovars in the USA are *icterohaemorrhagiae, canicola, autumnalis, hebdomadis, australis* and *pomona.*

3. **Occurrence**—Worldwide; in urban and rural, developed and primitive areas, except for polar regions. An occupational hazard to rice and sugar cane-field workers, farmers, sewer workers, miners, veterinarians, animal husbandmen, dairymen, abattoir workers, fish workers and military troops; outbreaks occur among those exposed to fresh river, canal or lake water contaminated by urine of domestic or wild animals, and to urine or

tissues of infected animals. A recreational hazard to bathers, campers and sportsmen in infected areas. Predominantly a disease of males, related to occupation.

4. Reservoir—Farm and pet animals, including cattle, dogs, horses and swine. Rats and other rodents act as the normal carrier host; wild animals, including deer, squirrels, foxes, skunks, raccoons, opossums, marine mammals (sea lions) and even reptiles and amphibians (frogs) may be infected. In Europe, field mice, voles, shrews and hedgehogs are common reservoir hosts. In carrier animals, an asymptomatic infection occurs in the renal tubules with leptospiruria persisting for long periods of time.

5. Mode of transmission—Contact of the skin, especially if abraded, or of mucous membranes with water, moist soil or vegetation contaminated with urine of infected animals, as in swimming or accidental or occupational immersion; direct contact with urine or tissues of infected animals; or occasionally through ingestion of food contaminated with urine of infected rats.

6. Incubation period—Usually 10 days with a range of 4–19 days.

7. Period of communicability—Direct transmission from person to person is rare. Leptospires may be excreted in the urine for usually 1 month but has been observed as long as 11 months after the acute illness.

8. Susceptibility and resistance—Susceptibility of man is general; immunity to the specific serovar follows infection or (sometimes) immunization but this may not protect against a different serovar.

9. Methods of control—

  A. Preventive measures:

    1) Protect workers in hazardous occupations by providing boots and gloves.
    2) Recognize potentially contaminated waters and soil and, when possible, drain such waters.
    3) Educate the public on modes of transmission, to avoid swimming or wading in potentially contaminated waters and to use proper protection when work requires such exposure.
    4) Rodent control in human habitations, especially rural and recreational. Burn cane fields before harvest.
    5) Segregate infected domestic animals; prevent contamination of man's living, working and recreational areas by urine of infected animals.
    6) Immunization of farm and pet animals prevents disease but not necessarily infection and renal shedding. The vaccine must contain the dominant local strains.

7) Immunization of man has been carried out against occupational exposures to specific serovars in Japan, China, Italy, Spain and Israel.

8) Doxycycline has been shown in Panamá to be effective in preventing leptospirosis when administered in an oral dose of 200 mg weekly during periods of high exposure.

B. *Control of patient, contacts and the immediate environment:*

1) Report to local health authority: Obligatory case report in many states and countries, Class 2B (see Preface).

2) Isolation: Blood/body fluid precautions.

3) Concurrent disinfection: Articles soiled with urine.

4) Quarantine: None.

5) Immunization of contacts: None.

6) Investigation of contacts: Search for exposure to infected animals or history of swimming in contaminated waters.

7) Specific treatment: Penicillin, streptomycin, tetracyclines and erythromycin are leptospirocidal in vitro. Doxycycline has been shown to be of value in the treatment of human disease when given within 4 days of onset. Peritoneal or renal dialysis may be required in case of renal failure.

C. *Epidemic measures:* Search for source of infection, such as a swimming pool; eliminate the contamination or prohibit use. Investigate industrial or occupational sources, including direct animal contact.

D. *Disaster implications:* A potential problem following flooding of certain areas with a high water table.

E. *International measures:* WHO Collaborating Centres (see Preface).

LISTERIOSIS

ICD-9 027.0

1. **Identification**—A bacterial disease usually manifested at the extremes of age, during pregnancy or among immunocompromised individuals as an acute meningoencephalitis with or without associated septicemia, less frequently septicemia only; very often neonatal. Onset of meningoencephalitis may be sudden with fever, intense headache, nausea, vomiting and signs of meningeal irritation, or may be subacute, particularly in an immunocompromised or elderly host. Delirium and coma may appear early; occasionally there is collapse and shock. Endocarditis, granulomat-

ous lesions in the liver and other organs, localized internal or external abscesses and pustular or papular cutaneous lesions may occur. Listeriosis in the normal host may be an acute, mild, febrile illness, sometimes with influenza-like symptoms. Infection in pregnant women may result in infection of the fetus and interrupted pregnancy. Infants may be stillborn, born with septicemia, or develop meningitis in the neonatal period, even though the mother is asymptomatic. The postpartum course of the mother is usually uneventful, but case fatality rate is 30% in newborn infants and approaches 50% when onset occurs in the first 4 days.

Diagnosis is confirmed by isolation of the infectious agent from CSF, blood, meconium, lochia, gastric washings and other sites of infection. Bacteriological methods are exacting, and care must be taken to distinguish *Listeria monocytogenes* from other gram-positive rods, particularly "diphtheroids." Isolations from contaminated specimens are more frequent after prolonged incubation at 4°C (39°F). Microscopic examination of CSF or meconium permits presumptive diagnosis; FA may be useful in visualizing the organisms in tissues and CSF. Serologic tests are unreliable because of cross reactions with other bacterial species.

2. Infectious agent—*Listeria monocytogenes,* a bacterium; types Ia, Ib, IVa, and IVb are most frequently isolated from man in USA.

3. Occurrence—An uncommonly diagnosed infection. Typically sporadic, rarely in outbreaks. Occurs in all seasons with a late summer/early autumn maximum, slightly more often in males than females. About 40% of clinical cases occur within the first 3 weeks of life; in adults infection occurs mainly after age 40. Nosocomial acquisition has been reported. Inapparent infections occur at all ages, although of consequence only during pregnancy. Abortion may occur, sometimes as early as the 2nd month of pregnancy but mainly in the 5th or 6th month; perinatal infection is acquired during the last trimester. Incidence unknown; in USA, a minimum estimate for illness requiring hospitalization is 1 case/million population/year. European studies have disclosed large numbers of human carriers.

4. Reservoir—Infected domestic and wild mammals, fowl and man; infection of foxes produces an encephalitis simulating rabies. Asymptomatic fecal carriage is common in man (up to 5%) and animals; asymptomatic vaginal carriage occurs in humans. The organism is frequently found free-living in water and mud. The seasonal use of silage as fodder is frequently followed by an increased incidence of listeriosis in animals.

5. Mode of transmission—In neonates, infection is transmitted from mother to fetus in utero or during passage through the infected birth canal. Papular lesions on hands and arms may occur from direct contact with infectious material or soil contaminated with infected animal feces. Listeriosis associated with ingestion of contaminated vegetables and presumed contaminated dairy products has been reported. Person-to-person transmission through venereal contact is possible, as is infection from inhalation of the organism. Nursery outbreaks attributed to spread via hands of medical and nursing staff have occurred.

6. Incubation period—Unknown; probably a few days to 3 wks. The fetus is usually infected within several days after maternal disease.

7. Period of communicability—Mothers of infected newborn infants may shed the infectious agent in vaginal discharges or urine for 7–10 days after delivery, rarely longer. Period of person-to-person communicability unknown.

8. Susceptibility and resistance—Fetuses and newborn infants are highly susceptible. Children and young adults generally are resistant, adults less so after age 40. Disease is frequently superimposed on other debilitating illnesses, especially in patients receiving steroids or other immunosuppressive agents. Little evidence of acquired immunity, even after prolonged severe infection.

9. Methods of control—

A. *Preventive measures:*

1) Pregnant women should avoid contact with potentially infective materials such as aborted animal fetuses on farms and with known infected persons.
2) Proper precautions by veterinarians and farmers in handling aborted fetuses.

B. *Control of patient, contacts and the immediate environment:*

1) Report to local health authority: Official report of clusters of cases required, Class 4 (see Preface).
2) Isolation: None.
3) Concurrent disinfection: None.
4) Quarantine: None.
5) Immunization of contacts: None.
6) Investigation of contacts and source of infection: Of no practical value except in outbreak situations.
7) Specific treatment: Penicillin or ampicillin together with aminoglycosides, ampicillin alone, the tetracyclines, and chloramphenicol may be effective. Ampicillin is preferred for maternal-fetal listeriosis; the tetracyclines are contraindicated for children less than 8 yrs.

C. *Epidemic measures:* Search for a common source of infection, and prevent further exposure to that source. A routine gram stain smear of meconium from all newborn infants should be examined for short gram-positive rods resembling *L. mono-cytogenes*. If positive, prophylactic antibiotics should be administered as a precaution.

D. **Disaster implications:** None.

E. **International measures:** None.

LOIASIS   ICD-9 125.2
(*Loa loa* infection, Eye worm disease of Africa)

1. Identification—A chronic filarial disease characterized by migration of the adult worm through subcutaneous or deeper tissues of the body, causing transient swellings several cm in size, located on any part of the body. These swellings may be preceded by localized pain accompanied by pruritus. Local names include "fugitive swelling" and "Calabar swelling." Migration under the bulbar conjunctivae may be accompanied by pain and edema. Allergic reactions with giant urticaria and fever may occur occasionally, particularly in Caucasians.

Infection with other filariae such as *Wuchereria bancrofti, Onchocerca volvulus,* or *Mansonella (Dipetalonema) perstans* requires differentiation in endemic areas.

Larvae (microfilariae) are present in peripheral blood during the daytime, and can be demonstrated in stained thick blood smears, stained sediment of laked blood or by membrane filtration. Eosinophilia is frequent. A travel history is very helpful in diagnosis.

2. Infectious agent—*Loa loa,* a nematode.

3. Occurrence—Widely distributed in tropical west and central Africa. In the Congo River basin up to 90% of indigenous inhabitants of some villages are infected.

4. Reservoir—An infected person harboring microfilariae in the blood.

5. Mode of transmission—Transmitted by a horsefly or deerfly of the genus *Chrysops. Chrysops dimidiata, C. silacea* and other species ingest blood containing microfilariae; the larvae develop within 10–12 days in the fat body of the fly. The developed larva migrates to the proboscis and is transferred to a human host by the bite of the infective fly.

6. Incubation period—Symptoms usually do not appear until several yrs after infection but may occur as early as 4 months. Microfilariae may appear in the peripheral blood 5–6 months after infection.

7. Period of communicability—The adult worm may live in man and microfilariae may be present in the blood as long as 17 yrs; in the fly, communicability is from 10–12 days after its infection and until all infective larvae have migrated or until the fly dies.

8. Susceptibility and resistance—Susceptibility is universal; repeated infections occur and immunity, if present, has not been demonstrated.

9. Methods of control—

A. Preventive measures:

1) Measures directed against the fly larvae are effective but have not proven practical, as the moist muddy breeding areas are usually too extensive.

2) Diethyltoluamide (Deet, detamide) or dimethyl phthalate applied to exposed skin are effective fly repellents.

3) Wearing long trousers; screening houses.

B. Control of patient, contacts and the immediate environment:

1) Report to local health authority: Official report not ordinarily justifiable, Class 5 (see Preface).

2) Isolation: Not practicable. So far as possible, patients with microfilaremia should be protected from *Chrysops* bites to reduce transmission.

3) Concurrent disinfection: None.

4) Quarantine: None.

5) Immunization of contacts: None.

6) Investigation of contacts: None; a community problem.

7) Specific treatment: Diethylcarbamazine (DEC, Hetrazan®) causes disappearance of microfilariae and may kill the adult worm with resulting cure; however, during therapy, hypersensitivity reactions commonly occur which are sometimes severe but controllable by steroids and/or antihistamines. Surgical removal of adult worm for relief of acute bulbar conjunctivitis is seldom indicated.

C. Epidemic measures: Not applicable.

D. Disaster implications: None.

E. International measures: WHO Collaborating Centres (see Preface).

LYME DISEASE   ICD-9 695.9, 716.59
(Lyme arthritis, Erythema chronicum migrans (ECM) with polyarthritis,
Tickborne meningopolyneuritis)

   1. **Identification**—This tickborne spirochetal zoonotic disease is characterized by a distinctive skin lesion (ECM), systemic symptoms,
polyarthritis, and neurological and cardiac involvement occurring in
varying combinations. This illness typically occurs in the summer and its
first manifestation, ECM, appears as a red macule or papule which expands
in an annular manner, sometimes with multiple similar lesions. The lesions
may be accompanied by malaise, fatigue, fever, headache, stiff neck,
myalgia, migratory arthralgias, or lymphadenopathy lasting several weeks;
these symptoms may precede the appearance of the skin lesions. Within
weeks to months after onset of ECM, neurological abnormalities (including
the clinical picture of aseptic meningitis, encephalitis, chorea, cerebellar
ataxia, cranial neuritis including facial palsy, motor or sensory radiculoneu-
ritis and myelitis) may develop; symptoms fluctuate and may last for
months. Cardiac abnormalities (including atrioventricular block, acute
myopericarditis or cardiomegaly) may occur within a few weeks after onset
of ECM. Weeks to years (usually about 4 weeks) after onset, swelling and
pain in large joints, especially the knees, may develop and recur for several
years; chronic arthritis may result. In Europe, the similar symptom
complex occurs in which arthritis or cardiac abnormalities occur less
frequently than in the USA cases.
   Diagnosis is currently based on clinical findings; serologic tests show a
rise in antibodies directed against the spirochete.

   2. **Infectious agent**—A spirochete first identified in 1982, for which the
name *Borrelia burgdorferi* has been proposed.

   3. **Occurrence**—In the USA, endemic foci exist along the coast from
Massachusetts to Virginia, in Wisconsin, Minnesota, California, and
Oregon; isolated cases have been reported from N Carolina, Georgia, Utah
and Arkansas. Elsewhere, it occurs in almost all of Europe, USSR and
Australia. Cases occur primarily during summer; distribution of cases
coincides with the distribution of *Ixodes dammini* ticks in eastern and
midwestern USA and with *I. pacificus* in western USA and, in Europe, with
the distribution of *I. ricinus*.

   4. **Reservoir**—Certain Ixodid ticks through transstadial transmission.
Deer, wild rodents and other animals maintain the cycle.

   5. **Mode of transmission**—Tickborne.

   6. **Incubation period**—From 3–32 days after tick exposure.

   7. **Period of communicability**—No evidence of natural transmission
from person to person.

8. Susceptibility and resistance—All persons are probably susceptible; age range of cases is 2–88 yrs. Reinfection has occurred.

9. Methods of control—

A. Preventive measures: See Rocky Mountain spotted fever, 9A, except for vaccine comments.

B. Control of patient, contacts and the immediate environment:

1)-5) See Rocky Mountain spotted fever, 9B.
6) Investigation of contacts: Studies to determine source of infection are indicated when cases occur outside a recognized endemic focus.
7) Specific treatment: Treatment of the ECM stage with tetracycline for adults or penicillin for children may prevent or lessen the severity of the major late cardiac, neurologic or arthritic complications.

C. Epidemic measures: See Rocky Mountain spotted fever, 9C.

D. Disaster implications: None.

E. International measures: None.

LYMPHOCYTIC CHORIOMENINGITIS   ICD-9 049.0
(LCM, Benign (or serous) lymphocytic meningitis)

1. Identification—A viral infection of animals, especially mice, transmissible to man with a marked diversity of clinical manifestations. At times it begins with an influenza-like attack followed by complete recovery; in some cases, meningeal symptoms appear after a brief remission, or the illness may begin with meningeal or meningoencephalomyelitic symptoms. Orchitis or parotitis occasionally occurs. The course is usually short; it is very rarely fatal and even with extremely severe disease (e.g., coma with meningoencephalitis) prognosis for recovery without sequelae is usually good. The CSF in cases with neurological involvement typically shows a pleocytosis and at times a low glucose level. The primary pathologic finding in the rare human fatality is diffuse meningoencephalitis. A few fatal cases of hemorrhagic fever-like disease have been reported.

Laboratory diagnostic methods include isolation of virus from blood, nasopharynx, or CSF early in the attack by intracerebral inoculation of LCM-free adult mice or tissue cultures; and rising titers of antibodies demonstrated by serological testing of paired sera. Requires differentiation from other aseptic meningitides.

2. **Infectious agent**—The virus of lymphocytic choriomeningitis, an arenavirus.

3. **Occurrence**—Uncommon. Localized foci of infection often persist over long periods of time, resulting in sporadic clinical disease. Outbreaks have occurred from hamsters sold as pets or from laboratory animals.

4. **Reservoir**—The infected house mouse, *Mus musculus;* natural infection in guinea pigs, hamsters, and monkeys has been documented.

5. **Mode of transmission**—Virus is excreted in urine, saliva and feces of infected animals, usually mice. Transmission to man is probably through virus-contaminated excreta, food or dust; no evidence of person-to-person spread by ordinary contact.

6. **Incubation period**—Probably 8–13 days; 15–21 days to meningeal symptoms.

7. **Period of communicability**—Not known to be directly transmitted from person to person. Naturally infected mice may carry and excrete the virus for life; the infected female transmits virus to offspring.

8. **Susceptibility and resistance**—Unknown. Sera of persons recovered from the disease neutralize virus, as occasionally do the sera of persons without a history of recognized attack.

9. Methods of control—

    A. *Preventive measures:* Clean home and place of work; eliminate mice and dispose of diseased animals. Virologic surveillance of commercial rodent breeding establishments, especially those producing hamsters and mice.

    B. *Control of patient, contacts and the immediate environment:*

        1) Report to local health authority: Obligatory report of outbreaks, no case report required, Class 4 (see Preface).

        2) Isolation: None.

        3) Concurrent disinfection: Of discharges from the nose and throat, of urine and feces, and of articles soiled therewith during acute febrile period. Terminal cleaning.

        4) Quarantine: None.

        5) Immunization of contacts: None.

        6) Investigation of contacts and source of infection: Search home and place of employment for presence of house mice or rodent pets.

        7) Specific treatment: None.

    C. *Epidemic measures:* Not applicable.

    D. *Disaster implications:* None.

E. *International measures:* None.

LYMPHOGRANULOMA VENEREUM   ICD-9 099.1
(Lymphogranuloma inguinale, Esthiomene, Climatic or tropical bubo)

1. Identification—A sexually acquired chlamydial infection beginning with a small painless evanescent erosion, papule, nodule or herpetiform lesion on the penis or vulva, frequently unnoticed. Regional lymph nodes undergo suppuration followed by extension of the inflammatory process to the adjacent tissues. In the male, inguinal buboes are seen which may become adherent to the skin, fluctuate and result in sinus formation. In the female, involvement is mainly of the pelvic nodes with extension to the rectum and rectovaginal septum, resulting in proctitis, stricture of the rectum and fistulae; more rarely, proctitis may result from rectal inter-course. Elephantiasis of the genitalia may occur in either sex. Fever, chills, headache, joint pains and anorexia are present. The disease course is often long and disability great, but generally not fatal. Rarely generalized sepsis with arthritis and meningitis occurs.

Diagnosis is made by demonstration of inclusion bodies in leukocytes of the bubo aspirate, by culture, or by specific micro-IF test. CF test may be of value.

2. Infectious agent—*Chlamydia trachomatis,* related to the organisms of trachoma and oculogenital chlamydial infections, but of immunotypes L-1, L-2 and L-3.

3. Occurrence—Worldwide, especially in tropical and subtropical areas; more common than ordinarily believed. Endemic in Asia and Africa and in some areas of southern USA, particularly among lower socio-economic classes. Age incidence is that of greatest sexual activity; sex differences not pronounced in countries with high endemicity; all races are affected. In temperate climate, found principally among male homosexuals.

4. Reservoir—Humans; often asymptomatic (particularly females).

5. Mode of transmission—Direct contact with open lesions of infected persons, usually during sexual intercourse.

6. Incubation period—Variable, with a range of 3–30 days for a primary lesion; if a bubo is the first manifestation, 10–30 days, to several months.

7. Period of communicability—Variable, from weeks to years, during presence of active lesions.

8. Susceptibility and resistance—Susceptibility is general; status of natural or acquired resistance unclear.

9. Methods of control—

   A.   *Preventive measures:* Except for measures which are specific for syphilis, preventive measures are those for sexually transmitted diseases. See Syphilis, 9A, and Granuloma Inguinale, 9A.

   B.   *Control of patient, contacts and the immediate environment:*

      1)   Report to local health authority: A reportable disease in selected endemic areas. Not a reportable disease in most countries. Class 3C (see Preface).

      2)   Isolation: None. Refrain from sexual contact until all lesions are healed.

      3)   Concurrent disinfection: None; care in disposal of discharges from lesions and of articles soiled therewith.

      4)   Quarantine: None.

      5)   Immunization of contacts: Not applicable; prompt treatment on recognition or clinical suspicion of infection.

      6)   Investigation of contacts: Search for sexual contacts of patient.

      7)   Specific treatment: Tetracycline antibiotics are effective for all stages, including buboes and ulcerative lesions. Administer orally for at least 2 weeks. Erythromycin or sulfonamides may be used when tetracycline is contraindicated. Do not incise buboes; drain by aspiration through healthy tissue.

   C.   *Epidemic measures:* Not applicable.

   D.   *Disaster implications:* None.

   E.   *International measures:* See Syphilis, 9E.

MALARIA   ICD-9 084

   1. Identification—The four human malarias can be sufficiently similar in their early symptoms to make differentiation difficult without laboratory studies. The most serious, falciparum malaria (malignant tertian), may present in a quite varied clinical picture including fever, chills, sweats and headache, and may progress to icterus, coagulation defects, shock, renal and liver failure, acute encephalopathy and coma. It is a possible cause of coma and other CNS symptoms, such as disorientation and delirium, in any person recently returned from a tropical area. Prompt treatment is essential even in mild cases since irreversible complications may appear suddenly; case fatality among untreated children and nonimmune adults considerably exceeds 10%.

The other human malarias, vivax (benign tertian), malariae (quartan), and ovale, generally are not life threatening except in the very young, the very old or in patients with concurrent disease. Illness may begin with indefinite malaise followed by a shaking chill and rapidly rising temperature, usually accompanied by headache and nausea and ending with profuse sweating. After an interval free of fever, the cycle of chills, fever, and sweating is repeated, either daily, every other day or every 3rd day. Duration of an untreated primary attack varies from a week to a month or longer. Relapses, seen with vivax and ovale infections, are common and may occur at irregular intervals for up to 2 and 5 years respectively; malariae infections may persist for as many as 50 years with recurrent febrile episodes.

Individuals who are partially immune or who have been taking prophylactic drugs may show an atypical clinical picture and a wide variation in the incubation period.

Laboratory confirmation is made by demonstration of malaria parasites in blood films. Repeated microscopic examinations may be necessary; parasites are often not demonstrable in films from patients recently or actively under treatment. Antibodies, demonstrable by IFA or other tests, appear after the first week of infection and may persist for years, indicating past malarial experience and not necessarily helpful for diagnosis of a present illness.

2. Infectious agents—*Plasmodium vivax, P. malariae, P. falciparum* and *P. ovale*. Mixed infections are not infrequent in endemic areas.

3. Occurrence—Endemic malarias no longer occur in many temperate zone countries but are a major cause of ill health in many parts of the tropics and subtropics. Falciparum and vivax malaria are found in many endemic areas; ovale malaria is seen mainly in west Africa where *P. vivax* is practically absent. *P. falciparum* strains, refractory to cure with the 4–aminoquinolines (such as chloroquine), occur in the tropical portions of both hemispheres. Current information on foci of drug-resistant malaria is published annually by the WHO and can be obtained from the Malaria Branch, CDC, Atlanta (see Preface).

4. Reservoir—Man is the only important reservoir of human malaria, although higher apes may harbor *P. malariae*. Nonhuman primates are naturally infected by many malarial species including *P. knowlesi, P. cynomolgi, P. brasilianum, P. inui, P. schwetzi* and *P. simium*, which can infect man but natural transmission is extremely rare.

5. Mode of transmission—By the bite of an infective female anopheline mosquito. Most species feed at dusk and during early night hours; some important vectors have biting peaks around midnight or the early hours of the morning. When a female *Anopheles* mosquito ingests blood containing the sexual stages of the parasite (gametocytes), male and female gametes are set free in the mosquito stomach where they unite and enter the stomach wall to form a cyst in which thousands of sporozoites develop; this requires 8–35 days, depending on species of parasite and the temperature to which the vector is exposed. These sporozoites migrate to various organs of the infected mosquito and some which reach the salivary glands mature and are infective when injected in man as the insect takes a blood meal.

In the susceptible host, the sporozoites enter hepatocytes and develop into exoerythrocytic schizonts. The hepatocytes rupture and asexual parasites (tissue merozoites) appear in the bloodstream and invade the erythrocytes to grow and multiply cyclically. Some will develop into asexual forms, from trophozoites to mature blood schizonts which rupture to liberate merozoites which invade other erythrocytes. Clinical symptoms coincide with the rupture of erythrocytic schizonts. Within some erythrocytes, the merozoite may develop into the male (microgametocyte) or the female (macrogametocyte) sexual forms. The period between the infective bite and the appearance of the parasite in the blood is the "prepatent period" and varies from 6–9 days with *P. falciparum*, *P. vivax* and *P. ovale*, and 12–16 days in the case of *P. malariae*. Gametocytes usually appear within 3 days of parasitemia with *P. vivax* or *P. ovale*, and after 12–14 days in *P. falciparum*. Some exoerythrocytic forms of *P. vivax* and probably *P. ovale* exist as dormant forms (hypnozoites) which remain in hepatocytes to mature months later and produce relapses. This phenomenon does not occur in falciparum nor in malariae malaria, and reappearance of disease is the result of inadequate treatment or of infection with drug-refractory strains. With *P. malariae* low levels of erythrocytic parasites may persist for many years to multiply at some future time to a level that may result again in clinical disease. The malarias may also be transmitted by injection or transfusion of blood of infected persons or by use of contaminated needles and syringes, as by drug addicts. Congenital transmission occurs rarely.

6. Incubation period—The time between the infective bite and the appearance of clinical symptoms is approximately 12 days for *P. falciparum*, 14 days for *P. vivax* and *P. ovale*, and 30 days for *P. malariae*. With some strains of *P. vivax*, mostly from temperate areas, there may be a protracted incubation period of 8–10 months and even longer with *P. ovale*. With infection by blood transfusion, incubation periods depend on the number of parasites infused; they are usually short but may range up to about 2 months.

7. Period of communicability—For infection of mosquitoes, as long as infective gametocytes are present in the blood of patients; this varies with species and strain of parasite and with response to therapy. Untreated or insufficiently treated cases may be a source of mosquito infection for more than 3 years in malariae, from 1–2 years in vivax, and generally not more than 1 year in falciparum malaria; the mosquito remains infective for life. Transmission by transfusion may occur as long as asexual forms remain in the circulating blood; with *P. malariae* this can continue for $\geqq 40$ yrs. Stored blood can remain infective for 16 days.

8. Susceptibility and resistance—Except in some with certain genetic traits, susceptibility is universal. Tolerance or refractoriness to disease is present in adults in highly endemic communities where exposure to infective anophelines is continuous over many years. Most black Africans show a natural resistance to infection with *P. vivax*, possibly associated with the absence of Duffy factor on their erythrocytes. Persons with sickle cell trait have relatively low parasitemia when infected with *P. falciparum*.

9. Methods of control—

   A. Preventive measures:

      1) Sanitary improvements, such as filling and draining areas of impounded water, which will result in permanent elimination or reduction of anopheline breeding habitats, should be encouraged. Larvicides and biological control with larvivorous fish may be useful.

      2) Application of residual insecticide on the inside walls of dwellings and on other surfaces upon which endophilic vector anophelines habitually rest will generally result in effective malaria control, except where vector resistance to these insecticides has developed or the vectors do not enter houses. Any use of residual insecticides should be preceded by a careful appraisal of the particular problem area, the development of specific plans, and their approval by the government concerned.

      3) Nightly spraying of screened living and sleeping quarters with a liquid or an aerosol preparation of pyrethrum or other insecticide is useful.

      4) In endemic areas, install screens and use bed nets.

      5) Insect repellents applied to uncovered skin of persons exposed to bites of vector anophelines are useful when applied repeatedly. The most effective repellent presently available is N,N diethyl-m-toluamide (Deet).

      6) Blood donors should be questioned for a history of malaria or possible exposure to the disease. In USA, blood donors who have not taken antimalarial drugs and have been free of symptoms may donate 6 months after return from an endemic area. If they have been on antimalarial prophylaxis or have had malaria or have immigrated or are visiting

from endemic areas, they may be accepted as donors 3 years after cessation of chemoprophylaxis or chemotherapy or departure from the endemic area if they have remained asymptomatic. A migrant or visitor from an area where malariae malaria is or was endemic may be a source of transfusion-induced infection for many years. Such areas include, but are not limited to, tropical Africa and countries such as Greece and Romania.

7) Prompt and effective treatment of acute and chronic cases is an important adjunct to malaria control.

8) Regular use of suppressive drugs in malarious areas.

   a) For suppression of malaria in nonimmunes temporarily residing in or traveling through endemic areas, chloroquine (Aralen®) 5 mg base/kg body weight (300 mg base or 500 mg chloroquine phosphate for the average adult) or amodiaquin (Camoquin®) at approximately the same dose level, once weekly. Pregnancy is not a contraindication. The drug must be continued on the same schedule for 6 weeks after leaving endemic areas.

   b) These chemosuppressive drugs do not eliminate intrahepatic parasites so that clinical relapses of vivax or ovale malaria may occur later after the drug is discontinued. Primaquine, 0.25 mg base/kg/d for 14 days (15 mg base or 26.3 mg of primaquine phosphate for the average adult), is effective and may be given concurrently with or following the suppressive drug; however, it can produce hemolysis in those with glucose-6-phosphate dehydrogenase (G-6-PD) deficiency. The decision to administer primaquine is made on an individual basis, considering the potential risk of adverse reactions. Larger daily doses (22.5 mg base) may be required for some SE Asian and southwest Pacific strains. Alternatively, primaquine 0.75 mg base/kg may be given once weekly for 8 doses (45 mg base or 79 mg primaquine phosphate for the average adult). If possible, prior to primaquine administration, the patient should be tested for possible G-6-PD deficiency. Primaquine should not be administered during pregnancy; chloroquine should be continued weekly for the duration of the pregnancy.

   c) In areas where the *P. falciparum* strains have become chloroquine-resistant (see section 3 above), adults should receive, in addition to their weekly chloroquine dose (which is needed to suppress infection with *P.*

vivax or *P. ovale*), a fixed combination of pyrimethamine (25 mg) and sulfadoxine (500 mg) (Fansidar®) for 6 wks after the last exposure. Strains resistant to this combination are becoming common. Fansidar should not be used during pregnancy nor in children under 2 years old, nor in those allergic to sulfonamides. There are no data on the effects of long-term administration of this triad. For toxic effects and revised recommendations, see MMWR 34:183–191, Apr. 12, 1985.

An alternative combination drug is Maloprim® (12.5 mg pyrimethamine and 100 mg dapsone). It is widely used in Australia and New Zealand. A new drug, mefloquine, to be available as the mono substance or combined with sulfadoxine and pyrimethamine, may become the suppressive drug of choice in areas with malaria resistant to other drugs.

B. *Control of patient, contacts and the immediate environment:*

1) Report to local health authority: Obligatory case report as a Disease under Surveillance by WHO, Class 1A (see Preface), in nonendemic areas preferably limited to smear-confirmed cases (USA); Class 3C is the more practical procedure in endemic areas.

2) Isolation: For hospitalized patients, blood/body fluid precautions. Patients should be in mosquito-proof areas at night.

3) Concurrent disinfection: None.

4) Quarantine: None.

5) Immunization of contacts: Not applicable.

6) Investigation of contacts: Determine history of previous infection or of exposure. If a history of needle sharing is obtained from the patient, investigate and treat all persons who shared the equipment. In transfusion-induced malaria, all donors must be located and their blood examined for malarial parasites and for antimalarial antibodies; parasite-positive donors should receive treatment.

7) Specific treatment for all forms of malaria:

a) The treatment of malarias due to infection with *P. vivax, P. malariae* and *P. ovale,* and with *P. falciparum* infections incurred in west Africa, is the oral administration of a total of 25 mg of chloroquine or amodiaquin base/kg administered over a 3-day period: 15 mg/kg the 1st day (10 mg/kg initially and 5 mg/kg 6 hours later; 600 and 300 mg doses for the average adult); 5 mg/kg the 2nd and 5 mg/kg the 3rd day.

b) For emergency treatment of adults with grave infections or for persons unable to retain orally administered medication, quinine dihydrochloride 650 mg (10 grains), diluted in 500 ml of normal saline, glucose or plasma administered by slow i.v. (over 2–4 hrs), repeated if needed in 6 hours but not more than 3 doses per 24 hours. Pediatric dosage is 25 mg/kg, half given over 1 hour and the other half 6–8 hours later if oral dose is not tolerated. If there is evidence of renal failure, quinine dosage should be reduced. In extremely severe falciparum infections, particularly those with parasitemia approaching or exceeding 50%, exchange transfusion should be considered. All parenteral drugs should be discontinued as soon as oral drug administration can be initiated.

c) For *P. falciparum* infections acquired in areas where chloroquine-resistant strains are present: Administer quinine 25 mg/kg/d divided into 3 doses, for 7–10 days; plus pyrimethamine 0.85 mg/kg/d administered in divided doses for 3 days. (For grave infections, administer quinine as described above). Follow the quinine administration with tetracycline 15 mg/kg given in 4 doses daily for 7 days. Fansidar® treatment failures are common in areas where the drug has been in use as a prophylactic. Mefloquine, a quinoline methanol, has been in use for several years in SE Asia, and treatment failures have been reported. Members of the phenanthrene methanol and quinazoline families, which may be effective against these refractory strains, are under active development.

d) For prevention of relapses in mosquito-acquired *P. vivax* and *P. ovale* infections, administer primaquine, as described in 9A8b above, upon completion of the treatment of an acute attack. It is desirable to test all patients (especially blacks, Asians and Mediterraneans) for G-6–PD deficiency to prevent drug-induced hemolysis. Many, particularly blacks, are able to tolerate the hemolysis, but consideration may have to be given to discontinuing primaquine, balancing the induced problem against the possible recurrence of malaria. Primaquine is not required in non-mosquito-transmitted disease (e.g., transfusion), since no liver phase was ever present.

C. *Epidemic measures:* Determine the nature and extent of the epidemic situation. Intensify control measures directed against adult and larval stages of the important vectors including elimination of breeding places, treatment of acute cases, use of personal protection and suppressive drugs. Mass treatment may be considered.

D. *Disaster implications:* Throughout history the malarias have been the concomitant or the result of wars and social upheavals. Any abnormal climatic change which increases the availability of mosquito-breeding sites in endemic areas can lead to an increase in malaria.

E. *International measures:*

1) Disinsection of aircraft, ships or other vehicles on arrival if the health authority at the place of arrival has reason to suspect importation of malaria vectors.

2) Disinsection of aircraft before departure or in transit using a space-spray application of an insecticide of a type to which the vectors are susceptible.

3) Enforce and maintain rigid antimosquito sanitation within the mosquito flight range of all ports and airports.

4) In special circumstances, administration of antimalarial drugs to potentially infected migrants, refugees, seasonal workers or persons taking part in periodic mass movement into an area or country where malaria has been eliminated. Primaquine, 30–45 mg base (0.5–0.75 mg/kg), given as a single dose renders the gametocytes of falciparum malaria noninfectious.

5) Malaria is a Disease under Surveillance by WHO, as it is considered an essential element of the world strategy of primary health care. National health administrations are expected to notify WHO twice a year of: those areas originally malarious with no present risk of infection, those malaria cases imported into areas in the maintenance phase of eradication, those areas with chloroquine-resistant strains of parasites, and those international ports and airports free of malaria. WHO Collaborating Centres (see Preface).

MEASLES

ICD-9 055

(Rubeola, Hard measles, Red measles and Morbilli)

1. **Identification**—An acute, highly communicable viral disease with prodromal fever, conjunctivitis, coryza, cough and Koplik spots on the buccal mucosa. A characteristic red blotchy rash appears on the 3rd to 7th day, beginning on the face, becoming generalized, lasting 4 to 7 days and sometimes ending in branny desquamation. Leukopenia is common. The disease is more severe in infants and adults. Complications from measles may result from viral replication or bacterial superinfection and include otitis media, pneumonia and encephalitis. In the USA, Canada and the UK, death from uncomplicated measles is rare; deaths that occur are from pneumonia, mainly in children less than 2 years old, especially the multi-handicapped; occasionally from encephalitis. Measles is a more severe disease among the very young and in malnourished children, associated with hemorrhagic measles, protein-losing enteropathy, mouth sores, dehydration and severe skin infections, with a case fatality rate of 5 to 10% or more. Both acute and delayed adverse effects on infant and child mortality have been documented. In children who are borderline nourished, measles often precipitates acute kwashiorkor. Subacute sclerosing panencephalitis (SSPE) develops very rarely (in the range of 1–5/1,000,000) several years after a measles infection as a late sequel of measles; over 50% of SSPE cases have had measles in the first two years of life.

In those who received inactivated measles vaccine (prior to 1968), infection with wild virus may cause severe atypical manifestations with pneumonitis, pleural effusion, peripheral edema and an atypical rash with predilection for the extremities resembling that of Rocky Mountain spotted fever.

Diagnosis is usually made on clinical and epidemiologic grounds; it can be confirmed by identification of viral antigen in nasopharyngeal aspirate using FA techniques, by virus isolation from blood, conjunctiva, nasopharynx or urine in tissue culture, or by a rise in antibody titers.

2. **Infectious agent**—Measles virus, a member of the genus *Morbillivirus* of family Paramyxoviridae.

3. **Occurrence**—Prior to widespread immunization, measles was common in childhood, so that over 90% of people had been infected by age 20; few persons went through life without an attack. Measles was endemic in large metropolitan communities, attaining epidemic proportions about every other year. In smaller communities and areas, outbreaks tended to be more widely spaced and somewhat more severe. With longer intervals between outbreaks, as in the Arctic and some island areas, measles often affected a large proportion of the population with a higher case fatality rate.

With effective childhood immunization programs, measles cases in the USA and Canada have dropped by 99% and are now generally limited to preschool children, adolescents, young adults and those refusing vaccination. In temperate climates measles occurs primarily in the late winter and early spring. In tropical countries measles occurs very early in life as maternal antibody decreases.

4. Reservoir—Man.

5. Mode of transmission—By droplet spread or direct contact with nasal or throat secretions of infected persons; less commonly by airborne spread or by articles freshly soiled with secretions of nose and throat. Measles is one of the most readily transmitted communicable diseases.

6. Incubation period—About 10 days, varying from 8–13 days from exposure to onset of fever; about 14 days until rash appears; uncommonly longer or shorter. IG, given later than the 3rd day of the incubation period for passive protection, may extend the incubation to 21 days instead of preventing disease.

7. Period of communicability—From slightly before the beginning of the prodromal period to 4 days after appearance of the rash; communicability is minimal after the second day of rash.

8. Susceptibility and resistance—Practically all persons who have not had the disease or been immunized are susceptible. Acquired immunity after disease is usually permanent. Infants born of mothers who have had the disease are ordinarily immune for approximately the first 6–9 months or more depending on the amount of residual maternal antibody at the time of pregnancy.

9. Methods of control—

   A. Preventive measures:

   1) Vaccination: Live attenuated measles vaccine is the agent of choice. Inactivated vaccines are no longer recommended. A single injection of live "further attenuated" measles vaccine, which may be combined with other live vaccines (mumps, rubella), induces active immunity in more than 95% of susceptible individuals, probably for life, by producing a mild or inapparent, noncommunicable infection. About 5–30% of vaccinees may develop malaise, fever to 39.4°C (103°F) 4–10 days post-vaccination, lasting 2–5 days but with little disability. Rash, coryza, mild cough and Koplik spots may occasionally occur. Seizures may occur without sequelae as a febrile response to vaccine in about 1:1,000 vaccinations, the highest incidence in children with a previous history, or a close

family history, of such reactions. CNS conditions, including encephalitis and encephalopathy, have been reported following measles vaccination (approximately 1 case per million doses administered).

a) Vaccine shipment and storage: Vaccination may not produce protection if the vaccine has been improperly handled or stored. Prior to reconstitution, frozen measles vaccine should be kept in the frozen state at a temperature of -10 to $-30°C$, $(14$ to $-22°F)$. Freeze-dried measles vaccine is relatively stable and can be stored at refrigerator temperatures $(2-8°C$ $(35.6-46.4°F))$ with safety for a year or more; for longer periods or for storage of large volumes, the freezing temperatures are recommended. Reconstituted vaccine should be kept at refrigerator temperatures and protected from light, which may inactivate the virus. Reconstituted vaccine unused after 8 hours should be discarded.

b) Indications for immunization: Measles vaccine is indicated for all individuals susceptible to measles, unless otherwise contraindicated (see 9A1d, below). The optimal age for vaccination of children varies from developed to developing countries and is related to the persistence of maternal antibodies that can be transferred to the child before birth (see section 8, above). In the USA, a single dose at 15 months of age or as soon as possible thereafter provides the greatest immunity. (Children susceptible to rubella or mumps can be given the measles vaccine combined with rubella or with both rubella and mumps vaccines). Studies conducted in developing countries (Africa and Latin America) have indicated that the optimal age for vaccination in those settings is at 9–10 months of age; the necessity for revaccination of these children has not been determined.

c) Revaccinations: In the USA, those given live measles vaccine before 12 months of age, those who are unsure of their age at vaccination, or who were vaccinated prior to 1968 with vaccine of unknown type should be revaccinated. In those who had received only inactivated measles vaccine before 1968, this may produce more severe reactions, such as local edema and induration, lymphadenopathy and fever; however, revaccination may protect against the atypical measles syndrome. Need for routine revaccination of those properly vaccinated has not been established.

d) Contraindications to the use of live vaccines: Pregnancy; purely on theoretical grounds, vaccine should not be given to pregnant women; others should be advised of the theoretical risk of fetal wastage if they become pregnant within the next month or two. Patients with immune deficiency diseases or suppressed immune responses from leukemia, lymphoma or generalized malignancy, or from therapy with corticosteroids, irradiation, alkylating drugs or antimetabolites should not receive live virus vaccine. Patients with a high fever or severe illness should have vaccination deferred until recovery; those with active tuberculosis should not be vaccinated until after anti-tuberculosis therapy has been initiated. Vaccination should be given 14 days before or deferred for 3 months after IG or blood transfusion.

2) Public education by health departments and private physicians should encourage measles vaccine for all susceptible infants, children, adolescents and adults; those for whom vaccine is contraindicated and who are exposed to measles in families or institutions, should be protected by IG.

3) The requirement of measles immunization for school attendance, from day-care centers through high school, is an important and effective means of measles control in the USA and some provinces of Canada. Immunity levels over 95% are probably needed for effective control.

B. *Control of patient, contacts and the immediate environment:*

1) Report to local health authority: Obligatory case report in most states and in many countries, Class 2B (see Preface). Early reporting provides opportunity for better outbreak control.

2) Isolation: Impractical in the community at large; children should be kept out of school for at least 4 days after appearance of the rash. In hospitals, respiratory isolation from onset of catarrhal stage of the prodromal period through 4th day of rash reduces the exposure of other children at high risk.

3) Concurrent disinfection: None.

4) Quarantine: Usually impractical. Quarantine of institutions, wards or dormitories for young children is of value; strict segregation of infants if measles occurs in an institution.

5) Protection of contacts: Live vaccine, if given within 72 hours of exposure, may provide protection. IG may be used within 6 days for susceptible household or other contacts for whom risk of complications is very high (contacts under 1 year of age), or for whom measles vaccine is contraindicated. The dose is 0.25 ml/kg (0.11 ml/lb) with a maximum of 15 ml. Live measles vaccine should be given 3 months later to those for whom vaccine is not contraindicated.

6) Investigation of contacts: A search for and immunization of exposed susceptible contacts should be done to limit the spread of disease. Carriers are unknown.

7) Specific treatment: None.

C. *Epidemic measures:*

1) Prompt reporting of suspected cases and comprehensive immunization programs to cover all potential susceptibles and limit spread.

2) In institutional outbreaks, new admissions should receive vaccine or IG.

3) In many less developed population groups and countries measles has a high fatality rate. If vaccine is available, prompt use at the beginning of an epidemic is essential to limit spread; if vaccine supply is limited, priority should be given to young children for whom the risk is greatest.

D. *Disaster implications:* Introduction of measles into disaster populations with a high proportion of susceptibles can result in a devastating epidemic with high fatality.

E. *International measures:* None.

MELIOIDOSIS   ICD-9 025

1. **Identification**—An uncommon disease with a range of clinical manifestations from inapparent infection or asymptomatic pulmonary consolidation to a rapidly fatal septicemia. It may simulate typhoid fever or, more commonly, tuberculosis, including pulmonary cavitation, empyema, chronic abscesses, and osteomyelitis.

Diagnosis depends upon isolation of the causative agent; a rising antibody titer in serologic tests is confirmatory. The possibility of melioidosis should be kept in mind in any unexplained suppurative disease, especially cavitating pulmonary disease, in a patient living in, or returned from SE Asia and other endemic areas.

2. **Infectious agent**—*Pseudomonas pseudomallei,* Whitmore's bacillus.

3. **Occurrence**—Clinical disease is uncommon, generally occurring in individuals who have had intimate contact with soil and surface water. It may appear as a complication of an overt wound or may follow aspiration of water. Cases have been recorded in, but probably not restricted to, SE Asia, the Philippines, Turkey, Iran, northeast Australia, Papua New Guinea, Guam, Burkina Faso (Upper Volta), Ecuador, Panamá, Mexico and Aruba. In certain of these areas, 5–20% of agricultural workers have demonstrable antibodies but no history of overt disease.

4. **Reservoir**—The organism is saprophytic in certain soils and waters. Various animals, including sheep, goats, horses, swine, monkeys and rodents (and a variety of animals in zoological gardens) can become infected. There is no evidence that they are important reservoirs except in transfer of the agent to new foci.

5. **Mode of transmission**—Usually by contact with contaminated soil or water through overt or inapparent skin wounds, by aspiration or ingestion of contaminated water or by inhalation of dust from soil.

6. **Incubation period**—Can be as short as 2 days. However, several months or years may elapse between the presumed exposure and the appearance of clinical disease.

7. **Period of communicability**—Person-to-person transmission is extremely rare; it has been reported only following sexual contact with an individual with prostatic infection. Laboratory-acquired infections are uncommon but occur, especially if procedures produce aerosols.

8. **Susceptibility and resistance**—Disease in man is uncommon even among persons in endemic areas who have close contact with soil or water containing the infectious agent. Many patients develop clinical disease following severe injuries or burns, or have a history of a systemic disease such as diabetes. These conditions may precipitate disease or recrudescence of disease in asymptomatically infected individuals.

9. **Methods of control**—

   A. *Preventive measures:* Unknown.

   B. *Control of patient, contacts and the immediate environment:*

      1) Report to local health authority; Optional report, Class 3B (see Preface).
      2) Isolation: Respiratory and sinus drainage precautions.
      3) Concurrent disinfection: Safe disposal of sputum and wound discharges.
      4) Quarantine: None.
      5) Management of contacts: None.

6) Investigation of contacts and source of infection: Human carriers are not known.

7) Specific treatment: The most effective agent is TMP-SMX. In vitro tests show susceptibility to sulfonamides, chloramphenicol, tetracyclines, many of the third generation cephalosporins and novobiocin. A favorable outcome may be expected in most subacute and chronic cases. The best treatment for septicemic cases has not been established, although recovery has been recorded following administration of multiple drugs; in chronic cases with positive cultures pulmonary resection may be considered.

C. *Epidemic measures:* Not applicable to man; a sporadic disease.

D. *Disaster implications:* None.

E. *International measures:* None. Introduction should be considered when animals are moved to areas where the disease is unknown.

GLANDERS   ICD-9 024

Glanders is a highly communicable disease of horses, mules and donkeys; it has disappeared from most areas of the world, although enzootic foci are believed to exist in Asia and some Eastern Mediterranean countries. Clinical glanders is not known to occur in the Western Hemisphere. Human infection has occurred rarely and sporadically and almost exclusively in those whose occupations involve contact with animals or work in laboratories. Infection with the etiological organism, *Pseudomonas mallei (Malleomyces mallei),* the glanders bacillus, cannot be differentiated serologically from *P. pseudomallei;* specific diagnosis can be made only by characterization of the isolated organism. Prevention depends on control of glanders in the equine species and care in handling causative organisms.

MENINGITIS
I. VIRAL MENINGITIS   ICD-9 047.9
(Aseptic meningitis, Serous meningitis, Nonbacterial or Abacterial meningitis)

1. **Identification**—A common, rarely fatal, clinical syndrome with multiple etiologies, most commonly viral, characterized by sudden onset of febrile illness with signs and symptoms of meningeal involvement, spinal fluid findings of pleocytosis (usually mononuclear but may be poly-

morphonuclear in early stages), increased protein, normal sugar, and absence of bacteria. A rash resembling rubella characterizes certain types caused by echoviruses and coxsackieviruses. Vesicular and petechial rashes may also occur. Active illness seldom exceeds 10 days. Transient paresis and encephalitic manifestations may occur; paralysis is unusual. Residual signs lasting a year or more may include weakness, muscle spasm, insomnia and personality changes. Recovery is usually complete. Gastrointestinal and respiratory symptoms may be associated with infection with enteroviruses.

Differential diagnosis: Various diseases caused by nonviral agents may mimic aseptic meningitis, such as inadequately treated pyogenic meningitis, tuberculous or cryptococcal meningitis or meningitis caused by other fungi, cerebrovascular syphilis and lymphogranuloma venereum. Postinfectious and postvaccinal reactions require differentiation, including sequelae to measles, mumps and varicella, and post-rabies and post-smallpox vaccination; these syndromes are usually encephalitic in type. Leptospirosis, listeriosis, syphilis, lymphocytic choriomeningitis, viral hepatitis, infectious mononucleosis, influenza and other diseases may produce the same clinical syndrome and are discussed in individual chapters.

Under optimal conditions, specific identification can be made in about half of the cases using serologic and isolation techniques and is indicated in case of epidemics. Viral agents may be isolated in early stages from throat washings or stool, and occasionally from CSF or blood, by tissue culture techniques or animal inoculation.

2. Infectious agents—Caused by a wide variety of infectious agents, many of which are associated with other specific diseases. Many viruses are capable of producing the syndrome. Half or more of the cases have no demonstrable agent. In epidemic periods, mumps may be responsible for over 25% of cases of established etiology. In the USA, enteroviruses (picornaviruses) cause most cases of known etiology; coxsackievirus group B types 1–6 cause roughly one-third and echovirus types 2, 5, 6, 7, 9 (most), 10, 11, 14, 18 and 30, about 50%. Poliovirus, coxsackievirus (group A types 2, 3, 4, 7, 9 and 10), arboviruses, measles, herpes simplex and varicella viruses, lymphocytic choriomeningitis virus, adenovirus and others are responsible for sporadic cases. The incidence of specific types varies with geographic location and time. Leptospira may be responsible for up to 20% of cases of "aseptic" meningitis in various areas of the world. (See Leptospirosis).

3. Occurrence—Worldwide, usually as sporadic cases, occasionally in epidemics as infections with coxsackievirus, echovirus or other viruses. Actual incidence is unknown. Commonly observed when other forms of meningitis are not present in the community; seasonal increase in late summer and early autumn due mainly to arboviruses and enteroviruses, and in late winter-spring due to mumps.

4. **Reservoir, 5. Mode of transmission, 6. Incubation period, 7. Period of communicability, 8. Susceptibility and resistance**—Vary with the specific infectious agent. (Refer to specific diseases).

9. Methods of control—

A. *Preventive measures:* Depend upon etiology. (See specific disease).

B. *Control of patient, contacts and the immediate environment:*

1) Report to local health authority: In selected endemic areas (USA); in many countries not a reportable disease, Class 3B (see Preface). If confirmed by laboratory means, specify the infectious agent; otherwise report as cause undetermined.

2) Isolation: Specific diagnosis depends upon laboratory data not usually available until after recovery. Therefore, enteric precautions are indicated for 7 days after onset of illness unless a nonenteroviral diagnosis is established.

3) Concurrent disinfection: Includes eating and drinking utensils and articles soiled by secretions and excretions of patients.

4) Quarantine: None.

5) Immunization of contacts: See specific diseases.

6) Investigation of contacts: Not usually indicated.

7) Specific treatment: None for the usual causative viral agents.

C. *Epidemic measures:* See specific diseases.

D. *Disaster implications:* None.

E. *International measures:* WHO Collaborating Centres (see Preface).

II. BACTERIAL MENINGITIS ICD-9 320

Neisseria meningitidis, Haemophilus influenzae, and *Streptococcus pneumoniae* account for the overwhelming majority of all reported cases of bacterial meningitis in the USA. Nearly 70% of all reported cases of bacterial meningitis occurred in children less than 5 years of age.

Other purulent meningitides are often secondary to systemic disease or parameningeal involvement originating from the nose, accessory nasal sinuses, middle ear or mastoid. The lungs, endocardium, joints, skin or other sites may be involved. Clinical signs and symptoms, including the rash, may be indistinguishable from those caused by meningococci. Differentiation is based on smears and bacteriologic studies. The more common infectious agents, which vary in frequency with age, are *H. influenzae* type b and rarely other types, *N. meningitidis, S. pneumoniae,* hemolytic and other streptococci (especially Group B), *Listeria monocytogenes, Escherichia coli;* less commonly, but increasing in frequency in recent years, members of the *Klebsiella-Enterobacter-Serratia* group, *Staphylococcus aureus, Salmonella, Pseudomonas aeruginosa,* and others. Several mycoses cause subacute and chronic meningitides. Aseptic meningitis, as well as meningismus due to other conditions, must be considered.

III. MENINGOCOCCAL MENINGITIS   ICD-9 036.0
(Meningococcal infection, Cerebrospinal fever, Meningococcemia)

1. **Identification**—An acute bacterial disease characterized by sudden onset with fever, intense headache, nausea and often vomiting, stiff neck, and frequently a petechial rash with pink macules or, very rarely, vesicles. Delirium and coma often appear; occasional fulminating cases exhibit sudden prostration, ecchymoses and shock at onset. Formerly case fatality rates exceeded 50% but with early diagnosis, modern therapy and supportive measures, the case fatality rate should be <10%.

Meningococcal infection may be restricted to the nasopharynx, asymptomatic or with only local symptoms; invasive with acutely ill septicemic patients, two-thirds of whom show a petechial rash, sometimes with joint involvement; or meningeal. In invasive disease, meningococcemia may occur without extension to the meninges and should be suspected in cases of otherwise unexplained acute febrile illness associated with petechial rash and leukocytosis. In fulminating meningococcemia the death rate remains high despite even prompt antibacterial treatment. Septic monarthritis occurs. In meningeal disease, the organisms have penetrated into the meninges to produce the classic disease.

Diagnosis is confirmed by the demonstration of typical organisms in a gram-stained smear of CSF and the recovery of meningococci from the CSF or blood. Microscopic examination of stained smears from petechiae may reveal organisms. Group-specific meningococcal polysaccharides may also be identified in CSF by latex agglutination, CIE, and coagglutination techniques.

2. **Infectious agent**—*Neisseria meningitidis,* the meningococcus. Group A organisms have caused the major epidemics in the USA and elsewhere; presently, Groups B and C are responsible for most cases. Additional serogroups have been recognized as pathogens in recent years, e.g., Groups W-135, X, Y and Z. Organisms belonging to some of these

serogroups may be less virulent, but fatal infections and secondary cases have occurred with all.

3. Occurrence—Meningococcal infections are common in both temperate and tropical climates, with sporadic cases throughout the year in both urban and rural areas; greatest incidence occurs during winter and spring. Epidemic waves occur at unexplained irregular intervals. Meningococcal disease, while primarily a disease of very small children, occurs commonly in children and young adults, in males more than in females, and more commonly in newly aggregated adults under crowded living conditions, such as in barracks and institutions. Large epidemics have occurred in hot dry regions; a broad area of high incidence has existed for many years in the sub-Saharan region of mid-Africa caused by Group A organisms, now being accompanied by Group C. Both groups A and C were associated with epidemic meningococcal disease in Brazil from 1974 to 1978. More recently, there was a major Group A epidemic in Finland.

4. Reservoir—Man.

5. Mode of transmission—By direct contact, including droplets and discharges from nose and throat of infected persons, more often from carriers than cases; usually causes only an acute nasopharyngitis or a subclinical mucosal infection; invasion sufficient to cause systemic disease is comparatively rare. Carrier prevalence of $\geqq 25\%$ may exist without cases of meningitis. During epidemics, over half the men in a military unit may be healthy carriers of pathogenic meningococci. Indirect contact is of questionable significance because the meningococcus is relatively susceptible to temperature changes and desiccation.

6. Incubation period—Varies from 2–10 days, commonly 3–4 days.

7. Period of communicability—Until meningococci are no longer present in discharges from nose and mouth. If the organisms are sensitive to sulfonamides, meningococci usually disappear from the nasopharynx within 24 hours after institution of treatment. Penicillin will temporarily suppress the organisms but they are usually not eradicated from the oro-nasopharynx by this drug.

8. Susceptibility and resistance—Susceptibility to the clinical disease is low and decreases with age; a high ratio of carriers to cases prevails. Those who are deficient in certain complement components are especially prone to recurrent disease. Group-specific immunity of unknown duration follows even subclinical infections.

9. Methods of control—

    A. Preventive measures:

        1)   Educate on personal hygiene and the necessity of reducing

direct contact or droplet infection and of maintaining good general health.

2) Prevent overcrowding in living quarters, public transportation, working places and especially in barracks, camps, ships and schools.

3) Vaccines containing Groups A, C, Y and W-135 meningococcal polysaccharides have been licensed in the USA and many other countries for use in adults and older children, and are available as monovalent or combined vaccines. Serogroup C vaccine is effective in adults and has been given to US military recruits since 1971; unfortunately, it is poorly immunogenic in children under 2 yrs old; when indicated, individuals older than 2 yrs are given 1 dose of either monovalent C or quadrivalent vaccine (which is currently given to US and Canadian military recruits). Serogroup A vaccine is effective in younger children; however, for those 3 months to 2 yrs old, 2 doses are given 3 months apart instead of the single dose given those over 2 yrs of age. Routine immunization of civilians is not recommended. The risk to travelers planning to have prolonged contact with the local populace in countries experiencing epidemic meningococcal A or C diseases will be reduced by immunization. No vaccine effective against Group B meningococci is currently available.

B. *Control of patient, contacts and immediate environment:*

1) Report to local health authority: Obligatory case report in most states and countries, Class 2A (see Preface).

2) Isolation: Respiratory isolation for 24 hours after start of chemotherapy.

3) Concurrent disinfection: Of discharges from the nose and throat and articles soiled therewith. Terminal cleaning.

4) Quarantine: None.

5) Protection of contacts: Close surveillance of household and other intimate contacts for early signs of illness, especially fever, to initiate appropriate therapy without delay. Consideration may be given to prophylactic administration of an effective agent to intimate contacts, such as persons sharing the same lodging. If the organisms in the outbreak have been shown to be sensitive to sulfadiazine, it may be given to adults and older children at a dosage of 1.0 g every 12 hours for 4 doses; for infants and children, the dosage is 125–150 mg/kg/d divided into 4 equal doses, on each of 2 consecutive days. If the organisms are

sulfonamide-resistant, rifampin can be used, giving adults 600 mg twice a day for 2 days, children over 1 month old 10 mg/kg doses and for those less than 1 month old 5 mg/kg. Health care personnel are rarely at risk even when caring for infected patients. Only if intimate exposure to nasopharyngeal secretions occurs (e.g., mouth-to-mouth resuscitation) would prompt prophylaxis be warranted. Vaccination of close household contacts is of no practical value.

6) Investigation of contacts: Routine throat or nasopharyngeal culture of contacts is usually impractical and not sufficiently sensitive or timely to alter decisions about prophylaxis.

7) Specific treatment: Penicillin given parenterally in adequate doses is the drug of choice for proven meningococcal disease; ampicillin and chloramphenicol are also effective. Treatment should begin immediately when the presumptive clinical diagnosis is made even before meningococci have been identified; in children, until the specific etiologic agent has been identified, therapy must be effective against *H. influenzae* as well as *S. pneumoniae*. While ampicillin is the drug of choice so long as the organisms are ampicillin-sensitive, it should be combined with chloramphenicol in the many places where ampicillin-resistant *H. influenzae* strains are known to occur. If the outbreak is caused by strains shown to be sulfonamide-sensitive, sulfadiazine may be given i.v.; however, sulfonamide-resistant strains of Groups B and C, and recently Group A, are commonplace in many parts of the world.

C. *Epidemic measures:*

1) When an outbreak occurs, major emphasis must be placed on careful surveillance, early diagnosis, and immediate treatment of suspected cases. A high index of suspicion is invaluable.

2) Separate individuals and ventilate living and sleeping quarters of all persons who are exposed to infection because of crowding, i.e., soldiers, miners or prisoners, or in congested living conditions.

3) When the epidemic strain is sulfonamide-sensitive, mass chemoprophylaxis of a closed community with sulfadiazine (0.5 g for children, 1.0 g for adults, every 12 hours, for 4 doses) reduces carrier rate and limits spread of the infection. Because of the current widespread prevalence of sulfonamide-resistant meningococcal strains throughout

the world, sulfonamide prophylaxis should not be instituted unless <5% of the strains obtained from cases or from a statistically valid sample of the carrier population show sulfonamide resistance (resistant strains are those resistant to more than 10 µg % of sulfadiazine). Rifampin (see 9B5, above) reduces the carrier rate and limits spread of infection when the entire community is treated; however, its use has been associated with the appearance of resistant strains so this drug is not recommended for mass prophylaxis. It may be advisable to administer prophylaxis to all intimate contacts (see 9B5, above).

4) The use of vaccine should be considered for the groups in which the cases due to Group A, C, W-135 or Y are occurring. (See 9A3, above).

D. *Disaster implications:* Epidemics may develop in situations of forced crowding.

E. *International measures:* WHO Collaborating Centres (see Preface).

IV. HAEMOPHILUS MENINGITIS   ICD-9 320.0
(Meningitis due to *Haemophilus influenzae*)

1. Identification—This is the most common bacterial meningitis in children 2 months to 5 years old in the USA. Otitis media or sinusitis may be a precursor. It is almost always associated with a bacteremia. The onset is usually sudden and symptoms are those of fever, vomiting, lethargy and meningeal irritation consisting of bulging fontanelle in infants or stiff neck and back in slightly older children. Progressive stupor or coma is common. Occasionally a patient will have low-grade fever for several days with more subtle CNS symptoms.

Diagnosis may be made by isolation of organisms from blood or CSF. Specific capsular polysaccharide may be identified by CIE or latex agglutination techniques.

2. Infectious agent—Most commonly *H. influenzae* type b. Other serogroups rarely cause meningitis.

3. Occurrence—Worldwide; most prevalent in the 2–month to 3–year age group, unusual over the age of 5 years. Secondary cases may occur in families and day-care centers.

4. Reservoir—Man.

5. Mode of transmission—By droplet infection and discharges from nose and throat during the infectious period. There may be a purulent rhinitis. The portal of entry is most commonly nasopharyngeal.

6. **Incubation period**—Probably short, 2–4 days.

7. **Period of communicability**—As long as organisms are present, which may be for a prolonged period even without nasal discharge. Noncommunicable within 24–48 hours after starting effective antibiotic therapy.

8. **Susceptibility and resistance**—Assumed to be universal. Immunity is associated with presence of circulating bactericidal or anticapsular antibody, either acquired transplacentally or from prior infection.

9. **Methods of control**—

    A. *Preventive Measures:*

        1) Monitor for cases occurring in susceptible population groups such as those in day-care centers and large foster homes.

        2) Educate parents regarding the risk of secondary cases in siblings under 4 years old and the need for prompt evaluation and treatment if any fever or other symptoms develop.

        3) An investigational capsular polysaccharide vaccine composed of repeating ribosyl-ribitol-phosphate (PRP) units has been shown to prevent meningitis in children ≧18 months of age. Protein-polysaccharide conjugate vaccines are being tested in younger children. (This vaccine was licensed in the USA in April 1985.)

    B. *Control of patient, contacts and immediate environment:*

        1) Report to local health authority: In selected endemic areas (USA), Class 3B (see Preface).

        2) Isolation: Respiratory isolation for 24 hours after start of chemotherapy.

        3) Concurrent disinfection: None.

        4) Quarantine: None.

        5) Protection of contacts: Rifampin prophylaxis (orally once daily for 4 days in a 20 mg/kg dose, maximal dose 600 mg/d) for all household contacts (including adults) in households where there are children (other than the index case) less than 4 years old. Rifampin prophylaxis of staff and children in day-care center classrooms may be considered when a case has occurred among the children.

        6) Investigation of contacts: Observe contacts under 6 years old, and especially infants, including those in household, day-care centers and nurseries, for signs of illness, especially fever.

        7) Specific treatment: Ampicillin has been the drug of choice

(parenteral 200–400 mg/kg/d). However, since 10–35% of strains are now resistant due to β-lactamase production, chloramphenicol is recommended concurrently or singly until antibiotic sensitivities are known. If there are household contacts under 4 years old, the patient should be given rifampin prior to discharge from the hospital to assure elimination of the organism.

C. *Epidemic measures:* Not applicable.

D. *Disaster implications:* None.

E. *International measures:* None.

PNEUMOCOCCAL MENINGITIS   ICD-9 320.1

This form of meningitis has a high case fatality rate. It is usually fulminant and occurs with bacteremia but not necessarily with another focus, although there may be otitis media or mastoiditis. The onset is usually sudden with high fever, lethargy or coma, and signs of meningeal irritation. A sporadic disease in young infants and elderly and in certain high-risk groups, including asplenic or hypogammaglobulinemic patients. Basilar fracture with persistent communication with nasopharynx is a predisposing factor. See Pneumonia, Pneumococcal.

NEONATAL MENINGITIS   ICD-9 320.8

Infants with neonatal meningitis develop lethargy, seizures, apneic episodes, poor feeding, hypo- or hyperthermia, and sometimes respiratory distress in their first week of life. The WBC count may be elevated or depressed. Culture of the CSF yields either Group B streptococci, *Listeria monocytogenes* (see Listeriosis) or *E. coli* K-1, acquired from the birth canal. Infants 2 weeks to 2 months of age may develop similar symptoms with recovery from the CSF of Group B streptococci or organisms of the *Klebsiella-Enterobacter-Serratia* group, acquired from the nursery environment. The meningitis in both groups is associated with septicemia. Treatment is with ampicillin plus an aminoglycoside until the etiologic organism has been identified and its antibiotic susceptibilities determined.

MENINGOENCEPHALITIS DUE TO *NAEGLERIA* AND *ACANTHAMOEBA*

ICD-9 136.2

(Naegleriasis, Primary amebic meningoencephalitis, Acanthamoebiasis)

1. **Identification**—A disease of the brain and meninges caused by free-living amebae that ordinarily are found in water, soil and decaying vegetation.

Two genera, *Naegleria* and *Acanthamoeba,* have been known to cause meningoencephalitis. *Naegleria* organisms invade the brain and meninges via the nasal mucosa and olfactory tissues, causing a typical syndrome of fulminating pyogenic meningoencephalitis with severe frontal headache, occasional olfactory hallucinations, nausea, vomiting, high fever, nuchal rigidity and somnolence, with death within 10 days, usually on the 5th or 6th day. The disease occurs mainly in active young people of both sexes. *Acanthamoeba* can invade the brain and meninges, probably secondary to entry through a skin lesion, without involvement of the nasal and olfactory tissues, causing a disease characterized by insidious onset and prolonged course.

Diagnosis of the *Naegleria*-type syndrome is made by microscopic examination of wet mount preparations of fresh CSF in which motile amebae may be seen, or by culture on non-nutrient agar seeded with *Escherichia coli, Klebsiella aerogenes* or other suitable *Enterobacter* spp. Amebae have been misidentified as macrophages or "gitter cells" and have been mistaken for *Entamoeba histolytica* when microscopic diagnosis is made under low magnification. The trophozoites of *Naegleria* may become flagellated after a few hours in water. The pathogenic *Naegleria (N. fowleri)* and *Acanthamoeba* spp. can be differentiated from each other morphologically and by immunological tests on CSF and brain tissue.

2. **Infectious agents**—*Naegleria fowleri* and *Acanthamoeba culbertsoni,* and other species of *Acanthamoeba (A. polyphaga, A. castellanii, A. astronyxis).*

3. **Occurrence**—Over 100 cases of meningoencephalitis caused by *Naegleria* have been reported from the USA (predominantly Virginia, Florida, California, Georgia, Texas), Europe (Belgium, Czechoslovakia, England, Ireland), Australia, New Zealand, Papua New Guinea, India, west Africa, Venezuela and Panamá. Cases in which *Acanthamoeba* invaded the CNS have been reported from Africa, India, Korea, Japan, Peru, Venezuela and the USA (Arizona, California, Louisiana, New York, Pennsylvania, S Carolina, Texas, Utah and Virginia).

4. **Reservoir**—The organisms are free-living in aquatic and soil habitats.

5. **Mode of transmission**—*Naegleria* infection is acquired by exposure

of the nasal passages to contaminated water, most commonly by diving or swimming in fresh water, especially somewhat stagnant ponds or lakes in areas of warm climate or during late summer, or in thermal springs or in bodies of water warmed by the effluent of industrial plants, or in hot tubs or spas. The *Naegleria* trophozoites colonize the nasal tissues, then invade the brain and meninges by extension along the olfactory nerves. *Acanthamoeba* trophozoites reach the CNS by hematogenous spread, probably from a skin lesion or other site of primary colonization, frequently in chronically ill or immunosuppressed patients, with no history of swimming or known source of infection.

6. Incubation period—From 3 to 7 days in documented cases of *Naegleria* infection; usually much longer in *Acanthamoeba* infection.

7. Period of communicability—No person-to-person transmission has been observed.

8. Susceptibility and resistance—Unknown. Apparently normal individuals develop *Naegleria* infection; immunosuppressed individuals are susceptible to infection with *Acanthamoeba*. *Naegleria* have not been found in asymptomatic individuals; *Acanthamoeba* have been found in the respiratory tract of healthy people.

9. Methods of control—

    A.   *Preventive measures:*

        1)   Protect the nasopharynx from exposure to water likely to contain *N. fowleri*. In practice this is difficult to accomplish since the amebae may occur in a wide variety of aquatic bodies, including swimming pools.

        2)   Educate the public to the dangers of swimming in lakes and ponds where infection is known or presumed to have been acquired and of allowing such water to be forced into the nose by diving or underwater swimming.

        3)   Swimming pools containing residual free chlorine of 1–2 parts per million are considered safe. No infection is known to have been acquired in a standard swimming pool in the USA.

    B.   *Control of patient, contacts and the immediate environment:*

        1)   Report to local health authority: Not reportable in most countries, Class 3B (see Preface).

        2)   Isolation: None.

        3)   Concurrent disinfection: None.

        4)   Quarantine: None.

        5)   Immunization of contacts: Not applicable.

        6)   Investigation of contacts and source of infection: History

of swimming or introducing water into the nose within the week prior to onset of symptoms may suggest the source of *Naegleria* infection.

7) Specific treatment: *N. fowleri* is sensitive to amphotericin B (Fungizone®); recovery has followed i.v. and intrathecal administration of amphotericin B and miconazole in conjunction with oral rifampin. Despite sensitivity of the organisms to antibiotics in laboratory studies, recoveries have been very rare.

C. *Epidemic measures:* Multiple cases may occur following exposure to an apparent source of infection. Any grouping of cases warrants prompt epidemiological investigation and the prohibition of swimming in implicated waters.

D. *Disaster implications:* None.

E. *International measures:* None.

ACANTHAMEBIASIS OF EYE AND SKIN

Species of *Acanthamoeba (A. polyphaga, A. castellanii)* have been associated with lesions of the conjunctiva, cornea and inner structures of the eye in the USA (Texas, New York, California, Ohio, Washington, Pennsylvania), England and the Netherlands. Chronic granulomatous lesions of the skin have been recorded in the USA (Arizona), Africa (Zambia) and Korea, with or without secondary invasion of the CNS. An infected mandibular bone graft has been recorded. The amebae in eye and skin lesions usually have been demonstrated in stained smears of scrapings, swabs, or aspirates; species identification has been based on immunodiagnostic tests on amebae in cultures, smears or tissue sections. No reliable treatment has been reported, but diamidines, pimaricin, rifampin and possibly neomycin have been suggested to be of possible benefit.

MOLLUSCUM CONTAGIOSUM   ICD-9 078.0

1. Identification—A viral disease of the skin which results in a smooth-surfaced, firm and spherical papule with umbilication of the vertex. The lesions may be flesh-colored, white, translucent or yellow. Most molluscum papules are 2–5 mm in diameter, but, giant cell molluscum, >15 mm in diameter, are occasionally seen. Lesions in adults are most often on the lower abdominal wall, pubis, genitalia and inner thighs; in

children lesions are most often on the face, trunk and proximal extremities. Occasionally the lesions itch and a linear orientation is seen, suggesting autoinoculation by scratching. Also, in some patients, 50–100 lesions may become confluent and form a single plaque.

Without treatment, molluscum contagiosum persists for 6 months to 2 years. Any one lesion has a life span of 2–3 months. Lesions may resolve spontaneously or as a result of the inflammatory response following trauma or secondary bacterial infection. Treatment, i.e., mechanically removing the molluscum lesions, may shorten the course of the illness.

Diagnosis can be made clinically, when multiple lesions are present. For confirmation, the core can be expressed onto a glass slide and examined by ordinary light microscopy for classic basophilic Feulgen-positive intracytoplasmic inclusions, the "molluscum bodies" or "Henderson-Paterson bodies." Electron microscopy can confirm the diagnosis.

2. Infectious agent—An unassigned poxvirus or one of Nakano's group 2 poxviruses.

3. Occurrence—Worldwide. Serological tests are not well standardized. Inspection of the skin is the only screening technique available. Therefore, epidemiologic studies of the disease have been limited. Population surveys have been conducted only in Papua New Guinea and in Fiji where the peak incidence of the disease is in children.

4. Reservoir—Man.

5. Mode of transmission—Usually by direct contact. Transmission is both sexual and nonsexual, the latter including spread via fomites. Also, autoinoculation is suspected.

6. Incubation period—For experimental inoculation, 19–50 days; clinical reports, 7 days to 6 months.

7. Period of communicability—Unknown, but probably as long as lesions persist.

8. Susceptibility and resistance—Any age may be affected, more often seen in children.

9. Methods of control—

A. Preventive measures: Avoid contact with affected patients.

B. Control of patient, contacts and the immediate environment:

1) Report to local health authority: Official report not ordinarily justifiable, Class 5 (see Preface).
2) Isolation: Generally not indicated. Infected children should be excluded from close contact sports such as wrestling.

3) Concurrent disinfection: None.
4) Quarantine: None.
5) Immunization of contacts: None.
6) Investigation of contacts and source of infection: Examination of sexual partners where applicable.
7) Specific treatment: Rarely indicated. Curettage with local anesthesia. Freezing with liquid nitrogen has some advocates.

C. *Epidemic measures:* Suspend close contact activities.

D. *Disaster implications:* None.

E. *International measures:* None.

MONONUCLEOSIS, INFECTIOUS ICD-9 075
(*Gammaherpesviral mononucleosis, EBV mononucleosis, Glandular fever)

1. **Identification**—An acute viral syndrome characterized clinically by fever, sore throat (often with exudative pharyngotonsillitis), and lymphadenopathy (especially posterior cervical); hematologically by mononucleosis and lymphocytosis of 50% or more, including 10% or more atypical cells; and serologically by the presence of heterophile and EBV antibodies. In children the disease is generally mild and more difficult to recognize. Jaundice occurs in about 4% of infected young adults and splenomegaly in 50 percent. Duration is from one to several weeks; very rarely fatal. A chronic form of the disease is suggested but not proven.

The causal agent, Epstein-Barr virus (EBV), is also closely associated with the pathogenesis of African Burkitt's lymphoma and nasopharyngeal cancer. (See Neoplasia, Malignant). Acute fatal immunoblastic sarcoma occurs with or without initial features of infectious mononucleosis in persons with an X-linked immunoproliferative disorder or an acquired defect in the immune system including AIDS. It involves a polyclonal expansion of EBV-infected B-lymphocytes.

A syndrome resembling infectious mononucleosis clinically and hematologically may be due to cytomegalovirus (another member of the herpesvirus group, see Cytomegalovirus Infections), acquired toxoplasmosis (q.v.), or certain other viral infections; differentiation depends on laboratory results; only EBV elicits the heterophile antibody. EBV accounts for over 90% of both heterophile-positive and heterophile-negative cases of the "mono" syndrome.

Laboratory diagnosis is based on finding a lymphocytosis exceeding 50%

(including 10% or more abnormal forms), abnormalities in liver function tests (SGOT) and an elevated heterophile antibody titer after absorption of the serum with guinea pig kidney. The absorbed horse-RBC test is the most sensitive, the beef-cell hemolysin test the most specific of the common tests. An immune adherence hemagglutination assay is also a highly sensitive and specific test. Young children may not show an elevation of the heterophile titer. If available, the IFA test for viral capsid IgM and IgA antibody or early antigen antibody against the causal virus is very helpful in diagnosis of heterophile-negative cases; anti-EB nuclear antibody (EBNA) is usually absent during the acute phase of illness.

2. **Infectious agent**—Epstein-Barr (EB) virus, human (gamma) herpesvirus 4, closely related to other herpes viruses morphologically, but distinct serologically; it infects and transforms B-lymphocytes.

3. **Occurrence**—Worldwide. Infection is common and widespread in early childhood in developing countries and in socioeconomically depressed population groups, where it is usually mild or asymptomatic. Typical clinical infectious mononucleosis occurs primarily in developed countries where the age of infection is delayed to older childhood and young adult age, so that it is most commonly recognized in high school and college students.

4. **Reservoir**—Man.

5. **Mode of transmission**—Person-to-person spread by oropharyngeal route via saliva. Young children may be infected by saliva on the hands of nurses or on toys; kissing facilitates spread among young adults. Spread may also occur via blood transfusion to susceptible recipients, but ensuing clinical disease is uncommon.

6. **Incubation period**—From 4 to 6 weeks.

7. **Period of communicability**—Prolonged; pharyngeal excretion may persist for a year after infection; 15–20% or more of EBV antibody-positive healthy adults are oropharyngeal carriers.

8. **Susceptibility and resistance**—Susceptibility is general. Infection confers a high degree of resistance; immunity from unrecognized childhood infection may account for low rates of clinical disease in lower socioeconomic groups.

9. **Methods of control**—

   A. *Preventive measures:* None known.

   B. *Control of patient, contacts and the immediate environment:*

      1) Report to local health authority: No individual case report, Class 4 (see Preface).

2) Isolation: None.
3) Concurrent disinfection: Of articles soiled with nose and throat discharges.
4) Quarantine: None.
5) Immunization of contacts: None.
6) Investigation of contacts: For the individual case, of little value.
7) Specific treatment: None. Steroids may be of some value in severe toxic cases.

C. *Epidemic measures:* None.

D. *Disaster implications:* None.

E. *International measures:* None.

MUMPS
(Infectious parotitis)

ICD-9 072

1. **Identification**—An acute viral disease characterized by fever, swelling and tenderness of one or more salivary glands, usually the parotid and sometimes the sublingual or submaxillary glands. Orchitis, usually unilateral, occurs in 15–25% of males and oophoritis in about 5% of females past puberty; sterility is an extremely rare sequel. The CNS is frequently involved, either early or late in the disease, usually as an aseptic meningitis. Permanent deafness is a rare complication. Orchitis and meningoencephalitis may occur without involvement of a salivary gland. Deafness (usually unilateral), pancreatitis, neuritis, arthritis, mastitis, nephritis, thyroiditis and pericarditis may occur. Death is a rare outcome. Mumps infection during the 1st trimester of pregnancy may increase the rate of spontaneous abortions, but there is no firm evidence that mumps during pregnancy causes congenital malformations.

Serological tests (CF, HI and neutralization) are of value in confirming diagnosis. Skin tests are unreliable. Virus may be isolated in chick embryo or cell cultures from saliva, blood, urine and CSF during the acute phase of the disease.

2. **Infectious agent**—Mumps virus, a member of the genus *Paramyxovirus,* antigenically related to the parainfluenza viruses.

3. **Occurrence**—Mumps occurs less regularly than other common communicable diseases of childhood, such as measles and chickenpox. About one-third of exposed susceptible persons have inapparent infections. Winter and spring are seasons of greatest prevalence. In the USA, incidence of mumps has declined dramatically since the wide use of mumps

vaccine began after its licensure in 1967. This decline has occurred in all age groups, but with effective pediatric and preschool immunization programs, the greatest risk of infection has shifted toward older children.

4. Reservoir—Man.

5. Mode of transmission—By droplet spread and by direct contact with saliva of an infected person.

6. Incubation period—About 2–3 wks, commonly 18 days.

7. Period of communicability—The virus has been isolated from saliva from 6 days before overt parotitis up to 9 days after; maximal infectiousness occurs about 48 hours before onset of illness. Urine may be positive for as long as 14 days after onset of illness. Inapparent infections can be communicable.

8. Susceptibility and resistance—Susceptibility is general. Immunity is generally lifelong and develops after inapparent as well as clinical attacks. Most adults are likely to have been infected naturally and may be considered to be immune, even if they did not have recognized disease.

9. Methods of control-

    A. *Preventive measures:* Live attenuated vaccine prepared in chick embryo cell culture is available either as a single vaccine or in combination with rubella and measles live virus vaccines. Fever may occur in 5% of recipients; other reactions have been reported rarely. More than 95% of recipients develop a solid immunity which is long lasting and may be lifelong. Vaccine may be administered any time after 1 yr of age; if given in combination with measles vaccine, it should ordinarily be given at or after 15 months of age. Special effort should be made to immunize all persons (especially males) with no definite history of mumps or vaccination before puberty. Vaccine is contraindicated in the immunocompromised; women known to be pregnant should not be given live vaccines. See Measles or Rubella for vaccine storage and transport, and for greater detail on contraindications.

    B. *Control of patient, contacts and the immediate environment:*

        1) Report to local health authority: Selectively reportable, Class 3C (see Preface).

        2) Isolation: Respiratory isolation and private room for 9 days from onset of swelling; less if swelling has subsided.

        3) Concurrent disinfection: Of articles soiled with nose and throat secretions.

        4) Quarantine: None.

5) Immunization of contacts: While immunization after exposure to natural mumps does not protect contacts, it is not contraindicated under such conditions. IG is not effective when administered following exposure.

6) Investigation of contacts: Susceptible contacts should be immunized.

7) Specific treatment: None.

C. Epidemic measures: Immunize susceptibles, especially those at risk of exposure; serological screening to identify susceptibles is unnecessary since there is no risk in vaccinating those who are already immune.

D. Disaster implications: None.

E. International measures: None.

MYALGIA, EPIDEMIC*   ICD-9 074.1
(Epidemic pleurodynia, Bornholm disease, Devil's grip)

1. Identification—An acute viral disease characterized by sudden onset of severe pain localized in the chest or abdomen which may be intensified by movement, usually accompanied by fever and frequently by headache. The pain tends to be more abdominal than thoracic in infants and young children, while the reverse applies in older children and adults. Most patients recover within one week of onset; frequently relapses may occur; no fatalities have been reported. Localized epidemics are characteristic. It is important to differentiate from more serious medical or surgical conditions. Complications occur relatively infrequently and include orchitis, pericarditis, pneumonia and aseptic meningitis. During outbreaks of epidemic myalgia, cases of group B coxsackievirus myocarditis of the newborn have been reported; while myocarditis in adults is a rare complication, the possibility should always be considered.

Diagnosis is supported by culture of the virus from throat washings and from feces, and by rise in titer of type-specific neutralizing antibodies in paired sera obtained early and late in illness, available in very few diagnostic laboratories at present.

2. Infectious agents—Group B coxsackievirus types 1–3, 5, 6 and echoviruses 1 and 6 are associated with the illness. Many group A and B coxsackieviruses and echoviruses have been associated with sporadic disease.

3. Occurrence—An uncommon disease occurring in summer and early autumn; usually seen in children and young adults ages 5–15, but all ages may be affected. Multiple cases in a household are frequent. Outbreaks have been reported in Europe, Australia, New Zealand and N America.

4. Reservoir—Man.

5. Mode of transmission—Directly by fecal-oral or respiratory droplet contact with an infected person or indirectly by contact with articles freshly soiled with feces or throat discharges of an infected person who may or may not have symptoms. Group B coxsackieviruses have been found in sewage and in flies, though the relationship to transmission of human infection is not clear.

6. Incubation period—Usually 3–5 days.

7. Period of communicability—Apparently during the acute stage of disease; stools may contain virus for several weeks.

8. Susceptibility and resistance—Susceptibility is probably general and presumably a type-specific immunity results from infection.

9. Methods of control—

   A. *Preventive measures:* None.

   B. *Control of patient, contacts and the immediate environment:*

   1) Report to local health authority: Obligatory report of epidemics, Class 4 (see Preface).
   2) Isolation: Ordinarily limited to enteric precautions. Because of the possibility of serious illness in the newborn, if a patient in a maternity unit or nursery develops an illness suggestive of group B coxsackievirus infection, precautions should be instituted at once. Similarly, individuals, including medical personnel, with suspected group B coxsackievirus infections should be excluded from visiting maternity and nursery units, women near term and infants.
   3) Concurrent disinfection: Prompt and safe disposal of respiratory discharges and of feces; wash or dispose of articles soiled therewith. Careful attention should be given to prompt handwashing when handling discharges, feces and articles soiled therewith.
   4) Quarantine: None.
   5) Immunization of contacts: None.
   6) Investigation of contacts: Of no practical value.
   7) Specific treatment: None.

   C. *Epidemic measures:* General notice to physicians of the presence of an epidemic and the necessity for differentiation from more serious medical or surgical emergencies.

D. *Disaster implications:* None.

E. *International measures:* None.

MYCETOMA
ACTINOMYCETOMA*

ICD-9 039

EUMYCETOMA
(Maduromycosis, Madura foot)

ICD-9 117.4

1. **Identification**—A clinical syndrome caused by a variety of aerobic actinomycetes and fungi, characterized by swelling and suppuration of subcutaneous tissues, and formation of sinus tracts with visible granules in the pus draining from the sinus tracts. Lesions usually are on the foot or lower leg, sometimes on the hand, shoulders and back, and rarely at other sites.

Mycetoma may be difficult to distinguish from chronic osteomyelitis and botryomycosis, the latter being a clinically and pathologically similar entity caused by a variety of bacteria including staphylococci and gram-negative bacteria.

Specific diagnosis depends on visualizing the granules in fresh preparations or histopathologic slices and isolation of the causative actinomycete or fungus in culture.

2. **Infectious agents**—Eumycetoma is caused principally by *Madurella mycetomatis, M. grisea, Pseudallescheria (Petriellidium) boydii, Scedosporium (Monosporium) apiospermum, Exophiala (Phialophora) jeanselmei, Acremonium (Cephalosporium) recifei, A. falciforme, Leptosphaeria senegalensis, Neotestudina rosatii,* and *Pyrenochaeta romeroi,* or several other species. Actinomycetoma is caused by *Nocardia brasiliensis, N. asteroides, N. caviae, Actinomadura madurae, A. pelletieri* or *Streptomyces somaliensis.*

3. **Occurrence**—Rare in continental USA; common in Mexico, northern Africa, southern Asia and other tropical and subtropical areas, especially where people go barefoot.

4. **Reservoir**—Soil and decaying vegetation.

5. **Mode of transmission**—Subcutaneous implantation of conidia or hyphal elements from a saprophytic source by penetrating wounds (thorns, splinters).

6. **Incubation period**—Usually months.

7. **Period of communicability**—Not transmitted from person to person.

8. **Susceptibility and resistance**—While etiologic agents are wide-spread in nature, clinical infection is rare, suggesting intrinsic resistance.

9. **Methods of control**—

A. *Preventive measures:* Protect against puncture wounds by wearing shoes or protective clothing.

B. *Control of patient, contacts and the immediate environment:*

1) Report to local health authority: Official report not ordinarily justifiable, Class 5 (see Preface).
2) Isolation: None.
3) Concurrent disinfection: None. Ordinary cleanliness.
4) Quarantine: None.
5) Immunization of contacts: None.
6) Investigation of contacts and source of infection: Not indicated.
7) Specific treatment: Some patients with eumycetoma may benefit from ketoconazole; some cases of actinomycetoma from sulfones, TMP-SMX or long-acting sulfonamides. Penicillin and other antibiotics are not useful. Resection of small lesions may be helpful, while amputation of an extremity with advanced lesions may be required.

C. *Epidemic measures:* Not applicable, a sporadic disease.

D. *Disaster implications:* None.

E. *International measures:* WHO Collaborating Centres (see Preface).

NEOPLASIA, MALIGNANT

Infectious agents are now recognized as causes or risk factors in malignant diseases. *Schistosoma haematobium* has been implicated in bladder cancer, *S. japonicum* in colorectal cancer in endemic areas in China, and *Clonorchis sinensis* in cholangiocarcinoma, possibly through chronic irritation. Several viruses have been implicated in the pathogenesis of various human malignancies, either directly or indirectly; these malignancies usually represent the late outcome of the viral infection. Co-factors, both external (environmental) and internal (genetic and physiologic at the immunological and molecular level), can be expected to play a rôle in each of these malignancies. Indeed, viruses and other causal factors appear to be part of a sequence of epidemiologic, immunologic and molecular events that ultimately lead to cancer. The virus is a necessary, but not by itself a sufficient, cause of the malignancy; viral transmission occurred some time in the past and the tumor itself is not transmissible. The implicated agents include both DNA and RNA viruses.

The 3 strongest DNA candidates are (1) Epstein-Barr virus (EBV) in relation to African Burkitt's lymphoma, nasopharyngeal cancer, and acute immunoblastic sarcoma and possibly Hodgkin's disease; some lymphomas occurring in immunosuppressed persons (renal transplant recipients, AIDS, X-linked lymphoproliferative disease) are also EBV-related; (2) hepatitis B virus (HBV) in relation to hepatocellular cancer (HCC); and (3) papilloma viruses and possibly herpes simplex virus in relation to cervical and vulvar cancer. All these viruses are worldwide, ubiquitous, and common agents that produce much more inapparent than apparent infection and most result in a latent virus state that is subject to reactivation. The associated malignancies are rare events that occur in special geographic and host settings. Primary infection very early in life and/or reactivation during immunosuppression are common features of most viral-related malignancies.

Among the RNA viruses the human T-cell leukemia virus (HTLV-I) and related retroviruses (HTLV-II) are the strongest candidates for causing human T-cell leukemia/lymphoma. In contrast to the DNA viruses, the RNA viruses are less ubiquitous, and more geographically localized; infection appears to occur later in life. A similar retrovirus (HTLV-III) is involved in human AIDS.

The elements of proof relating these viruses to cancer include: (1) serologic evidence that there is a higher frequency and/or higher titer of antibody (or of antigen for HBV) in cases than in controls and demonstration in prospective studies that these markers precede the disease; (2) virologic evidence that the virus, its genome, or viral-specific sequences are present in the malignant cells (and not in normal cells or other forms of cancer) and that in vitro oncogenicity can be shown, as in transformation of normal cells; (3) experimental evidence that the virus or viral infected cells can induce a similar malignant disease in animals, especially nonhuman primates, can be demonstrated in the malignant cells, and can be passed serially to other animals; and (4) protective evidence that removal of the virus, or immunization against it, reduces the incidence of the tumor. It cannot be expected that all morphological examples of a single tumor will have the same cause in all geographic settings or age groups. This section will provide brief summaries of the 5 more important associations.

I. BURKITT'S LYMPHOMA   ICD-9 200.2
(African Burkitt's lymphoma, Endemic Burkitt's lymphoma, Burkitt's tumor)

1. Identification—Burkitt's lymphoma (BL) is a monoclonal tumor of B cells, usually involving children, in whom jaw involvement is common. The pathological and morphological features have been strictly defined. The tumor may also develop in immunosuppressed patients (renal transplant patients, familial and X-linked immunodeficiency, and AIDS). These may be monoclonal, polyclonal or mixed; not all are Burkitt-type but are acute lymphoblastic sarcomas.

2. Infectious agent—Epstein-Barr virus (EBV), a herpesvirus which produces the clinical picture of infectious mononucleosis in young adults in developed countries, plays an important pathogenic role in about 97% of BL cases in Africa and Papua New Guinea where EBV infection occurs in infancy and where malaria, a co-factor, is holoendemic. Both are B-cell mitogens and induce a polyclonal B-cell proliferation. EBV is regarded as the initiator and malaria as the promotor of the tumor. EBV is also associated with BL in about 30% of nonendemic, nonmalarial areas (American BL). The evidence for the relationship of EBV to African BL consists of: (1) higher antibody titers to several EBV antigens in cases than in age- and sex-matched indigenous controls, but not to other herpes viruses. A prospective study has shown that the IgG antibody to viral capsid antigen precedes the development of the tumor by 7–72 months and that high antibody titers increase the risk of BL 30–fold; (2) the presence of EBV genome in tumor cells; (3) the in vitro "immortalization" or transformation of B cells by EBV; and (4) experimental reproduction of a malignant lymphoma by EBV in cotton-top marmosets and owl monkeys.

Typical chromosomal changes, usually from chromosome 8 to 14, are a characteristic of both EBV and non-EBV related BL cells. The tumor is monoclonal. The activation of oncogenes, especially *c-myc*, and perhaps a second one (Ha-*ras*, B-lymphoma) by EBV or other agents appears to be involved in the malignant process.

3. Occurrence—Tumor is worldwide but is hyperendemic in highly malarial areas such as tropical Africa and lowland Papua New Guinea. These areas have heavy rainfall (usually >40 inches/yr) and are below 3,000 feet elevation.

4. Reservoir—Man and perhaps other primates.

5. Mode of transmission—See Mononucleosis, section 5. For the development of BL, primary infection usually occurs early in life or involves immunosuppression and reactivation of EBV later. Malaria may be an important co-factor in Africa.

6. Incubation period—Estimated at 2–12 yrs from primary EBV infection; peak onset of tumor after about 6 yrs.

7. Period of communicability—See Mononucleosis, section 7. The tumor is not communicable.

8. Susceptibility and resistance—Susceptibility to EBV is general; however, tumor development is rare and may occur when infection is early in life, usually in the presence of malaria, of immunosuppression or in genetically susceptible persons.

9. Methods of control—Prevention of EBV infection early in life or malaria control (see Malaria) might reduce tumor incidence in Africa and Papua New Guinea. Cases should be reported to a tumor registry. Chemotherapy is usually effective.

II. NASOPHARYNGEAL CARCINOMA (NPC)   ICD-9 147.9

1. Identification—This is a malignant tumor of the epithelial cells of the nasopharynx usually involving adults between 20 and 40 yrs. There is an approximate tenfold higher incidence in certain groups of Chinese descent in Southern China and Taiwan or in those who have moved elsewhere, including the USA, than in the general population.

IgA antibody to the viral capsid antigen of EBV in both serum and nasopharyngeal secretions is a characteristic feature and has been used in China as a screening test for the tumor.

2. Infectious agent—The tumor is strongly associated with Epstein-Barr virus (EBV). The serologic and virologic evidence relating EBV to NPC is similar to that found in African Burkitt's lymphoma (high EBV antibody titer, genome present in tumor cells) and this relationship has been found irrespective of the geographic origin of the patient. NPC has not been reproduced in experimental animals. Chromosomal changes seen in Burkitt's lymphoma cells have not been found in NPC cells.

3. Occurrence—Worldwide but highest in Southern China, SE Asia, north and east Africa, and in the Arctic region. Males outnumber females about 2:1. Chinese persons with HLA-2 and SIN-2 antigen profiles have about a fivefold higher risk.

4. Reservoir—Only man is known to have the tumor.

5. Mode of transmission—EBV is probably transmitted via saliva. Infection occurs early in life in settings where NPC is most common, yet the tumor does not appear until ages 20–40, suggesting the occurrence of some secondary, reactivating factor with epithelial invasion later in life. The method of entry of EBV into epithelial cells is not clear as it can not infect such cells in vitro; repeated respiratory infections or chemical irritants may play a rôle. The tumor itself is not transmissible.

6. Incubation period—Unknown. The tumor occurs in adults; primary EBV infection probably in early childhood.

7. Period of communicability—For communicability of etiological virus, see Mononucleosis, section 7.

8. Susceptibility and resistance—Persons of Chinese descent, especially with certain HLA haplotypes, are more susceptible to the tumor. The higher frequency of the tumor in persons of southern Chinese origin irrespective of later residence and the association with certain HLA haplotypes suggests a genetic susceptibility; however a lower incidence among those migrating to the USA and elsewhere suggests a possible environmental (e.g., plant mitogen) factor.

9. Methods of control—None known. Early detection by careful clinical study of individuals with EBV IgA antibodies to viral capsid antigen would permit early treatment. Cases should be reported to tumor registry; chemotherapy after early recognition is the only specific therapy.

III. HEPATOCELLULAR CARCINOMA   ICD-9 155.0
(HCC, Primary liver cancer, Primary hepatocellular carcinoma)

1. Identification—Primary hepatocellular cancer (PHC) or hepatocellular carcinoma (HCC) occurs in highest frequency in young males in certain African and Asian countries but is recognized worldwide. Infection with hepatitis B virus (HBV) very early in life and persistent antigenemia are important causal factors.

2. Infectious agent—Hepatitis B antigenemia occurs more commonly both in geographic areas and in individuals with HCC than in low incidence areas or in controls. In these high incidence areas the frequency is 10–15 times higher than in controls. Prospective studies in Taiwan have shown a 230–fold higher risk of HCC in persons with HBV antigenemia than in those without. Preliminary evidence indicates viral DNA in some HCC tumor cells. HBV viral sequence has been shown to be integrated into host hepatic DNA in patients with HCC. In addition, recent work suggests that HBV replicates through an RNA intermediate, requiring reverse transcriptase activity reminiscent of retroviruses. The tumor has not been experimentally reproduced in animals but the woodchuck hepatitis virus, which is immunologically related to HBV, produces a hepatoma in the woodchuck. Aflatoxins (see Aspergillosis, section 1), genetic susceptibility, alcohol and other factors may be involved.

3. Occurrence—HCC occurs with highest frequency among Chinese (especially in coastal areas of China), Africans, and Filipinos. In Taiwan and

Mozambique it is the most common tumor of young men; it may be the most common cancer overall. The geographic areas of high prevalence of the tumor such as SE Asia and sub-Saharan Africa have high prevalence of hepatitis B antigenemia but there is variation from region to region.

4. **Reservoir**—Man and certain nonhuman primates (chimpanzee).

5. **Mode of transmission**—HBV is transmitted through blood and body fluids (see Viral Hepatitis B, section 5). Most patients go through a stage of liver cirrhosis before the tumor appears. Early perinatal infection is an important risk factor; for HCC, presence of antigenemia, and especially of e antigen in the mother (resulting in early infection of the infant during passage through the birth canal or later) is an important factor leading to antigen persistence, cirrhosis and the late development of the tumor.

6. **Incubation period**—Unknown for tumor. HBV infection in infancy leading to the tumor in young adults suggests a 15–25 yr induction period.

7. **Period of communicability**—HBV antigenemia may persist for a lifetime and in the presence of HBV e antigen is highly infectious. The tumor itself is not communicable.

8. **Susceptibility and resistance**—All are susceptible to HBV. Early infection and aflatoxin exposure increases the risk of the tumor; alcohol consumption may be a co-factor.

9. **Methods of control**—See Viral Hepatitis B. Interruption of transmission of HBV infection from mother to infant offers hope of prevention of the tumor, by administration of HB vaccine and HBIG. Cases should be reported to a tumor registry.

IV. CERVIX UTERI, MALIGNANT NEOPLASM OF   ICD-9 180
(Carcinoma of the uterine cervix, Cervical cancer)

1. **Identification**—Cervical cancer occurs worldwide with a higher incidence in women with a history of early and frequent intercourse, multiple sex partners, and often in the lower socioeconomic groups. Papilloma virus and herpesvirus have been implicated in its causation but the evidence for both is much weaker than that of EBV to African Burkitt's lymphoma and nasopharyngeal carcinoma, and that of HBV to hepatocellular cancer.

2. **Infectious agents**—Human papilloma virus (HPV) has been implicated in the etiology of cervical cancer. While usually the cause of benign warts or verrucae (see Warts, Viral). evidence of types 16 and 18 viruses

have been found in tumor tissue from cervical neoplasia; other types were associated with acuminate warts, but only infrequently with true neoplasia.

Herpes simplex virus types 1 and 2 (HSV-1, 2), especially in primary genital infections, have been implicated in a causal rôle mostly on serological grounds. However, serological differentiation of HSV-1 and HSV-2 has been unreliable. Since HSV-1 is usually acquired early in life and HSV-2 at the age of starting sexual activity, there is almost always HSV-1 present when testing for HSV-2. Despite this, most seroepidemi-ological surveys have shown a higher frequency of HSV-2 antibody in cases than in controls; however, in a few geographic areas the frequency has been higher in controls than in cases. One cohort study has not demonstrated conclusively that persons with HSV-2 antibody are at higher risk than those without; indeed, one large prospective study failed to find any correlation between the two. The evidence of viral genome in cervical tumor tissue is inconclusive as is evidence of experimental reproduction of the tumor.

3. Occurrence—Worldwide but higher in certain countries such as Colombia, Chile, and Poland. Scandinavian countries and the USA are at intermediate risk; Israel and New Zealand are at low risk. Within each area, women with a history of early onset of sexual activity, frequent intercourse and multiple sexual partners are at highest risk. However, occurrence in nonpromiscuous women in some geographic areas suggests that sexual activity of males may be a critical determinant of the partner's risk of cancer. Persons at low socioeconomic levels have more cervical cancer. In the USA, Jews and Amish have a lower incidence, while blacks and Puerto Ricans a higher one.

4. Reservoir; 5. Mode of transmission; 6. Incubation period; 7. Period of communicability; 8. Susceptibility and resistance; 9. Methods of control—See Herpes Simplex and Warts, Viral. Tumors should be reported to a tumor registry. Treatment is based on early detection by Papanicolaou (Pap) smears and surgical excision.

V. LYMPHATIC TISSUE, MALIGNANT   ICD-9 200-208 NEOPLASM OF

(Adult T-cell leukemia (ATL), T-cell lymphosarcoma (TLCL), peripheral T-cell lymphoma (Sézary's disease), Hairy cell leukemia, Non-Hodgkin's lymphoma)

1. Identification—Leukemias and lymphomas of T-cell origin exist under the name adult T-cell leukemia (ATL) in Japan; T-cell lymphoma sarcoma-cell leukemia (TLCL) in the Caribbean; and peripheral T-cell lymphoma (Sézary's disease) in the USA. They involve primarily adults and seem to represent similar clinical syndromes, some cases of which are

associated with the family of retroviruses termed the human T-cell lymphotrophic viruses (HTLV).

2. **Infectious agent**—At least 3 retrovirus serotypes have been identified. HTLV-I has been implicated in causation of leukemia/lymphoma by both serologic and virologic evidence. Antibody to HTLV-I in healthy adults is uncommon except in areas where the malignancy occurs. Both the time of acquisition of the antibody and the appearance of the tumors seem to be in adult life. In southern Japan, where ATL is common, antibody prevalence rates of 5–30% are present in the normal population, higher in relatives of ATL patients, and highest in the cases themselves. The virus has been isolated from affected T-cells of cases and viral sequences identified in such cells. One isolate in the USA (HTLV-II) was obtained from a patient with hairy cell leukemia, and there is virologic and serologic evidence of a related virus HTLV-III, in the acquired immunodeficiency syndrome (see AIDS), with or without Kaposi's sarcoma. The French isolate, lymphadenopathy virus (LAV) is identical or closely related to HTLV-III.

3. **Occurrence**—Human T-cell leukemia/lymphoma cases related to HTLV-I have been recognized most commonly in Southern Japan and less commonly in the Caribbean Islands, equatorial Africa and southern USA. Adult Japanese and blacks are at highest risk, males more often than females.

4. **Reservoir**—Human and probably other primates are infected with HTLV strains; the tumor has been found only in man.

5. **Mode of transmission**—Currently unknown but transmission of the virus by blood and blood products seems possible. The occurrence of both the infection and of the tumor primarily in adults supports the possibility of sexual transmission, although other epidemiological possibilities exist.

6. **Incubation period**—Unknown.

7. **Period of communicability**—Unknown.

8. **Susceptibility and resistance**—The occurrence of the tumor in Japanese and blacks suggests genetic susceptibility, but environmental causes have not been excluded.

9. **Methods of control**—Not known. Report to a tumor registry.

NOCARDIOSIS   ICD-9 039.9

1. **Identification**—A chronic disease usually originating in the lungs, which may spread by the blood to produce abscesses of brain, subcutaneous tissue and other organs; fatality rate is high in other than subcutaneous involvement. The frequent isolation of *Nocardia asteroides* from patients with other chronic pulmonary diseases may represent cases of a mild form of nocardiosis. Several species of *Nocardia,* particularly *N. brasiliensis* also cause mycetoma (q.v.).

Microscopic examination of stained smears of sputum, pus or CSF reveals gram-positive, weakly acid-fast, branching filaments; culture confirms the identity of the organism. Biopsy or autopsy establishes involvement in causing disease.

2. **Infectious agents**—*Nocardia asteroides, N. caviae* and *N. brasiliensis,* aerobic actinomycetes.

3. **Occurrence**—An occasional sporadic disease in man and animals in all parts of the world. No evidence of age, sex, or racial differences.

4. **Reservoir**—Soil.

5. **Mode of transmission**—*Nocardia* spp. are presumed to enter the body principally by inhalation of contaminated dust into the lung.

6. **Incubation period**—Uncertain; probably a few days to a few weeks.

7. **Period of communicability**—Not directly transmitted from man or animals to man.

8. **Susceptibility and resistance**—Unknown. Endogenous or iatrogenic adrenal hypercorticism, lipoid pneumonia and pulmonary alveolar proteinosis probably predispose to infection. *Nocardia* species may cause "opportunistic infection" in patients with compromised immunity.

9. **Methods of control**—

   A. Preventive measures: None.

   B. Control of patient, contacts and the immediate environment:

      1) Report to local health authority: Official report not ordinarily justifiable, Class 5 (see Preface).
      2) Isolation: None.
      3) Concurrent disinfection: Of discharges and contaminated dressings.
      4) Quarantine: None.
      5) Immunization of contacts: None.
      6) Investigation of contacts: Not indicated.

7) Specific treatment: Sulfonamides in high doses are effective in systemic infections if given early and for prolonged periods. Some isolates of *Nocardia* are sensitive in vitro to ampicillin, minocycline, erythromycin, amikacin, fusidic acid or other antibiotics; one of these drugs is sometimes given in addition to a sulfonamide. Trimethoprim has also been used in combination with a sulfonamide.

C. **Epidemic measures:** Not applicable, a sporadic disease.

D. **Disaster implications:** None.

E. **International measures:** None.

ONCHOCERCIASIS
(River blindness)

ICD-9 125.3

1. **Identification**—A chronic, nonfatal filarial disease with fibrous nodules in subcutaneous tissues, particularly of the head and shoulders (America) or pelvic girdle and lower extremities (Africa). The adult parasites are found in these nodules and also in deep-seated bundles lying against the periosteum of bones or near joints. The female worm discharges microfilariae which migrate through the skin, often causing intense pruritic rash, altered pigmentation, edema and atrophy of the skin. Loss of skin elasticity may result in "hanging groin." Microfilariae frequently reach the eye, causing visual disturbances and blindness; they may be found in organs and tissues other than skin and eye but their clinical significance is not yet clear; in heavy infections they may also be found in the blood, tears, sputum and urine.

Laboratory diagnosis is made by superficial skin biopsy with demonstration of microfilariae in fresh preparations by microscopic examination; by excising nodules and finding adult worms; in ocular manifestations, by slit-lamp observation of microfilariae in cornea, anterior chamber or vitreous body; or by finding microfilariae in the urine. In the Mazzotti reaction, oral administration of 25 mg of diethylcarbamazine citrate produces characteristic pruritis; it may occur in low density infections when microfilariae are difficult to demonstrate. Differentiation from other filarial diseases, including filariasis (q.v.), is required in endemic areas.

2. **Infectious agent**—*Onchocerca volvulus,* a nematode.

3. **Occurrence**—Geographical distribution in the Western Hemisphere is limited to Guatemala (principally on the western slope of the Continental Divide), southern Mexico (states of Chiapas and Oaxaca), Venezuela, small

areas in Colombia and Ecuador and in the state of Amazonas in Brazil; in Africa south of the Sahara in an area extending from Senegal to Ethiopia down to Angola in the west and Malawi in the east; also in Yemen. In some areas, especially in west Africa, almost all of the population is infected and visual impairment and blindness are serious problems.

4. Reservoir—Infected persons. Can be experimentally transmitted to chimpanzees and has been found rarely in nature in gorillas. Other species found in animals rarely infect man.

5. Mode of transmission—By the bite of infected female blackflies of the genus *Simulium;* in Central America mainly *S. ochraceum;* in S America, *S. metallicum* complex, *S. sanguineum/amazonicum* complex, *S. quadrivittatum* and possibly other species; in Africa, *S. damnosum* complex and *S. neavei* complex. Microfilariae, ingested by a blackfly feeding on an infected person, penetrate thoracic muscles of the fly, develop into infective larvae, migrate to the cephalic capsule and are liberated on the skin and enter the bite wound during a subsequent bloodmeal.

6. Incubation period—Microfilariae are found in the skin usually 1 year or more after infection. In Guatemala they have been found in children as young as 6 months of age. In Africa, vectors are infective after 6 days; in Guatemala measurably longer, up to 14 days because of lower temperatures.

7. Period of communicability—Man can infect flies as long as living microfilariae occur in the skin, i.e., for 10–15 years if untreated. Not directly transmitted from person to person.

8. Susceptibility and resistance—Susceptibility is universal; reinfection may occur; severity of disease depends on cumulative effects of the infections.

9. Methods of control—

    A. *Preventive measures:*

        1) Avoid bites of *Simulium* flies by wearing protective clothing and headgear as much as possible or by use of an insect repellent such as diethyltoluamide (Deet).

        2) Identify the vector species and its breeding sites; control the larvae, which usually develop in rapidly running streams and in artificial waterways, by use of biodegradable insecticides such as temephos (Abate®). Aerial spraying may be used to ensure coverage of breeding places in large-scale control operations such as in Africa; because of the mountainous terrain such procedures generally are not feasible in Central America. Elimination of crabs on which immature stages of *S. neavei* develop has been effective.

3) Provide facilities for diagnosis and treatment.

B. *Control of patient, contacts and the immediate environment:*

1) Report to local health authority: Official report not ordinarily justifiable, Class 5 (see Preface).
2) Isolation: None.
3) Concurrent disinfection: None.
4) Quarantine: None.
5) Immunization of contacts: None.
6) Investigation of contacts: A community problem.
7) Specific treatment: Diethylcarbamazine citrate (DEC, Hetrazan®) is useful but may cause severe reactions due to destruction of microfilariae; these reactions may respond to corticosteroids. DEC does not kill adult worms. Suramin (Bayer 205, Naphuride, Antrypol), which is available in the USA from CDC, Atlanta (see Preface), kills the adult worms and leads to gradual disappearance of microfilariae; nephrotoxicity and other undesirable reactions may occur so its use requires close medical supervision. Neither drug is suited to mass treatment. Newer drugs are under investigation. In Central America where nodules commonly occur on the head, their excision may reduce symptoms and prevent blindness.

C. *Epidemic measures:* In areas of high prevalence make concerted effort to reduce incidence, taking measures listed under 9A.

D. *Disaster implications:* None.

E. *International measures:* A coordinated program, the Onchocerciasis Control Program in the Volta River Basin of west Africa supported by the World Bank, UNDP, FAO and WHO, has been joined by neighboring countries where the disease is endemic, based mainly on anti-blackfly measures applied systematically over large enough ecological zones to limit reinvasion of flies (some of which have a flight range of over 100 miles) from untreated areas. WHO Collaborating Centres (see Preface).

ORF VIRUS DISEASE ICD-9 051.2
(Contagious pustular dermatitis, Human orf, Ecthyma contagiosum)

1. **Identification**—Primarily a proliferative cutaneous viral disease of sheep and goats, transmissible to man by contact. The lesion in man, usually solitary and located on hands, arms or face, is maculopapular or pustular, progressing to a weeping nodule with central umbilication. There may be several lesions, each measuring up to 3 cm in diameter, lasting 3–6 wks. With secondary bacterial infection, lesions may become pustular. Regional adenitis occurs in a minority of cases. Erythema multiforme and erythema multiforme bullosum are rare complications. Disseminated disease and serious ocular damage have been reported. Fatal human cases have been claimed but these were not laboratory confirmed. The disease has been confused with cutaneous anthrax and malignancy.

Diagnosis is made by history of contact with sheep or goats and, in particular, their young; EM demonstration of typical virus particles in the lesion; negative conventional bacteriology; growth of the virus on tissue cultures of ovine, bovine or primate origin; and positive results by IFA or CF tests.

2. **Infectious agent**—Orf virus, a DNA virus belonging to the *Parapoxvirus* genus of Poxviruses. The causative agent is closely related to "milker's nodule virus."

3. **Occurrence**—Probably worldwide among farm workers, shepherds, veterinarians and abattoir workers in areas producing sheep or goats; an important occupational disease in New Zealand.

4. **Reservoir**—Probably in sheep, goats, reindeer and musk oxen. The virus is very resistant to physical factors, except ultraviolet light, and may persist in the environment or on animal coats.

5. **Mode of transmission**—By direct contact with the mucous membranes of infected animals, with lesions on udders of nursing dams, or through intermediate passive transfer as from apparently normal animals contaminated by contact, knives, shears, stall sides or manger, trucks, or clothing. One instance of person-to-person transmission has been claimed. Human infection may follow production and administration to animals of attenuated vaccines.

6. **Incubation period**—Generally 3–6 days.

7. **Period of communicability**—Unknown. Human lesions show a decrease in the number of virus particles as the disease progresses.

8. **Susceptibility and resistance**—Susceptibility is probably universal with recovery producing only relative immunity.

9. **Methods of control**—

A. *Preventive measures:* Good personal hygiene and washing the exposed area with soap and water. All herds should be considered to be potential sources of infection. General cleanliness of animal housing areas. The value of attenuated virus vaccine in animals has not been determined.

B. *Control of patient, contacts and the immediate environment:*

1) Report to local health authority: Not required, but desirable when a human case occurs in areas not previously known to have the infection, Class 5, (see Preface).
2) Isolation: None.
3) Concurrent disinfection: Incinerate or bury dressings.
4) Quarantine: None.
5) Immunization of contacts: None.
6) Investigation of contacts and source of infection: Important to secure history of contact.
7) Specific treatment: None.

C. *Epidemic measures:* None.

D. *Disaster implications:* None.

E. *International measures:* None for man.

PARACOCCIDIOIDOMYCOSIS   ICD-9 116.1
(South American blastomycosis, Paracoccidioidal granuloma)

1. Identification—A serious and at times fatal chronic mycosis characterized by patchy pulmonary infiltrates and/or ulcerative lesions of the mucosa (oral, nasal, gastrointestinal) and of the skin. Lymphadenopathy is frequent. In disseminated cases all viscera may be affected; the adrenal gland is especially susceptible.

Keloidal blastomycosis (Lobo's disease), a disease with only skin involvement, formerly confused with paracoccidioidomycosis, is caused by *Loboa loboi,* a fungus known only in its tissue form and not yet grown in culture.

Diagnosis is confirmed histologically or by cultivation of the infectious agent. Serological techniques may assist in diagnosis.

2. Infectious agent—*Paracoccidioides brasiliensis,* a dimorphic fungus.

3. Occurrence—Endemic in the tropical and subtropical regions of S America and, to a lesser extent, of Central America and Mexico. Workers in contact with soil such as farmers, laborers and construction workers are especially at risk. Highest incidence is in adults aged 30–50 yrs; much more common in males than in females.

4. **Reservoir**—Presumably soil or fungus-laden dust.

5. **Mode of transmission**—Presumably acquired through inhalation of contaminated soil or dust.

6. **Incubation period**—Highly variable, from 1 month to many years.

7. **Period of communicability**—Direct transmission of clinical disease from person to person is not known.

8. **Susceptibility and resistance**—Unknown.

9. **Methods of control**—

    A.   *Preventive measures:* None.

    B.   *Control of patient, contacts and the immediate environment:*

        1)   Report to local health authority: Official report not ordinarily justifiable, Class 5 (see Preface).

        2)   Isolation: None.

        3)   Concurrent disinfection: Of discharges and contaminated articles. Terminal cleaning.

        4)   Quarantine: None.

        5)   Immunization of contacts: None.

        6)   Investigation of contacts: Not indicated.

        7)   Specific treatment: Ketoconazole appears to be the drug of choice for all but the patients ill enough to require hospitalization, who should receive i.v. amphotericin B (Fungizone®) followed by prolonged therapy with ketoconazole. Sulfonamides are cheaper but less effective than ketoconazole.

    C.   *Epidemic measures:* Not applicable, a sporadic disease.

    D.   *Disaster implications:* None.

    E.   *International measures:* None.

PARAGONIMIASIS   ICD-9 121.2
(Pulmonary distomiasis, Lung fluke disease)

1. **Identification**—Clinical manifestations of this trematode disease depend on the path of migration and the organs invaded. Lungs are most frequently involved; symptoms are cough and hemoptysis. Worms become

surrounded by an inflammatory reaction which eventually organizes into a fibrous, cystic lesion. Localization in other organs is not infrequent, with worms in such sites as the brain, subcutaneous tissues, intestinal wall, lymph nodes, or genitourinary tract. Infection usually lasts for years, and the infected person may appear essentially well. It may be mistaken for tuberculosis on chest x-rays of Asian immigrants.

The sputum generally contains orange-brown flecks, sometimes diffusely distributed, in which masses of eggs are seen microscopically, establishing the diagnosis. However, acid-fast staining for tuberculosis destroys the eggs and precludes diagnosis. The eggs are swallowed and thus are found in feces, especially when a good concentration method is used. Serological tests are helpful, but cross reactions occur, especially with clonorchiasis (q.v.).

2. Infectious agents—*Paragonimus westermani* and other species in Asia; *P. africanus* and *P. uterobilateralis* in Africa, and *P. mexicanus (P. peruvianus)* and other species in the Americas.

3. Occurrence—Extensive in Asia, particularly Korea, Japan and Taiwan; scattered foci in the Philippines, parts of mainland China, SE Asia, Siberia, west and central Africa, and in S America (Brazil, Colombia, Ecuador, Peru, Venezuela), in Central America (Costa Rica) and in Mexico.

4. Reservoir—Man, dog, cat, pig and wild carnivores are definitive hosts and act as reservoirs.

5. Mode of transmission—Infection occurs when the raw or partially cooked flesh of fresh water crabs such as *Eriocheir* and *Potamon* and of crayfish such as *Cambaroides* containing infective larvae (metacercariae) are eaten. The larvae emerge in the duodenum, then penetrate the intestinal wall, migrate through the tissues, become encapsulated, usually in the lungs, and develop into egg-producing adults. Eggs leave the definitive host via sputum and feces, gain access to fresh water, and embryonate in 2–4 weeks. A larva (miracidium) hatches, penetrates a suitable fresh water snail *(Semisulcospira, Thiara, Aroapyrgus* or other species) and undergoes a cycle of development of approximately 3 months. Larvae (cercariae) emerge from the snail and penetrate and encyst in fresh water crabs and crayfish. Pickling of these crustaceans in wine, brine or vinegar, a common practice in Asia, frequently does not kill the encysted larvae.

6. Incubation period—Flukes mature and begin to lay eggs approximately 6 wks after man ingests infective larvae. The interval until symptoms appear is long, variable, poorly defined and depends on the organ invaded and the number of worms involved.

7. Period of communicability—Eggs may be discharged by infected people for 20 yrs or more; duration of infection in mollusc and crustacean hosts is indefinite. Not directly transmitted from person to person.

8. Susceptibility and resistance—Susceptibility is general. Increased resistance possibly develops as a result of infection.

9. Methods of control—

   A. Preventive measures:

      1) Educate people in endemic areas about the life cycle of the parasite.

      2) Stress thorough cooking of crustacea.

      3) Sanitary disposal of sputum and feces.

      4) Control of snails by molluscicides is feasible in some areas.

   B. Control of patient, contacts and the immediate environment:

      1) Report to local health authority: Official report not ordinarily justifiable, Class 5 (see Preface).

      2) Isolation: None.

      3) Concurrent disinfection: Of sputum and feces.

      4) Quarantine: None.

      5) Immunization of contacts: None.

      6) Investigation of contacts: None.

      7) Specific treatment: Bithionol gives good results; praziquantel (Biltricide®) seems to be equally effective and less toxic.

   C. Epidemic measures: In an endemic area, occurrence of small clusters of cases or even sporadic infections is an important signal for examination of local waters for infected snails, crabs and crayfish and determination of reservoir mammalian hosts to establish appropriate controls.

   D. Disaster implications: None.

   E. International measures: None.

PARATYPHOID FEVER   ICD-9 002.1-002.3

1. **Identification**—A bacterial enteric infection, often with abrupt onset, continued fever, malaise, headache, enlargement of spleen, sometimes rose spots on trunk, usually diarrhea, and involvement of lymphoid tissues of the mesentery and intestines. While clinically similar, the fatality

rate is much lower than for typhoid fever. Mild and asymptomatic infections occur. Relapses may occur in approximately 3.5% of cases. (See Salmonellosis).

Laboratory confirmation and identification of infecting species are by bacteriologic examination especially of blood, but also of feces and urine.

2. Infectious agents—Three main groups are recognized: (1) *Salmonella paratyphi A (S. enteritidis* serotype paratyphoid A), (2) *S. paratyphi B (S. enteritidis* serotype paratyphoid B, *S. schottmülleri),* and (3) *S. paratyphi C (S. enteritidis* serotype paratyphoid C, *S. hirschfeldii).* All are predominantly of human origin; a number of phage types can be distinguished.

3. Occurrence—Sporadically or in limited outbreaks. Probably more frequent than reports suggest. In the USA and Canada, paratyphoid fever is infrequently identified; of the 3 varieties, serotype paratyphoid B is most common, A less frequent and C extremely rare.

4. Reservoir—Usually man; rarely domestic animals. In one outbreak in England, dairy cows excreted *S. paratyphi B* organisms in milk and feces.

5. Mode of transmission—Direct or indirect contact with feces or rarely urine of patient or carrier. Spread is often by food, especially milk, milk products and shellfish, usually contaminated by hands of a carrier or case. Under some conditions, flies are thought to be possible vectors. Multiplication of the bacilli frequently occurs in the contaminated food. A few outbreaks are related to water supplies.

6. Incubation period—One to 3 weeks for enteric fever; 1–10 days for gastroenteritis.

7. Period of communicability—As long as the infectious agent persists in excreta, which is from appearance of prodromal symptoms, throughout illness, and for periods up to several weeks or months but commonly 1-2 wks after recovery. Some infected persons may become permanent carriers.

8. Susceptibility and resistance—Susceptibility is general. Some species-specific immunity usually follows recovery.

9. Methods of control—

    A. Preventive measures: Same as those listed under typhoid fever, 9A, 1–10. Standard vaccines against paratyphoid fever have not proven to be effective.

    B. Control of patient, contacts and the immediate environment:

        1) to 4): Same as for typhoid fever, 9B.
        5)   Immunization of contacts: None.
        6)   Investigation of contacts: Bacteriological investigation is

indicated, especially of household contacts. Close contacts should not be employed as foodhandlers until at least two cultures of fecal specimens taken at least 24 hours apart are found to be free of *Salmonellae*.

7) Specific treatment: For overt enteric fever or septicemia, chloramphenicol, ampicillin or TMP-SMX are the drugs of choice. With these or other antibiotics, sensitivity tests should be performed. Defervescence may not occur for 5 days or longer following institution of antibiotic therapy.

C. *Epidemic measures:* Those for typhoid fever, 9C.

D. *Disaster implications:* Those for typhoid fever, 9D.

E. *International measures:* WHO Collaborating Centres (see Preface).

PEDICULOSIS   ICD-9 132

1. **Identification**—Infestation of the head, the hairy parts of the body or clothing (especially along the seams of inner surfaces), with adult lice, larvae, or nits (eggs), which results in severe itching and excoriation of the scalp or body. Secondary infection may occur with ensuing cervical lymphadenitis. Crab lice usually infest the pubic area; they may infest facial hair (including eye lashes), axillae and body surface.

2. **Infesting agents**—*Pediculus capitis,* the head louse, *P. humanus,* the body louse, and *Phthirus pubis,* the crab louse. Only the body louse is of major medical importance as the vector of epidemic typhus, trench fever, and louseborne relapsing fever. Lice of lower animals do not infest man, although they may be present transiently.

3. **Occurrence**—Worldwide. Outbreaks of head lice are common among children in schools and institutions.

4. **Reservoir**—Infested persons.

5. **Mode of transmission**—For head and body lice, direct contact with an infested person. For body lice and to a lesser extent for head lice, indirect contact with their personal belongings, especially sharing clothing and headgear. While other means are possible, crab lice are most frequently transmitted through sexual contact. Lice leave a febrile host; fever and overcrowding increase transfer from person to person.

6. **Incubation period**—Under optimal conditions the eggs of lice hatch

in a week, and sexual maturity is reached approximately 8–10 days after hatching.

7. Period of communicability—As long as lice or eggs remain alive on the infested person or in clothing.

8. Susceptibility and resistance—Any person may become louse infested under suitable conditions of exposure. Repeated infestations often result in dermal hypersensitivity.

9. Methods of control—

A. Preventive measures:

1) Avoid physical contact with infested individuals and their belongings, especially clothing and bedding.
2) Health education of the public in the value of laundering clothing and bedding in hot water (55°C or 131°F for 20 min.) or dry cleaning to destroy nits and lice.
3) Regular direct inspection of all primary school children for head lice and, when indicated, of body and clothing, particularly of children in schools, institutions, nursing homes and summer camps.

B. Control of infested persons, contacts and the immediate environment:

1) Report to local health authority: Official report not ordinarily justifiable; school authorities should be informed, Class 5 (see Preface).
2) Isolation: Contact isolation until 24 hours after application of effective insecticide.
3) Concurrent disinfection: With body lice in members of a family or group, to include clothing, bedding and other appropriate vehicles of transmission (e.g., cosmetic articles), treated by laundering in hot water, by dry cleaning or by application of an effective chemical insecticide and ovicide (see 9B7, below). After chemical treatment has been completed, clothes and laundry facilities should be rinsed adequately.
4) Quarantine: None.
5) Immunization of contacts: Does not apply.
6) Investigation of contacts: Examination of household and other close personal contacts, with concurrent treatment as indicated.
7) Specific treatment: For head and pubic lice, 1% gamma benzene hexachloride lotions (Lindane, Kwell®) (not recommended for infants, young children and pregnant or

lactating women), pyrethrins synergized with piperonyl butoxide (A-200 Pyrinate®, RID® and XXX®), 0.5% malathion (Prioderm®) carbaryl and benzyl benzoate are effective. Retreatment after 7–10 days is recommended to assure that no eggs have survived. For body lice: Clothing and bedding should be washed with the hot cycle of an automatic washing machine, or, if not available, dusted with powders containing 1% lindane or, preferably, in view of widespread resistance to lindane, 1% malathion or pyrethrins with piperonyl butoxide or carbaryl, and then laundered before using. Abate® (temephos) as a 2% dusting powder is also effective and is recommended by WHO for use in areas where strains of body lice are resistant to malathion.

C. *Epidemic measures:* Mass treatment as recommended in 9B7.

D. *Disaster implications:* Diseases for which *P. humanus* is a vector are particularly prone to occur at times of social upheaval (see Typhus Fever, Epidemic).

E. *International measures:* None.

PERTUSSIS
(Whooping cough, Parapertussis)

ICD-9 033

1. Identification—An acute bacterial disease involving the respiratory tract. The initial catarrhal stage has an insidious onset with an irritating cough which gradually becomes paroxysmal, usually within 1 to 2 weeks, and lasts for 1 to 2 months. Paroxysms are characterized by repeated violent coughs; each series of paroxysms has many coughs without intervening inhalation and may be followed by a characteristic crowing or high pitched inspiratory whoop; paroxysms frequently end with the expulsion of clear, tenacious mucus. Young infants and adults often do not have the typical whoop or cough paroxysm. Fatality in the USA is low; approximately 75% of deaths are among children under 1 year of age, most in those under 6 months. Morbidity and mortality are higher in females than males. In unimmunized populations, especially those with underlying malnutrition and multiple infections, pertussis is among the most lethal diseases of infants and young children.

Parapertussis is a similar but usually milder disease clinically indistinguishable from pertussis. It is usually seen in school-age children, and occurs relatively infrequently. Identification is by culture, biochemical and immunologic differences between *Bordetella parapertussis* and *B. pertussis*.

A similar clinical syndrome has been reported in association with viruses, especially adenoviruses.

Diagnosis is based on the recovery of the etiological organism from nasopharyngeal swabs obtained during the catarrhal and early paroxysmal stages. Direct FA staining of nasopharyngeal secretions provides rapid presumptive diagnosis, but requires an experienced laboratory. Strikingly high total WBC counts with a strong preponderance of lymphocytes are found as the whooping stage develops; this may not occur in young infants.

2. Infectious agent—*Bordetella pertussis,* the pertussis bacillus.

3. Occurrence—A disease common to children everywhere, regardless of race, climate, or geographic location. There has been a marked decline in incidence and mortality rates during the past four decades, chiefly in communities fostering active immunization and where good nutrition and medical care are available. From 1979–83 an average of 1750 cases was reported annually in the USA; it is likely that many more cases were unidentified or unreported. In recent years incidence rates have increased in countries where immunization levels have fallen.

4. Reservoir—Infected persons.

5. Mode of transmission—Primarily by direct contact with discharges from respiratory mucous membranes of infected persons by the airborne route, probably by droplets. Frequently brought home by an older sibling.

6. Incubation period—Commonly 7 days, almost uniformly within 10 days, and not exceeding 21 days.

7. Period of communicability—Highly communicable in the early catarrhal stage before the paroxysmal cough stage. Thereafter, communicability gradually decreases and becomes negligible for ordinary nonfamilial contacts in about 3 weeks, despite persisting spasmodic cough with whoop. For control purposes, the communicable stage extends from the early catarrhal stage to 3 weeks after onset of typical paroxysms in patients not treated with antibiotics; when treated with erythromycin or TMP-SMX, the period of infectiousness usually extends only 5 to 7 days after onset of therapy.

8. Susceptibility and resistance—Susceptibility is general; there is no clear evidence of effective transplacental immunity in infants. Predominantly a childhood disease; incidence rates are highest under 5 years of age. Numerous milder and missed atypical cases occur. One attack confers definite and prolonged immunity, although second attacks can occasionally occur. Cases occurring in adolescents and adults in the USA, particularly among health workers and parents, reflect incomplete immunization coverage in these age groups or perhaps waning of vaccine-induced immunity.

9. Methods of control—

A. *Preventive measures:*

1) Active immunization is recommended with a vaccine consisting of a suspension of killed bacteria adsorbed on aluminum salts. There is no advantage to nonadsorbed ("plain") preparations, either for primary immunization or booster shots. The schedule of immunization is that recommended for diphtheria for those under 7 years of age (see Diphtheria); some countries recommend different ages for specific doses or a different number of injections. In general, pertussis vaccine is not given to persons 7 years of age or older since the disease is usually milder and reactions to the vaccine more marked in older children and adults. Vaccinees who experience severe reactions such as convulsions, a persistent or unusual severe screaming, collapse, a temperature of $>40.5°C$ ($>105°F$), or an encephalopathy should not receive a further dose of pertussis-containing vaccines. Less serious systemic and local reactions follow a large proportion of DTP doses and are not contraindications to further pertussis vaccine doses. Pertussis vaccine may not provide complete or permanent immunity; active immunization started after exposure will not protect against disease resulting from that exposure. Best protection is obtained by adhering to the recommended schedule. Passive immunization is of no proven value in pertussis, even if given immediately after exposure. Pertussis IG is no longer available.

2) When there is an outbreak, protection of health workers at high risk of exposure by the administration of a booster dose of 0.25 ml pertussis vaccine (available from Biologic Products Division, Michigan Department of Health, P.O. Box 30035, Lansing, MI 48909) or a 14-day course of erythromycin may be considered; local policies may vary.

3) Education of the public, and particularly parents of infants, to the dangers of whooping cough and to the advantages of initiating immunization at 2–3 months of age and adhering to the immunization schedule is important. This is increasingly important because of the wide publicity of the relatively rare adverse reactions.

B. *Control of patient, contacts and the immediate environment:*

1) Report to local health authority: Case report obligatory in most states and countries, Class 2B (see Preface). Early reporting permits better outbreak control.

2) Isolation: Respiratory isolation for known cases. Exclude suspected cases from the presence of young children and infants, especially unimmunized infants, until the cases have received at least 5 days of a minimum 14–day course of antibiotics.

3) Concurrent disinfection: Discharges from nose and throat and articles soiled therewith. Terminal cleaning.

4) Quarantine: Inadequately immunized household contacts less than 7 years old should be excluded from schools, day-care centers and public gatherings for 14 days after last exposure or until the cases and contacts have received 5 days of a minimum 14–day course of antibiotics.

5) Protection of contacts: Passive immunization is not effective, and it is too late for the initiation of active immunization to protect against a prior exposure. Close contacts less than 7 years old who have not received 4 DTP doses or have not received a DTP dose within 3 years should be given a DTP dose as soon after exposure as possible. It may be prudent to consider a 14–day course of erythromycin or TMP-SMX for close contacts less than 1 year old, regardless of immunization status, and for unimmunized close contacts less than 7 years of age.

6) Investigation of contacts: A search for early, missed or atypical cases is indicated where a nonimmune infant or young child is or might be at risk.

7) Specific treatment: Antibiotics (e.g., erythromycin or TMP-SMX) may shorten the period of communicability, but often have little effect on symptomatology.

C. *Epidemic measures:* A search for unrecognized and unreported cases is indicated to protect preschool children from exposure and to assure adequate preventive measures for exposed children less than 7 years old. Accelerated immunization with the 1st dose at 6 wks of age, the 2nd and 3rd at 4-wk intervals, may be indicated; complete immunization for those already started.

D. *Disaster implications:* Pertussis could become a problem if introduced into crowded refugee camps with many unimmunized children.

E. *International measures:* Assure completion of primary immunization of infants and young children before they travel to other countries; review need for a booster dose. WHO Collaborating Centres (see Preface).

PINTA
(Carate)

ICD-9 103

1. **Identification**—An acute and chronic nonvenereal treponemal skin infection. A scaling papule with satellite lymphadenopathy appears within 1–8 weeks after infection, usually on the hands, legs or dorsum of the feet. In 3–12 months a maculopapular, erythematous secondary rash appears and may evolve into tertiary splotches of altered skin pigmentation (dyschromic) of variable size. These treponema-containing macules pass through stages of blue to violet to brown pigmentation, finally becoming treponema-free depigmented (achromic) scars. Lesions are in different stages of evolution and are most common on the face and extremities. Organ systems are not involved; physical disability and death do not occur.

Spirochetes are demonstrable in dyschromic (but not achromic) lesions by darkfield examination. Serologic tests for syphilis usually become reactive before or during the secondary rash and thereafter behave as in venereal syphilis.

2. **Infectious agent**—*Treponema carateum,* a spirochete.

3. **Occurrence**—Found in the Western Hemisphere among isolated rural populations living under crowded unhygienic conditions in tropical areas of Central and S America. Predominantly a disease of older children and adults. Frequent in some Amazonian populations wearing little clothing in the hot humid climate.

4. **Reservoir**—Man.

5. **Mode of transmission**—Presumably person-to-person transmission by direct and prolonged contact with initial and early dyschromic skin lesions; the location of primary lesions suggests that trauma provides a portal of entry. Various biting and sucking arthropods, especially blackflies, have been suspected but not proven as biological vectors.

6. **Incubation period**—Usually 2–3 weeks.

7. **Period of communicability**—Unknown; potentially communicable while dyschromic skin lesions are active, sometimes for many years.

8. **Susceptibility and resistance**—Undefined; presumably as in other treponematoses.

9. **Methods of control**—

   A. *Preventive measures:* Those applicable to other nonvenereal treponematoses apply to Pinta; see Yaws, 9A.

   B. *Control of patient, contacts and the immediate environment:*

1) Report to local health authority: In selected endemic areas; in most countries not a reportable disease, Class 3B (see Preface).

2) through 7): Same as for Yaws, 9B.

C. *Epidemic measures:* See Yaws, 9C.

D. *Disaster implications:* None.

E. *International measures:* See Yaws, 9E.

PLAGUE
(Peste)

ICD-9 020

1. Identification—A specific zoonosis involving rodents and their fleas which transfer the infection to various animals including man. The initial response is commonly a lymphadenitis in the nodes receiving drainage from the site of the flea bite. This is bubonic plague and occurs more often in lymph nodes in the inguinal area and less commonly in those in the axillary or cervical areas. The involved nodes are swollen, inflamed and tender and may suppurate. Fever is usually present. All forms, including instances in which lymphadenopathy is not apparent, may progress to septicemic plague with dissemination by the blood to diverse parts of the body including the meninges. Secondary involvement of the lungs results in pneumonia; mediastinitis or pleural effusion may develop. This secondary pneumonic plague is of special significance since aerosolized droplets of sputum may serve as the source of primary pneumonic or of pharyngeal plague. Further person-to-person transfer can result in localized outbreaks or in devastating epidemics.

Untreated bubonic plague has a case fatality rate commonly reported to be about 50%; rarely it is no more than a localized infection of short duration (pestis minor). Plague organisms have been recovered from throat cultures of asymptomatic contacts of pneumonic plague patients. Untreated primary septicemic plague and pneumonic plague are invariably fatal. Modern therapy markedly reduces fatality from bubonic plague; pneumonic and septicemic plague also respond if recognized and treated early.

A rapid presumptive diagnosis of plague can be made by visualizing bipolar-staining, ovoid, gram-negative organisms in direct microscopic examination of material aspirated from a bubo, sputum or CSF. Examination by FA test is more specific and is particularly useful in sporadic cases. An antigen-capture ELISA test promises to permit an early rapid diagnosis in acute cases. Diagnosis is confirmed by culture and identification of the causal organism from fluid aspirated from buboes, blood, CSF or sputum, or by a fourfold rise or fall in antibody titer. The passive hemagglutination test (PHA) using *Yersinia pestis* Fraction-1 antigen is most frequently used for serodiagnosis.

2. Infectious agent—*Yersinia pestis,* the plague bacillus.

3. Occurrence—Plague continues to be dangerous because of vast areas of persistent wild rodent infection; contact of wild rodents with domestic rats occurs frequently in some enzootic areas. Wild rodent plague exists in the western third of the USA, large areas of S America, northcentral, eastern and southern Africa, the Near East, Iranian Kurdistan and along the frontier between Yemen and Saudi Arabia, central and SE Asia and Indonesia. There are several natural plague foci within the USSR. Urban plague has been controlled in most of the world; human plague has occurred recently in several countries in Africa (Angola, Kenya, Malagasy, Namibia, S Africa, Tanzania, Uganda, Zimbabwe, Zaire). Plague is endemic in Burma and also in S Vietnam where thousands of cases of bubonic plague, both urban and rural, with scattered outbreaks of pneumonic plague, were reported between 1962 and 1972. In the Americas, foci in northeastern Brazil and in the Andean region (Bolivia, Ecuador and Peru) continue to produce sporadic cases and occasional outbreaks. Human plague in the USA is sporadic, with only single cases or small common source clusters in an area, usually following exposure to wild rodents or their fleas. Between 1974 and 1983, cases were reported from 9 western states. In 1983, 40 human cases occurred; 26 were exposed in New Mexico and ten in Arizona. No human-to-human transmission has occurred in the USA since 1924.

4. Reservoir—Wild rodents are the natural reservoir of plague. Lagomorphs (rabbits and hares) and carnivores may be a source of infection to humans.

5. Mode of transmission—Plague in people occurs as a result of human intrusion into the zoonotic (also termed sylvatic or rural) cycle during or following an epizootic or by the entry of sylvatic rodents or their infected fleas into man's habitat. Domestic pets may carry plague-infected wild rodent fleas into homes. Contact by commensal rodents and their fleas with plague among sylvatic rodents may result in the development of a rat epizootic and epidemic plague. The most frequent source of exposure resulting in human disease worldwide has been the bites of infected fleas (especially *Xenopsylla cheopis,* the oriental rat flea). Other important sources include the handling of tissues of infected animals, especially rodents and rabbits but also carnivores; airborne droplets from humans or household pets with plague pneumonia; and careless manipulation of laboratory cultures. Certain occupations and lifestyles carry an increased risk of exposure. Man-to-man transmission by *Pulex irritans* fleas is important in the Andean region of S America and in other places where plague occurs and this "human" flea is abundant.

6. Incubation period—From 2–6 days; may be a few days longer in vaccinated individuals. For primary plague pneumonia, 1–6 days, usually short.

7. Period of communicability—Fleas may remain infective for months under suitable conditions of temperature and humidity. Bubonic plague is not usually transmitted directly from person to person unless there is a complicating pneumonia or contact with pus from suppurating buboes. Pneumonic plague may be highly communicable under appropriate climatic conditions; overcrowding facilitates transmission.

8. Susceptibility and resistance—Susceptibility is general. Immunity after recovery is relative; it may not protect against a large inoculum.

9. Methods of control—

A. *Preventive measures:* The basic objective is to reduce the likelihood of humans being bitten by infected fleas or of being exposed to pneumonic plague patients.

   1) Educate the public in enzootic areas on the modes of human exposure; the importance of preventing access to food and shelter by domestic rodents through appropriate storage and disposal of food, garbage and refuse; and on the importance of avoiding flea bites by use of insecticides and repellents. In sylvatic or rural plague areas, the public should be warned not to camp near rodent burrows and to avoid handling, but to report, dead or sick rodents to health authorities. Dogs and cats in such areas should be treated periodically with appropriate insecticides.

   2) Periodic surveys of rodent populations to determine the effectiveness of sanitary programs or to evaluate the potential for epizootic plague. Rat suppression by poisoning (see 9B6, below) may be necessary to augment basic environmental sanitation measures; rat control should always be preceded or accompanied by measures to control fleas. Surveillance of natural foci by bacteriologic testing of sick or dead wild rodents and by serologic studies of wild carnivore and feral dog populations in order to define areas of plague activity. Collection and testing of fleas from rodents, nests and burrows may also be appropriate.

   3) Rat control on ships and docks and in warehouses by rat-proofing or periodic fumigation, combined when necessary with destruction of rats and their fleas in vessels and

in cargoes, especially containerized cargoes, before shipment and upon arrival from plague locations.

4) Active immunization with a vaccine of killed bacteria confers protection in most recipients for at least several months when administered in a primary series of 2 or 3 doses; booster injections are necessary. Vaccination of persons living in areas of high incidence and of laboratory and field workers handling plague bacilli or infected animals is justifiable but should not be relied upon as the sole preventive measure. Live attenuated vaccines are used in some countries but they produce more reactions and there is no evidence that they are more protective.

B. Control of patient, contacts and the immediate environment:

1) Report to local health authority: Case report of suspect and confirmed cases universally required by International Health Regulations, Class 1 (see Preface).

2) Isolation: Rid patient, and especially his clothing and baggage, of fleas using an insecticide effective against local fleas and known to be safe for people; hospitalize if practical. For patients with bubonic plague, if there is no cough and the chest x-ray is negative, drainage/ secretion precautions are indicated for 3 days after start of effective therapy. **For patients with pneumonic plague, strict isolation with precautions against airborne spread is required** until 3 full days of appropriate antibiotic therapy have been completed and there has been a favorable clinical response. (See 9B7, below).

3) Concurrent disinfection: Of sputum and purulent discharges and articles soiled therewith. Terminal cleaning. Bodies of persons dying of plague should be handled with strict aseptic precautions.

4) Quarantine: Those who have been in household or face-to-face contact with patients with pneumonic plague should be provided chemoprophylaxis (see 9B5) and placed under surveillance for 7 days; those who refuse chemoprophylaxis should be maintained in strict isolation with careful surveillance for 7 days.

5) Protection of contacts: In epidemic situations, contacts of bubonic plague cases, particularly where human fleas are known to be involved, should be disinfested with an appropriate insecticide. All close contacts should be evaluated for chemoprophylaxis. Close contacts of confirmed or suspected plague pneumonia cases (including medical personnel) should be provided chemoprophylaxis using

tetracycline (15–30 mg/kg) or sulfonamides (40 mg/kg) daily in 4 divided doses for one week.

6) Investigation of contacts and source of infection: Search for persons with household or face-to-face exposure to pneumonic plague and for sick or dead rodents and their fleas. Flea control must precede or coincide with antirodent measures. Dust rodent runs, harborages and burrows in and about known or suspected plague foci with an insecticide labeled for flea control and known to be effective against local fleas. If nonburrowing wild rodents are involved, insecticide bait stations can be used. If urban rats are involved, disinfest by dusting the houses, outhouses and household furnishings; dust the persons and clothing of all residents in the immediate vicinity. Suppress rat populations by well-planned and energetic campaigns of poisoning and with vigorous concurrent measures to reduce rat harborages and food sources.

7) Specific treatment: Streptomycin, tetracyclines and chloramphenicol used early (within 8–24 hours after onset of pneumonic plague) are highly effective. After a satisfactory response to drug therapy, some patients will have a self-limited brief febrile episode on the 5th or 6th day, unaccompanied by any other evidence of illness. Reappearance of fever may result from a secondary infection or a suppurative bubo which may require incision and drainage.

C. Epidemic measures:

1) Investigate all possible plague deaths, with autopsy and laboratory examinations when indicated. Develop and carry out case-finding. Establish the best possible facilities for diagnosis and treatment. Alert existing medical facilities to report cases immediately and utilize diagnostic and therapeutic services fully.

2) Attempt to mitigate public hysteria by appropriate informational and educational releases through the press and news media.

3) Institute intensive flea control in expanding circles from known foci.

4) Implement rodent destruction within affected areas only **after satisfactory flea control has been accomplished.**

5) Protect all contacts as noted in 9B5, above.

6) Protect field workers against fleas; dust clothing with insecticide powder and use insect repellents daily.

D. *Disaster implications:* Plague could become a significant problem in endemic areas when there are social upheavals, crowding and unhygienic conditions. See preceding and following paragraphs for appropriate actions.

E. *International measures:*

1) Telegraphic notification by governments to WHO and to adjacent countries of the first imported, first transferred or first nonimported case of plague in any area previously free of the disease. Report newly discovered or reactivated foci of plague among rodents.

2) Measures applicable to ships, aircraft, and land transport arriving from plague areas are specified in International Health Regulations (1969), Third Annotated Edition, 1983, WHO, Geneva.

3) All ships should be free of rodents or periodically de-ratted.

4) Ratproof buildings at seaports and airports; apply appropriate insecticide; de-rat with effective rodenticide.

5) International travelers: International regulations require that prior to their departure on an international voyage from an area where there is an epidemic of pulmonary plague, those suspect shall be placed in isolation for 6 days after last exposure. On arrival of an infected or suspected ship or an infected aircraft, travelers may be disinsected and kept under surveillance for a period of not more than 6 days from the date of arrival. Vaccination against plague cannot be required as a condition of admission to a territory.

6) WHO Collaborating Centres (see Preface).

PNEUMONIA
I. PNEUMOCOCCAL PNEUMONIA   ICD-9 481

1. Identification—An acute bacterial infection characterized typically by sudden onset with a shaking chill, fever, pleural pain, dyspnea, a cough productive of "rusty" sputum and leukocytosis. Onset may be less abrupt, especially in the elderly, and x-rays may provide the first evidence of pneumonia. In infants, vomiting and convulsions may be the initial manifestations. Consolidation may be bronchopneumonic, especially in children and the aged, rather than segmental or lobar. Pneumococcal pneumonia is an important cause of death in infants and the aged. Fatality, formerly 20–40% among hospitalized patients, has fallen to 5–10% with antimicrobial therapy, but remains 20–40% among patients with substantial underlying disease.

Early etiologic diagnosis is important for treatment. The diagnosis can be suspected from the presence of many gram-positive diplococci together with polymorphonuclear leukocytes in smears of sputum; it can be confirmed by isolation of pneumococci from blood or from secretions aspirated from the lower respiratory tract.

2. Infectious agent—*Streptococcus pneumoniae* (pneumococcus). Twenty-three capsular types out of 83 known serologic types account for approximately 90% of infections in the USA.

3. Occurrence—A disease of continuing endemicity, particularly in infancy, old age and alcoholics; more frequent in industrial cities and lower socioeconomic groups. It occurs in all climates and seasons; incidence is highest in winter and spring in temperate zones. Usually sporadic in the USA, it may occur in epidemics in closed populations and during rapid urbanization. Recurring epidemics have been described in S African miners; incidence is high in certain geographic areas, e.g., Papua New Guinea. An increased incidence often accompanies epidemics of viral respiratory disease, especially influenza.

4. Reservoir—Man. Pneumococci are commonly found in the upper respiratory tract of healthy persons throughout the world.

5. Mode of transmission—By droplet spread; by direct oral contact; or indirectly, through articles freshly soiled with respiratory discharges. Person-to-person transmission of the organisms is common, but illness among casual contacts and attendants is infrequent.

6. Incubation period—Not well determined; believed to be 1–3 days.

7. Period of communicability—Presumably until discharges of mouth and nose no longer contain virulent pneumococci in significant numbers. Penicillin will render the patient noninfectious within 24–48 hours.

8. Susceptibility and resistance—Resistance is generally high but may be lowered by any process affecting the anatomic or physiologic integrity of the lower respiratory tract, including viral respiratory infection, pulmonary edema of any cause, aspiration following alcoholic intoxication or other causes, chronic lung disease or exposure to irritants in the air. Resistance is also reduced in those who have functional or surgical asplenia. Immunity, specific for the infecting capsular serotype, usually follows an attack and may last for years.

9. Methods of control—

A. *Preventive measures:*

1) Avoid crowding in living quarters whenever practical, particularly in institutions, barracks or ships.

2) Administer polyvalent vaccine containing the capsular polysaccharides of the 23 pneumococcal types causing 90% of all bacteremic pneumococcal infection in the USA, to those at high risk of fatal infection, including individuals over 65 yrs of age. (The vaccine in use in the UK contains the capsular polysaccharides of the 14 most frequently occurring types.) High-risk persons include those with anatomic or functional asplenia, sickle cell disease, or a variety of chronic systemic illnesses including heart and lung disease, cirrhosis of the liver, renal insufficiency and diabetes. Because risk of infection and the case fatality rates increase with age, benefits of immunization increase with increasing age. Pneumococcal vaccine **should be given only once to adults** because local and systemic reactions are more frequent and more severe among adults revaccinated with a second dose. Those who have received the 14–valent vaccine need not be revaccinated with the 23–valent vaccine. The vaccine is less effective in those under 2 years of age.

B. *Control of patient, contacts and the immediate environment:*

1) Report to local health authority: Obligatory report of epidemics; no individual case report, Class 4 (see Preface).

2) Isolation: None. If antimicrobial-resistant pneumococci are prevalent, contact isolation is warranted.

3) Concurrent disinfection: Of discharges from nose and throat. Terminal cleaning.

4) Quarantine: None.

5) Immunization of contacts: None. (See 9C, below.)

6) Investigation of contacts: Of no practical value.

7) Specific treatment: Penicillin G, parenterally; use eryth-

romycin for those hypersensitive to penicillin. Because pneumococci relatively resistant to penicillin and other antimicrobials have been recognized, the sensitivities of strains isolated from blood or CSF should be determined.

C. *Epidemic measures:* In outbreaks in institutions or in other closed population groups, immunization with a polysaccharide vaccine against the prevailing pneumococcal types should be carried out if available.

D. *Disaster implications:* None.

E. *International measures:* None.

II. MYCOPLASMAL PNEUMONIA ICD-9 483
(Primary atypical pneumonia)

1. **Identification**—Predominantly a febrile lower respiratory infection; less often a pharyngitis that sometimes progresses to bronchitis or pneumonia. Onset is gradual with headache, malaise, cough often paroxysmal, and usually substernal pain (not pleuritic). Sputum, scant at first, may increase later. Early patchy infiltration of the lungs is often more extensive on x-ray than clinical findings suggest. In severe cases the pneumonia may progress from one lobe to another. Leukocytosis occurs after the first week in approximately one-third of cases. Duration of illness varies from a few days to a month or more. Secondary bacterial infection and other complications such as CNS involvement are infrequent and fatalities are rare.

Differentiation is required from pneumonitis due to many other agents: bacteria, adenoviruses, influenza, parainfluenza, measles, Q fever, psittacosis, certain mycoses and tuberculosis.

Diagnosis is based on a rise in antibody titers between acute and convalescent sera. The ESR is almost always very high. Development of cold hemagglutinins (CA) or of agglutinins for *Streptococcus MG,* or both, supports the diagnosis and may occur in one-half to two-thirds of hospitalized cases. The heights of CA titers reflect the severity of the disease. The infectious agent may be cultured on special media.

2. **Infectious agent**—*Mycoplasma pneumoniae,* bacteria of the family of Mycoplasmataceae.

3. **Occurrence**—Worldwide; sporadic, endemic and occasionally epidemic, especially in institutions and military populations. Attack rates vary from 5 to >50/1000/yr in military populations and 1–3/1000/yr in civilians. The incidence is greatest during fall and winter months in temperate climates, with much variation from year to year and in different geographic areas. No selectivity for race or sex. It occurs at all ages but is asymptomatic

or very mild in children under 5 years; recognized disease is most frequent among school-age children and young adults.

4. **Reservoir**—Man.

5. **Mode of transmission**—Probably by droplet inhalation, direct contact with an infected person (probably including those with subclinical infections) or with articles freshly soiled with discharges of nose and throat from an acutely ill and coughing patient. Secondary cases of pneumonia among contacts, family members and attendants are frequent.

6. **Incubation period**—Six to 23 days.

7. **Period of communicability**—Probably less than 10 days; occasionally longer with persisting febrile illness or persistence of the organism in convalescence (as long as 13 weeks is known).

8. **Susceptibility and resistance**—Clinical pneumonia occurs in about 3 to 30% of infections with *M. pneumoniae*, depending on age. Attack varies from mild afebrile pharyngitis to febrile illness involving the upper or lower respiratory tract. Duration of immunity is uncertain. Second attacks of pneumonia may occur. Resistance has been correlated with humoral antibodies which remain for 1 or more years.

9. **Methods of control**—

A. *Preventive measures:* Avoid crowding in living and sleeping quarters whenever possible, especially in institutions, in barracks and on shipboard.

B. *Control of patient, contacts and the immediate environment:*

1) Report to local health authority: Obligatory report of epidemics; no individual case report, Class 4 (see Preface).
2) Isolation: None. Respiratory secretions may be infectious.
3) Concurrent disinfection: Of discharges from nose and throat. Terminal cleaning.
4) Quarantine: None.
5) Immunization of contacts: None.
6) Investigation of contacts: Valuable in detecting treatable clinical disease among family members.
7) Specific treatment: Erythromycin or a tetracycline in severe mycoplasmal pneumonia. Erythromycin is preferred for children under 8 years of age to avoid tetracycline staining of immature teeth. Neither antibiotic eliminates organisms from the pharynx; during treatment erythromycin-resistant mycoplasms may be selected.

C. *Epidemic measures:* No reliably effective measures for control are available.

D. *Disaster implications:* None.

E. *International measures:* WHO Collaborating Centres (see Preface).

III. PNEUMOCYSTIS PNEUMONIA ICD-9 136.3
(Interstitial plasma-cell pneumonia)

1. Identification—An acute to subacute, often fatal pulmonary disease, especially in malnourished, chronically ill or premature infants. In older children and adults it occurs as an opportunistic infection associated with the use of immunosuppressants and diseases of the immune system. It is a major disease problem for persons with acquired immunodeficiency syndrome (see AIDS). Clinically, there is progressive dyspnea, tachypnea and cyanosis; fever may not be present. Auscultatory signs, other than râles, are usually minimal or absent. Chest x-ray typically shows bilateral interstitial infiltrates. Postmortem examination reveals heavy airless lungs, thickened alveolar septa, and foamy material containing clumps of parasites in the alveolar spaces.

Diagnosis is established by demonstration of the causative agent in material from open lung biopsy or lung aspirates or in smears of tracheobronchial mucus. Organisms are stained by methenamine silver, toluidine blue, or Giemsa methods. There are no satisfactory culture or serologic diagnostic methods in routine use at present.

2. Infectious agent—*Pneumocystis carinii,* a protozoan parasite.

3. Occurrence—The disease has been recognized on all continents; may be endemic and epidemic in debilitated, malnourished or immunosuppressed infants. It affects approximately 60% of patients with AIDS.

4. Reservoir—Man. Organisms have been demonstrated in rodents, cattle, dogs and other animals, but the public health significance of these potential sources of infection is unknown.

5. Mode of transmission—Animal-to-animal transmission via the airborne route has been demonstrated in rats. The mode of transmission in man is not known. In one study, approximately 75% of normal individuals were reported to have humoral antibody to *P. carinii* by the age of 4 years, suggesting that subclinical infection is common. Pneumonitis in the compromised host may result from either a reactivation of latent infection, or a newly acquired infection.

6. Incubation period—Unknown. Analysis of data from institutional outbreaks and animal studies indicates that the onset of disease often occurs 1 to 2 months after the institution of immunosuppression.

7. Period of communicability—Unknown.

8. Susceptibility and resistance—Susceptibility is enhanced by prematurity, by chronic debilitating illness, or by disease or therapy in which immune mechanisms are impaired.

9. Methods of control—

A. *Preventive measures:* Prophylaxis with TMP-SMX has proven to be effective (as long as the patient is on the drug) in preventing endogenous reactivation in immunosuppressed patients, especially those treated for lymphatic leukemia and bone marrow transplant patients.

B. *Control of patient, contacts and the immediate environment:*

   1) Report to local health authority: Official report not ordinarily justifiable, Class 5 (see Preface). However, cases occurring in persons with no known underlying cause of immune deficiency should be reported as possible AIDS.

   2) Isolation: None.

   3) Concurrent disinfection: Insufficient knowledge.

   4) Quarantine: None.

   5) Immunization of contacts: None.

   6) Investigation of contacts: None.

   7) Specific treatment: TMP-SMX is the drug of choice. An alternate drug is pentamidine.

C. *Epidemic measures:* Knowledge of source of organism and mode of transmission is so incomplete that there are no generally accepted measures.

D. *Disaster implications:* None.

E. *International measures:* None.

IV. CHLAMYDIAL PNEUMONIA   ICD-9 483
(Pertussoid eosinophilic pneumonia)

1. Identification—A subacute pulmonary disease occurring in early infancy among infants of mothers with infection of the uterine cervix. Clinically the disease is characterized by insidious onset, cough (characteristically staccato), lack of fever, patchy infiltrates on chest x-ray with hyperinflation, eosinophilia, elevated IgM and IgG. A history of neonatal conjunctivitis is present in about 50%. Duration of illness is commonly one to three weeks, but may extend as long as 2 months. No fatalities have been recorded.

Diagnosis is established by cell culture isolation of the causative agent from the posterior nasopharynx. Definitive diagnosis requires demonstration of specific serum antibody at a titer of 1:32 or higher by micro-IF. A high titer of specific IgG antibody supports the diagnosis.

2. Infectious agent—*Chlamydia trachomatis* of immunotypes D-K (excluding immunotypes that cause lymphogranuloma venereum).

3. Occurrence—Probably the worldwide distribution of genital chlamydial infection. The disease has been recognized in the USA and a number of European countries. Epidemics have not been recognized.

4. Reservoir—Man. Experimental infection with *C. trachomatis* has been induced in nonhuman primates and mice, but is not known to occur in nature.

5. Mode of transmission—Transmitted from the infected cervix to an infant during birth, with resultant nasopharyngeal infection (and occasionally chlamydial conjunctivitis). Direct contact or respiratory transmission has not been established.

6. Incubation period—Not known but pneumonia may occur in infants from one to 18 weeks of age (more commonly between 4 and 12 weeks). Nasopharyngeal infection is usually not recognized before 2 weeks of age.

7. Period of communicability—Unknown.

8. Susceptibility and resistance—Unknown. Maternal antibody does not protect the infant from infection.

9. Methods of control—

   A. *Preventive measures:* Same as for Conjunctivitis, Chlamydial.

   B. *Control of patient, contacts and the immediate environment:*

   1) Report to local health authority: Official report not ordinarily justifiable, Class 5 (see Preface).
   2) Isolation: Drainage/secretion precautions.
   3) Concurrent disinfection: Of discharges from nose and throat.
   4) Quarantine: None.
   5) Immunization of contacts: None.
   6) Investigation of contacts: Examine parents for infection and treat if positive.
   7) Specific treatment: Oral erythromycin (50 mg/kg/day) is the drug of choice. Sulfisoxazole is a possible alternative.

   C. *Epidemic measures:* No epidemic occurrence recognized.

   D. *Disaster implications:* None.

   E. *International measures:* None.

OTHER PNEUMONIAS   ICD-9 480, 482

Among the known viruses, the adenoviruses, respiratory syncytial virus, the parainfluenza viruses and probably others as yet unidentified may induce a pneumonitis. Because these infectious agents cause upper respiratory disease more often than pneumonia, they are presented under Respiratory Disease, Acute Viral. Viral pneumonia occurs in measles, influenza and chickenpox. Pneumonia is also caused by infection with chlamydia (psittacosis), rickettsiae (Q fever) and *Legionella*. It can also be associated with the invasive phase of nematode infections such as ascariasis and with mycoses such as aspergillosis, histoplasmosis and coccidioidomycosis.

Various pathogenic bacteria commonly found in the mouth, nose and throat such as *Staphylococcus aureus, Klebsiella pneumoniae, Haemophilus influenzae, Streptococcus pyogenes* (group A hemolytic streptococci), *Neisseria meningitidis* (notably group Y), *Bacteroides* spp. and anaerobic cocci may produce pneumonia, especially in association with viral infections such as influenza, as superinfection following broad-spectrum antibiotic therapy, as complications of chronic pulmonary disease, and after aspiration of gastric contents or tracheostomy. With increased use of antimicrobial and immunosuppressive therapy, pneumonias caused by enteric gram-negative bacilli have become more common, especially those caused by *Escherichia coli, Pseudomonas aeruginosa,* and *Proteus* spp. Management depends on the specific organism involved.

POLIOMYELITIS, ACUTE   ICD-9 045
(Polioviral fever*, Infantile paralysis)

1. Identification—An acute viral infection with severity ranging from inapparent infection to a nonparalytic febrile illness, to an aseptic meningitis, to paralytic disease and possible death. Symptoms include fever, malaise, headache, nausea and vomiting, excruciating muscle pain and spasms, and stiffness of neck and back with or without flaccid paralysis, the hallmark of the disease. Virus multiplies in the alimentary tract; viremia may then follow with invasion of the CNS and selective involvement of motor cells resulting in flaccid paralysis, most commonly of the lower extremities. Paralysis of muscles of respiration and swallowing frequently threatens life. The site of paralysis depends upon location of nerve cell destruction in spinal cord or brain stem, but is characteristically asymmetrical. Nonparalytic poliomyelitis is sometimes manifested as aseptic meningitis (see Meningitis). The incidence of inapparent infections and "minor" illness usually exceeds that of paralytic cases by more than a

hundredfold or even more when infection occurs very early in life. Fatality rates for paralytic cases vary from 2–10% in epidemics and increase markedly with age. Some evidence suggests further weakness may occur infrequently many years after the acute attack.

Paralytic poliomyelitis can usually be recognized on clinical grounds but can be confused with post-infectious polyneuritis and other paralytic conditions. Other enteroviruses (echovirus type 71, and sometimes type 70; coxsackieviruses, especially group A, type 7) can cause illness simulating paralytic poliomyelitis, though usually less severe and with fewer common signs and negligible residual paralysis. Tick-bite paralysis occurs uncommonly but worldwide, manifested by a flaccid ascending motor paralysis which usually disappears promptly when the tick is removed. Guillain-Barré syndrome may resemble paralytic poliomyelitis but fever, headache, nausea, vomiting and pleocytosis are usually absent. Postencephalitic syndromes, cerebral palsy, trauma and some drugs may result in lameness or a flaccid paralysis simulating the residua of poliomyelitis.

The differential diagnosis of acute nonparalytic poliomyelitis includes other forms of acute nonbacterial meningitis, purulent meningitis, brain abscess, tuberculous meningitis, leptospirosis, lymphocytic choriomeningitis, infectious mononucleosis, the encephalitides, and toxic encephalopathies.

The laboratory diagnosis is made by isolation of the virus by inoculating various cell culture systems of human or monkey origin (primate cells) with CSF, fecal material or oropharyngeal secretions. Antibodies may rise so early after paralysis occurs that significant titer rises may not be demonstrable in paired sera; neutralizing antibody tests are generally more helpful than CF antibody tests. Differentiation of "wild" from vaccine strains should be made in developed countries, and other viral causes, such as enteroviruses 70 and 71, excluded.

2. Infectious agent—Poliovirus types 1, 2 and 3; all types cause paralysis. Type 1 is the most paralytogenic, type 3 less frequently, type 2 uncommonly. Most vaccine-associated cases are due to type 2 or 3.

3. Occurrence—Worldwide. Before large-scale immunization programs were carried out, the highest incidence of clinically recognized disease was in temperate zones and in the more developed countries, occurring as sporadic cases and in small epidemics; more common during summer and early autumn in temperate climates but with wide variations from year to year and from region to region. Characteristically a disease of children and adolescents, depending on socioeconomic level. Improvement in living standards may be associated with emergence of paralytic poliomyelitis in older individuals by reducing the frequency of asymptomatic infantile infections and subsequent immunity; this has been observed as rising polio rates where infant mortality rates were falling. In the absence of natural or artificial immunity, adults are affected and their risk of paralysis is greater than in children. Epidemics, formerly uncommon in less developed areas, now occur with increasing frequency, mainly involving infants and young children. In such areas, antibodies to all 3 types of poliovirus are generally present by school age and most paralytic disease occurs before age 3. In countries where polio vaccines have been used extensively, paralytic cases occur chiefly among groups not reached by the immunization program, mainly preschool children of lower social classes and members of religious groups who object to immunization. During 1978 and 1979, poliomyelitis appeared in one such religious group in the Netherlands, then in Canada, and finally affected members of this group within the USA. The use of both live and killed virus vaccines has resulted in a marked decrease in worldwide overall incidence of paralytic disease. During 1976-81 a yearly average of 154 was reported in industrialized Europe. From 1976 to 1983 an annual average of 12 cases was reported in the USA. Many of the cases in developed countries, where wild poliomyelitis transmission has been essentially eradicated, are associated with vaccine virus.

4. **Reservoir**—Man only, most frequently persons with inapparent infections, especially children. Long-term carriers have not been found.

5. **Mode of transmission**—Direct contact through close association. In rare instances milk, foodstuffs and other fecally contaminated materials have been incriminated as vehicles. No reliable evidence of spread by insects or virus-contaminated sewage; water is rarely, if ever, involved. Fecal-oral is the major route of transmission where sanitation is poor, but during epidemics and where sanitation is good, pharyngeal spread becomes relatively more important. Virus is more easily detectable, and for a longer period, in feces than in throat secretions.

6. **Incubation period**—Commonly 7–14 days for paralytic cases, with a range of 3 to possibly 35 days.

7. **Period of communicability**—Not accurately known. Poliovirus is demonstrable in throat secretions as early as 36 hours and in the feces 72 hours after exposure to infection in both clinical and inapparent cases, and virus persists in the throat for approximately 1 week and in the feces for 3–6 weeks or longer. Cases are probably most infectious during the first few days before and after onset of symptoms.

8. **Susceptibility and resistance**—Susceptibility to infection is general but paralytic infections are rare, increasing in frequency with age at the time of infection. Type-specific resistance of lifelong duration follows both clinically recognizable and inapparent infection. Second attacks are rare and result from infection with poliovirus of a different type. Infants born of immune mothers have transient passive immunity to paralysis. Tonsil-

lectomy increases the risk of bulbar involvement; injection of precipitated antigens or certain other insoluble substances may provoke paralysis in an already infected but symptom-free person, the paralysis tending to be localized in the affected limb or appearing there first. Excessive muscular fatigue in the prodromal period may likewise predispose to paralytic involvement of the exercised limb. An increased susceptibility to paralytic poliomyelitis is associated with pregnancy.

9. Methods of control—

A. *Preventive measures:*

1) Currently both noninfectious inactivated poliovirus vaccine (IPV) given by injection, and live attenuated poliovirus vaccine (OPV) preparations given orally are commercially available and in wide use. Their use varies in different countries: some use IPV alone, some OPV alone, a few use a combination. In the USA, OPV is preferred because it simulates natural infection and induces both circulating antibody and intestinal resistance and by secondary spread protects susceptible contacts. In some developing countries poor serologic response to OPV has been reported; this may be due to breaks in the cold chain (so that the vaccine was permitted to warm and deteriorate), presence of diarrhea that excretes the virus before it can attach to the mucosal cell, interference with intestinal infection by other enteroviruses, or other unknown factors. IPV blocks pharyngeal excretion but does not prevent intestinal infection though it may limit its duration. Its use in combination with diphtheria-tetanus-pertussis (DTP) vaccine has been suggested as an alternative to or in addition to OPV in developing countries where vaccine failures have been observed after vaccination with OPV. The WHO currently recommends OPV for routine use in the Expanded Program of Immunization.

a) OPV—In the USA, recommendations for trivalent, live, oral poliovirus vaccine (OPV) for primary immunization in infants are integrated with DTP immunization so that the first dose is given with the first DTP inoculation at 6–12 wks of age. A second dose should be given about 2 months later; a 3rd dose 6–12 months after the second usually provides protection against all 3 poliovirus types in most recipients. An additional OPV dose is recommended for children on entry into elementary school to ensure that all are protected. No additional "boosters" are currently recommended except in situations of possible increased exposure to wild poliovirus, such as in travelers to endemic areas. In endemic areas, such as tropical and developing countries, the basic course should be given to infants during the first 14 weeks of life because true "infantile paralysis" usually occurs in the 6–21 month age group in these settings. For children and adolescents (up to the 18th birthday) in nonendemic areas, primary immunization consists of 2 doses of OPV at 8–wk intervals and a third dose 6 months to a year later.

Contraindications to OPV include individuals with immune deficiency states (B-lymphocyte deficiency, thymic dysplasia), those receiving current immunosuppressive therapy, those in disease states associated with immunosuppresssion (lymphoma, leukemia, generalized malignancy), or siblings of an immunodeficient individual. (IPV can be used in such persons.) Diarrhea should not be considered a contraindication to OPV, but the dose should not be counted and another dose given at the first opportunity, since the diarrhea might have interfered with immunization. Cases of paralytic poliomyelitis have been associated with the vaccine strains in vaccine recipients or their healthy contacts. This occurs approximately once per 3 million OPV doses distributed. In the USA, twice as many OPV-associated cases have occurred among contacts of recipients as among recipients; the incidence is higher in adults than in children.

b) IPV—Formalin-inactivated vaccine (IPV) containing all 3 polio types is given parenterally. In infancy, the primary schedule is usually integrated with DTP immunization by use of a combined vaccine or by concurrent injection. The first 3 doses are given at 1–2 month intervals and the 4th dose 6–12 months after the 3rd. IPV is indicated for those with contraindications to OPV (see 9A1a, above). Booster doses every 5 yrs are necessary for the IPV licensed in the USA. A more potent vaccine has been licensed in France which might require fewer doses.

c) Immunization of adults: Routine immunization for adults residing in the continental USA and Canada is not considered necessary but a completed series of

OPV or a dose of IPV is advised for adults traveling to developing countries, for members of communities or population groups in which poliovirus disease is present, for laboratory workers who may handle specimens containing poliovirus, and for health care workers who may be exposed to patients excreting polioviruses. Because of the slightly higher risk of vaccine-associated paralysis, IPV is preferred for primary immunization of adults, giving 2 doses of the current vaccine with a 1–2 month interval. Those who have previously completed a course of immunization and now will be under increased risk of exposure may be given an additional dose of either IPV or OPV. If OPV is to be used in a household with documented nonimmune adults, consideration should be given to the administration of 1 or preferably 2 doses of IPV one month apart to these adults before the infant is immunized, provided the immunization of the infant is assured and is not unnecessarily delayed.

2) Educate the public on the advantages of immunization in early childhood, and on modes of spread.

B. Control of patient, contacts and the immediate environment:

1) Report to local health authority: Obligatory case report of paralytic cases as a Disease under Surveillance by WHO, Class 1A. Each case is to be designated as paralytic. Supplemental reports giving vaccine history and vaccine lot number if vaccine-associated, virus type, severity and persistence of residual paralysis 60 days or longer after onset are necessary measures for effective control. Nonparalytic cases, Class 2A (see Preface).

2) Isolation: Enteric precautions in hospital. Of little value under home conditions because the greatest risk of spread of infection had been in the prodromal period.

3) Concurrent disinfection: Of throat discharges and feces and of articles soiled therewith. In communities with modern and adequate sewage disposal systems, feces and urine can be discharged directly into sewers without preliminary disinfection. Terminal cleaning.

4) Quarantine: Of no community value because of large numbers of unrecognized infections in the population.

5) Protection of contacts: Vaccination of familial and other close contacts contributes little to immediate control; ordinarily the virus has already infected susceptible contacts by the time the first case is recognized. In countries

with zero or near zero prevalence, occurrence of a single non-vaccine-associated paralytic case in a community should prompt an immediate investigation. If wild poliovirus is implicated and at least 2 cases are associated by time and place, an immunization program designed to contain spread should be initiated, using a trivalent OPV.

6) Investigation of contacts: Thorough search for sick persons, especially children, to assure early detection and to facilitate control and permit appropriate treatment of unrecognized and unreported cases. Foot drop, scoliosis and other deformities resulting in functional impairment may be late manifestations of initially mild or inapparent illness.

7) Specific treatment: None; attention during the acute illness to the complications of paralysis requires expert knowledge, especially for patients in need of respiratory assistance.

C. *Epidemic measures:*

1) Institute mass vaccination with oral vaccine at the earliest indication of an outbreak. Trivalent vaccines are fully effective in controlling outbreaks and should be put into use immediately. Seek to achieve the most rapid and complete immunization of epidemiologically relevant groups, especially younger children in developing countries. Establish vaccination centers in relation to population densities, taking advantage of normal social patterns; schools often meet these criteria.

2) With the use of mass immunization, it is no longer necessary to disrupt community activities by closing schools and other places of population aggregation.

3) Postpone elective surgery, especially nose and throat operations, and elective immunizations until after the epidemic has ended.

4) Provide strategically located centers for specialized medical care of acutely ill patients and rehabilitation of those with significant paralysis.

D. *Disaster implications:* Overcrowding of nonimmune groups, together with inadequate sewage disposal facilities, poses a threat of an epidemic outbreak.

E. *International measures:*

1) Poliomyelitis is a Disease under Surveillance by WHO. National health administrations are expected to inform

WHO of outbreaks promptly by telegram or telex, and to supplement these reports as soon as possible with details of the source, nature and extent of the epidemic and of the identity of the type of epidemic virus involved.

2) International travelers visiting areas of prevalence should be adequately immunized.

3) WHO Collaborating Centres (see Preface).

PSITTACOSIS
(Ornithosis, Parrot fever)

ICD-9 073

1. Identification—An acute generalized chlamydial disease with variable clinical presentations; fever, headache, myalgia, chills and upper or lower respiratory tract disease are common. Respiratory symptoms are often disproportionately mild compared to the extensive pneumonia demonstrable by x-ray. Cough is initially absent or non-productive; when present, sputum is mucopurulent, not copious; pleuritic chest pain and splenomegaly occur infrequently; the pulse is usually slow in relation to temperature. Lethargy, encephalitis, myocarditis, and thrombophlebitis are occasional complications; occasional relapses occur. Although often mild or moderate in character, human infections may be severe, with high case fatality rates, especially in untreated older persons.

Laboratory diagnosis is made by demonstrating significant increase in specific antibodies during convalescence; or, under suitably safe laboratory conditions only, by isolation of the infectious agent from sputum, blood or postmortem tissues in mice, eggs, or tissue culture. Recovery of the agent may be difficult, especially if the patient has received broad-spectrum antibiotics.

2. Infectious agent—*Chlamydia psittaci.*

3. Occurrence—Worldwide. Often associated with sick or healthy-looking pet birds. Outbreaks occasionally occur in individual households, pet shops, aviaries and pigeon lofts. Turkey and duck farms and processing and rendering plants have been sources of occupational disease. Most human cases are sporadic; infections are probably frequently not recognized.

4. Reservoir—Parakeets, parrots, pigeons, turkeys, ducks and other birds. Apparently healthy birds can be carriers and occasionally shed the infectious agent, particularly when subjected to the stresses of crowding and shipping.

5. Mode of transmission—Infection is usually acquired by inhaling the agent from desiccated droppings and secretions of infected birds in an enclosed space or directly from infected birds or squab, turkey and duck farms and in poultry processing plants. Turkeys are usually involved but ducks and pigeons are occasionally responsible for human disease. Geese have been known to be infected in Europe. Household birds are a frequent source; laboratory infections have occurred. Transmission from person to person is rare; personnel attending patients with paroxysmal coughing may be infected.

6. **Incubation period**—From 4–15 days, commonly 10 days.

7. **Period of communicability**—Diseased as well as seemingly healthy birds may shed the agent intermittently and sometimes continuously for weeks or months. The rare person-to-person transmission can occur with paroxysmal coughing during the acute illness.

8. **Susceptibility and resistance**—Susceptibility is general; older adults have a more severe illness; immunity following infection is incomplete and transitory. No evidence that persons with antibody at any given level have protection.

9. **Methods of control**—

   A. Preventive measures:

   1) Regulate importing, raising and trafficking of birds of the parrot family to prevent or eliminate infections by quarantine and appropriate antibiotic treatment.

   2) Psittacine birds offered in commerce should be raised under psittacosis-free conditions and handled in such manner as to prevent infection. Tetracycline can be effective in controlling disease in parakeets, parrots and pigeons if properly administered to ensure adequate intake.

   3) Surveillance of pet shops and aviaries where psittacosis has occurred or where birds epidemiologically linked to cases were obtained, and of farms or processing plants to which human psittacosis was traced epidemiologically. Infected birds should be treated or destroyed and the room or area where they had been housed thoroughly cleaned and disinfected with a phenolic compound.

   4) Educate the public in the danger of household or occupational exposure to infected birds of the parrot family. Medical personnel responsible for occupational health in processing plants should be aware that pneumonic disease among the workers may be psittacosis.

   B. Control of patient, contacts and the immediate environment:

1) Report to local health authority: Obligatory case report in most states and countries, Class 2A (see Preface).
2) Isolation: None. Coughing patients should be instructed to cough into paper tissue.
3) Concurrent disinfection: Of all discharges. Terminal cleaning.
4) Quarantine: Of infected farms or premises with infected pet birds until diseased birds have been destroyed or adequately treated with tetracycline and the buildings disinfected.
5) Immunization of contacts: None.
6) Investigation of contacts and source of infection: Trace origin of suspected birds. Kill suspect birds and immerse bodies in 2% phenolic or equivalent disinfectant. Place in plastic bag, close securely, and ship frozen (on dry ice) to nearest competent laboratory. If suspect birds cannot be killed, swab-cultures of their cloacae or droppings should be shipped to the laboratory in appropriate transport media and shipping container.
7) Specific treatment: Antibiotics of the tetracycline group, continued for 10–14 days after temperature returns to normal.

C. *Epidemic measures:* Epidemics related to infected aviaries or bird suppliers may be difficult to recognize but may be extensive. Reported cases are usually sporadic or confined to family outbreaks, but should be investigated if more extensive outbreaks or epizootics among birds are to be recognized. Report outbreaks of psittacosis in flocks of turkeys to state agriculture and health authorities. Large doses of tetracyclines will suppress but may not eliminate infection in poultry flocks and may complicate investigations.

D. *Disaster implications:* None.

E. *International measures:* Reciprocal compliance with national regulations to control importation of psittacine birds.

Q FEVER
(Query fever)

ICD-9 083.0

1. Identification—An acute febrile rickettsial disease; onset may be sudden with chills, retrobulbar headache, weakness, malaise and severe

sweats; much variation in severity and duration. A pneumonitis occurs in many cases with cough, scanty expectoration, chest pain and minimal physical findings. Acute pericarditis, acute hepatitis and generalized infections have been reported. Chronic endocarditis can occur in those with damaged heart valves or valve replacements. Inapparent infections occur. Case fatality rate in untreated cases is <1% and with treatment is negligible except in elderly persons and individuals who develop endocarditis or hepatitis.

Laboratory diagnosis is made by demonstration of rise in specific antibodies between acute and convalescent stages by IF, microagglutination or CF; high titers of Phase I antibodies may indicate chronic infection such as subacute rickettsial endocarditis. Recovery of the infectious agent from blood of patients is diagnostic but poses a hazard to laboratory workers.

2. **Infectious agent**—*Coxiella burnetii (Rickettsia burneti)*, an organism with unusual stability in the free state.

3. **Occurrence**—Reported from all continents; the incidence is greater than that reported because of limited clinical suspicion and few laboratories testing for it. It is endemic in many areas, affecting veterinarians, meat workers, dairy workers and farmers. Explosive epidemics have occurred among workers in stockyards, meat packing and rendering plants, in diagnostic laboratories, in medical centers which use sheep in research and also where no direct animal contact can be demonstrated. Cases are very common among researchers working with *C. burnetii*. Casual visitors often become infected.

4. **Reservoir**—Cattle, sheep, goats, ticks and some wild animals (bandicoots) are natural reservoirs. Infected domestic animals are usually asymptomatic but shed massive numbers of organisms at parturition.

5. **Mode of transmission**—Commonly by airborne dissemination of rickettsiae in dust from premises contaminated by placental tissues, birth fluids and excreta of infected animals, in establishments processing infected animals or their by-products, and in necropsy rooms. Airborne particles containing organisms may be carried downwind for a considerable distance (half a mile or more). Also contracted by direct contact with infected animals or other contaminated materials such as wool, straw, fertilizer and the laundry of exposed persons. Raw milk from infected cows has been responsible for some cases.

6. **Incubation period**—Depends on the size of the infecting dose; usually 2–3 weeks.

7. **Period of communicability**—Direct transmission from person to person is very rare, but may occur in cases of pneumonia.

8. Susceptibility and resistance—Susceptibility is general. Immunity following recovery from clinical illness is probably lifelong.

9. Methods of control—

A. *Preventive measures:*

1) Health education on sources of infection and the necessity for adequate disinfection and disposal of animal products of conception and strict hygienic measures in cow and sheep sheds and barns and in laboratories (dust, urine, feces, rodents) and for hygienic practices such as pasteurization of milk.

2) Pasteurization of milk from cows, goats and sheep at 62.8°C (145°F) for 30 minutes or at 71.7°C (161°F) for 15 seconds, or boiling, inactivates rickettsiae.

3) Immunization with inactivated vaccine prepared from *C. burnetii* (Phase I)-infected yolk sac is useful in protecting laboratory workers and is strongly recommended for those working with live *C. burnetii*. It might also be considered for others in hazardous occupations. Vaccine should not be used in individuals with a positive CF or a history suggestive of Q fever unless preceded by a sensitivity skin test with a small dose of vaccine to avoid severe local reactions. Vaccine may be obtained by contacting the commanding officer, US Army Medical Research Institute of Infectious Diseases, Frederick MD, 21701.

4) Research workers using sheep should be immunized and should manage the animals and the research studies with the assumption that the sheep are excreting rickettsiae; preferably in facilities away from populated areas and allowing no visitors. Vaccination of sheep has been reported to reduce markedly the shedding of rickettsiae.

B. *Control of patient, contacts and the immediate environment:*

1) Report to local health authority: In the USA, in areas where disease is endemic; in many countries not a reportable disease, Class 3B (see Preface).

2) Isolation: None.

3) Concurrent disinfection: Of sputum and blood and articles freshly soiled therewith. Precautions at postmortem examination of suspected cases in humans or animals.

4) Quarantine: None.

5) Immunization of contacts: Unnecessary.

6) Investigation of contacts and source of infection: Search for history of contact with cattle, sheep or goats on farms

or in research facilities, consumption of raw milk, or direct or indirect association with a laboratory which handles *C. burnetii.*

7) Specific treatment: Tetracyclines administered orally and continued for several days after the patient is afebrile; reinstitute if relapse occurs. Chloramphenicol and rifampicin may be effective. For chronic endocarditis, tetracycline combined with lincomycin may be effective.

C. *Epidemic measures:* Outbreaks are generally of short duration; control measures are limited essentially to elimination of sources of infection, observation of exposed persons and antibiotic therapy for those becoming ill.

D. *Disaster implications:* None.

E. *International measures:* Control of importation of goats, sheep and cattle. WHO Collaborating Centres (see Preface).

RABIES   ICD-9 071
(Hydrophobia, Lyssa)

1. **Identification**—An almost invariably fatal acute viral encephalomyelitis; onset is with a sense of apprehension, headache, fever, malaise, and indefinite sensory changes often referred to the site of a preceding animal bite wound. The disease progresses to paresis or paralysis; spasm of muscles of deglutition on attempts to swallow leads to fear of water (hydrophobia); delirium and convulsions follow. Usual duration is 2 to 6 days, sometimes longer; death is often due to respiratory paralysis.

Other diseases resulting from animal bites include pasteurellosis *(Pasteurella multocida* and *P. haemolytica)* from cat and dog bites; B-virus *(Herpesvirus simiae)* from monkey bites; encephalitis, especially due to other rhabdoviruses such as Duvenhage virus; tularemia; rat-bite fever; cat-scratch fever; plague; and tetanus, as well as pyogenic infections.

Diagnosis is confirmed by specific FA staining of brain tissue or by virus isolation in mouse or tissue culture systems. Presumptive diagnosis may be made by specific FA staining of frozen skin sections, corneal impressions, or mucosal scrapings. Serologic diagnosis is based on neutralization tests in mice or tissue culture, or by CF test.

2. **Infectious agent**—Rabies virus, a rhabdovirus. Related viruses that exist in Africa (Mokola and Duvenhage) and Europe (Duvenhage) are associated with fatal rabies-like human illness. Some of these illnesses might be diagnosed as rabies by the standard FA test.

3. **Occurrence**—Worldwide. Uncommon in man. In the five years 1979–1983, 9 deaths occurred in the USA; 5 cases were acquired within the country, 3 were acquired elsewhere and the place of acquisition of the last case was not clearly defined. In 1984, three deaths had occurred by October 15, two indigenous and one imported. Rabies is primarily a disease of animals. The only areas free of rabies in the animal population at present include Australia, New Zealand, Japan, Hawaii, Taiwan and other Pacific Islands, UK, Ireland, Spain, Portugal, mainland Norway, Sweden, and some of the West Indies and Atlantic islands. Urban rabies is a problem of dogs and cats; sylvatic or rural rabies is a disease of wild carnivores and bats, with sporadic disease among dogs, cats, and livestock. In the USA and Canada wildlife rabies is increasing in raccoons; in Europe, fox rabies is widespread.

4. **Reservoir**—Many wild and domestic Canidae, including dogs, foxes, coyotes, wolves and jackals; also cats, skunks, raccoons, mongooses, and other biting mammals. Vampire, fruit-eating, and insectivorous bats are infected in Central and S America and Mexico, while infected insectivorous bats are found in the USA, Canada and Europe. In the lesser developed countries, dogs remain the principal reservoir. Rabbits, squirrels, chipmunks, rats and mice are rarely infected and their bites rarely, if ever, call for rabies prophylaxis.

5. **Mode of transmission**—Virus-laden saliva of a rabid animal is introduced by a bite (or into a fresh break in the skin or rarely through intact mucous membranes) or very rarely by a scratch. Transmission from person to person is possible since the saliva of the infected human may contain virus, but has been documented only via corneal transplants taken from persons dying of undiagnosed CNS disease. Airborne spread has been demonstrated in caves where millions of bats were roosting and in laboratory settings, but this occurs very rarely. In Latin America, transmission from infected vampire bats to domestic animals is common. In the USA the rôle of indigenous bats in the transmission of rabies to other animals in the wild has not been established.

6. **Incubation period**—Usually 2 to 8 weeks, occasionally as short as 10 days or as long as a year or more; depends on the severity of the wound, site of the wound in relation to richness of nerve supply and distance from the brain, amount of virus introduced, protection provided by clothing and other factors.

7. **Period of communicability**—In dogs and cats, for 3 to 5 days before onset of clinical signs and during the course of the disease. Very rarely, longer periods of excretion before onset of symptoms have been observed; the significance of these observations is unknown. Bats may shed virus for 2 weeks before evidence of illness.

8. Susceptibility and resistance—All warm-blooded mammals are susceptible. Natural immunity in man is unknown.

9. Methods of control—

   A.   Preventive measures:

      1)   Registration and licensing of all dogs; collection and destruction of ownerless animals and strays may be indicated. Preventive vaccination of all dogs and cats. Education of pet owners and the public that restrictions for dogs and cats are necessary, e.g., leashed in congested areas when not confined on owner's premises; that strange-acting or sick animals of any species, domestic or wild, may be dangerous and should not be picked up or handled; that it is necessary to report such animals and animals that have bitten a person or another animal to the police and/or the local health department; that confinement and observation of such animals is a preventive measure against rabies; and that wild animals should not be kept as pets.

      2)   Ten-day detention and clinical observation of dogs and cats known to have bitten a person or showing suspicious signs of rabies; alternatively, unwanted dogs and cats may be killed immediately and examined for rabies by fluorescent microscopy. Valuable dogs or cats need not be killed until existence of rabies is reasonably established by clinical signs. If the animal were infective at the time of the bite, signs of rabies will follow usually within 5 days, with a change in behavior, and excitability or paralysis, followed by death. Wild animals should be sacrificed immediately and the brain examined for evidence of rabies. In the case of bites by a normal-behaving very valuable zoo animal, it may be appropriate to consider postexposure prophylaxis for the victim as an alternative to sacrificing the animal.

      3)   Immediate submission to a laboratory of intact heads packed in ice (not frozen) of animals that die of suspected rabies for testing for viral antigen by FA staining, or, if not available, by microscopy for Negri bodies.

      4)   Unvaccinated dogs or cats bitten by known rabid animals should be destroyed immediately; if detention is elected, hold the animal in an approved pound or kennel for at least 6 months and vaccinate against rabies 30 days before release. If previously vaccinated, revaccinate and detain (leashing and confinement) for at least 90 days.

      5)   Institution of cooperative programs with wildlife conservation authorities to reduce fox, skunk, and other terrestrial

wildlife hosts of sylvatic rabies in enzootic areas near campsites or areas of human habitation.

6) Individuals at high risk, e.g., veterinarians and wildlife conservation personnel in enzootic areas, staff of quarantine kennels, laboratory and field personnel working with rabies, should receive preexposure immunization. One type of vaccine is currently available in the USA—human diploid cell rabies vaccine (HDCV), an inactivated virus vaccine prepared from virus grown in human diploid cells. HDCV is given in three 1–ml i.m. doses on days 0, 7 and 21 or 28; this regimen has been so satisfactory that routine postvaccination serology is not recommended. If risk of exposure continues, either single booster doses are given or serum tested for neutralizing antibody every 2 years. Intradermal administration of three 0.1–ml doses of HDCV manufactured by Merieux can be substituted for the three 1–ml doses used for preexposure immunization. Results in the USA have generally been good, but the mean antibody response is somewhat lower and may be of shorter duration than with the 1.0–ml dose given i.m. Antibody response in some groups given intradermal vaccine outside the USA has been erratic for unknown reasons and therefore intradermal immunization should not be used unless facilities are available for testing sera for development of neutralizing antibodies.

7) Prevention of rabies after animal bites is based on physical removal of the virus by proper management of the bite wound and on specific immunological protection.

a) Treatment of bite wound: The most effective rabies prevention is immediate thorough cleansing and flushing with soap or detergent and water of all wounds caused by an animal bite or scratch. The wound should not be sutured unless unavoidable for cosmetic or tissue support reasons. Sutures should be placed after local infiltration of antiserum (see 9A7b, below), should be loose, and should not interfere with free bleeding and drainage.

b) Immunologic prevention of rabies in man is by administering rabies immune globulin (RIG) to neutralize the virus in the bite wound, and by giving vaccine as soon as possible after exposure to develop active immunity.

Passive immunization: RIG should be used in a single dose of 20 I.U./kg; half should be infiltrated around the bite wound if possible, and the rest given i.m. If serum of animal origin is used, an intradermal or s.c. test dose should precede its administration to detect allergic sensitivity and the dose increased to a total of 40 I.U./kg.

Vaccine: Preferably HDCV in five 1–ml i.m. doses in the deltoid region; the first as soon as possible after the bite (at the same time as the single dose of RIG is given) and the other doses 3, 7, 14 and 28 days after the first dose. In individuals with possible immunodeficiency, a serum specimen should be collected at the time the last dose of vaccine is administered and forwarded for testing for rabies antibodies. A reinforcing dose is recommended by WHO on day 90. If sensitization reactions appear in the course of immunization, consult health department or infectious disease consultants for guidance. If the person has had a previous full course of antirabies inoculations with HDCV, or had developed neutralizing antibody after preexposure immunization (9A6, above), or other postexposure regimen, only 2 doses of HDCV need to be given, one immediately and the second 3 days later. No RIG is given with this regimen.

c) The following is a guide to prophylaxis in different circumstances: If a bite were unprovoked, the animal not apprehended, and rabies is present in that species in the area, administer RIG and vaccine. Bites of wild carnivorous mammals or bats would be considered potential rabies exposures unless negated by laboratory tests. If available, the biting animal may be killed immediately (with the owner's and health authorities' concurrence) and its brain examined by the FA technique to determine whether antirabies treatment is necessary. Dogs or cats may be confined and observed for 10 days (see 9A2, above). The decision to administer RIG and vaccine immediately after exposure or during the observation period should be based on the behavior of the animal, the presence of rabies in the area, and the circumstances of the bite.

d) Rabies vaccination carries a very small risk of post-vaccinal encephalitis; only 2 cases of transient neuroparalytic illness have been reported. Local reactions such as pain, erythema, swelling or itching at the injection site were reported in 25% of those receiving five 1.0–ml doses. Mild systemic reactions of headache, nausea, muscle aches, abdominal pain and dizziness were reported by about 20%. "Serum sickness-like" reactions, including primarily urticaria with generalized itching, and wheezing were reported infrequently.

However, among those receiving booster doses for preexposure prophylaxis, hypersensitivity reactions occurring 2 to 21 days after HDCV presenting as a generalized pruritic rash, urticaria, possible arthralgia, arthritis, angioedema, nausea, vomiting, fever and malaise, have increased in frequency, occurring in approximately 7% of recipients. These symptoms have responded to antihistamines; a few have required corticosteroids or epinephrine, and indicate that booster injections should be given in facilities equipped to handle anaphylactic reactions. Persons who have been exposed to rabies who develop these symptoms should complete the required number of injections but in a setting where such a reaction can be treated. No significant reactions have been attributed to RIG; antiserum from a nonhuman source produces serum sickness in up to 40% of recipients. These risks must be weighed against the risk of contracting rabies. No antirabies treatment is indicated unless the skin is broken or a mucosal surface has been contaminated by the animal's saliva.

e) Management of an animal bite, adapted from the Sixth Report of the WHO Expert Committee on Rabies, the Working Group 2, WHO, 1978, and from the USPHS Advisory Committee on Immunization Practices (1984), is:

CHECKLIST OF TREATMENTS FOR ANIMAL BITES

1. Cleanse and Flush Wound Immediately (First Aid).
2. Thorough Wound Cleansing Under Medical Supervision.
3. Rabies Immune Globulin and/or Vaccine as Indicated.
4. Tetanus Prophylaxis and Antibacterial Treatment When Required.
5. No Sutures or Wound Closure Advised Unless Unavoidable.

B. *Control of patient, contacts and the immediate environment:*

1) Report to local health authority: Obligatory case report required in most states and countries, Class 2A (see Preface).
2) Isolation: Contact isolation for respiratory secretions for duration of the illness.
3) Concurrent disinfection: Of saliva and articles soiled

RABIES POSTEXPOSURE PROPHYLAXIS GUIDE*

The following recommendations are only a guide. In applying them, take into account the animal species involved, the circumstances of the bite or other exposure, vaccination status of the animal and presence of rabies in the region. Local or state health officials should be consulted if questions arise about the need for rabies prophylaxis.

SPECIES	CONDITION OF ANIMAL AT TIME OF ATTACK	TREATMENT
Domestic dog and cat	Healthy and available for 10 days of observation	None, unless animal develops rabies[1]
	Rabid or suspected rabid	RIG[2] & HDCV[3]
	Unknown (escaped)	Consult public health official. If treatment is indicated, give RIG[2] & HDCV[3]
Wild carnivores skunk, fox, bat, coyote, bobcat, raccoon	Regard as rabid unless proven negative by laboratory tests[4]	RIG[2] & HDCV[3]
Other livestock, rodents and lagomorphs (hares and rabbits)	Consider individually. Local and state public health officials should be consulted on questions about the need for rabies prophylaxis. Bites of squirrels, hamsters, guinea pigs, gerbils, chipmunks, rats, mice, other rodents, rabbits, and hares almost never call for antirabies prophylaxis.	

* All bites and wounds should immediately be thoroughly cleansed with soap and water. If antirabies treatment is indicated, both RIG and HDCV should be given as soon as possible, regardless of the interval from exposure.

[1] During the usual holding period of 10 days, begin treatment with RIG and HDCV at first sign of rabies in a dog or cat that has bitten someone. The symptomatic animal should be killed immediately and tested to confirm the diagnosis.

[2] If RIG is not available, use antirabies serum, equine. Do not use more than the recommended dosage.

[3] Local reactions to vaccines are common and do not contraindicate continuing treatment. Discontinue vaccine if FA tests of the animal are negative.

[4] The animal should be killed and tested as soon as possible. Holding for observation is not recommended.

Adapted from recommendations of the Immunization Practices Advisory Committee (ACIP), MMWR 33:393, 1984.

therewith. Although transmission to attending personnel has not been documented, immediate attendants should be warned of the potential hazard of infection from saliva and should wear rubber gloves, protective gowns, and some protection to avoid exposure from patient coughing saliva in attendant's face.

4) Quarantine: None.

5) Immunization of contacts: Contacts with an open wound or mucous membrane which has been exposed to the patient's saliva should receive antirabies specific treatment (see 9A7b, above).

6) Investigation of contacts and source of infection: Search for rabid animal and for persons and other animals bitten.

7) Specific treatment: For clinical rabies, intensive supportive medical care.

C. *Epidemic (epizootic) measures:* Applicable only to animals; a sporadic disease in man.

1) Establish area control under authority of state laws, public health regulations and local ordinances, in cooperation with appropriate wildlife conservation and animal health authorities.

2) Widespread mass vaccination of dogs through officially sponsored intensified programs providing immunization at temporary and emergency stations. For protection of other domestic animals, approved vaccines appropriate for each animal species must be used.

3) Strict enforcement of regulations requiring collection, detention and destruction of ownerless or stray dogs, and of unvaccinated dogs found off owner's premises.

4) Encourage reduction in the dog population by castration, spaying or drugs.

D. *Disaster implications:* A potential problem if the disease is freshly introduced or enzootic in an area where there are many stray dogs.

E. *International measures:*

1) Strict compliance by common carriers and by travelers with national laws and regulations that institute quarantine or require vaccination of animals, certificates of health and origin, etc.

2) WHO Collaborating Centres (see Preface).

RAT-BITE FEVER ICD-9 026

Two diseases rare in the USA are included under the general term of rat-bite fever; one, streptobacillary fever is caused by *Streptobacillus moniliformis,* and spirillary fever by *Spirillum minor.* Because they have clinical and epidemiological similarities, only streptobacillary fever is presented in detail; variations manifested by *Spirillum minor* infection (which is rarer in the USA) are noted in a brief summary.

STREPTOBACILLARY FEVER ICD-9 026.1
(Haverhill fever, Epidemic arthritic erythema, Rat-bite fever due to *Streptobacillus moniliformis*)

1. Identification—Usually there is a history of a rat bite within 10 days which healed normally. An abrupt onset with chills and fever, headache and muscle pain is followed shortly by a maculopapular or sometimes petechial rash most marked on the extremities. One or more large joints usually then become swollen, red and painful. Relapses are common. Bacterial endocarditis and focal abscesses may occur late in untreated cases, with a case fatality rate of 7–10%.

Laboratory confirmation is made by isolation of the organism by inoculation of material from the primary lesion, lymph node, blood, joint fluid, or pus into the appropriate bacteriological medium or into laboratory animals (guinea pigs or mice which are not naturally infected). Serum antibodies may be detected by agglutination tests.

2. Infectious agent—*Streptobacillus moniliformis (Streptothrix muris rattus, Haverhillia multiformis, Actinomyces muris).*

3. Occurrence—Worldwide, but uncommon in N and S America and most European countries. Recent cases in the USA have followed bites by laboratory rats.

4. Reservoir—An infected rat, rarely other animals (squirrel, weasel).

5. Mode of transmission—Infection is transmitted by secretions of mouth, nose or conjunctival sac of an infected animal, most frequently introduced by biting. Sporadic cases occur without a history of a bite. Blood from an experimental laboratory animal has infected man. Contact with rats is not necessary; infection has occurred in persons working or living in rat-infested buildings. In outbreaks, contaminated milk or water has usually been suspected as the vehicle of infection.

6. Incubation period—Three to 10 days, rarely longer.

7. **Period of communicability**—Not directly transmitted from person to person.

8. **Susceptibility and resistance**—No information.

9. **Methods of control**—

A. *Preventive measures:* Reduce rat populations and ratproof dwellings.

B. *Control of patient, contacts and the immediate environment:*

1) Report to local health authority: Obligatory report of epidemics; no case report required, Class 4 (see Preface).
2) Isolation: Blood/body fluid precautions for 24 hours after start of effective therapy.
3) Concurrent disinfection: None.
4) Quarantine: None.
5) Immunization of contacts: None.
6) Investigation of contacts and source of infection: Only to establish whether there are additional unrecognized cases.
7) Specific treatment: Penicillin or tetracyclines. Treatment should continue for 7 to 10 days.

C. *Epidemic measures:* Grouped cases presenting the typical symptoms require search for a common source, possibly a milk supply.

D. *Disaster implications:* None.

E. *International measures:* None.

SPIRILLARY FEVER   ICD-9 026.0
(Sodoku, Rat-bite fever due to *Spirillum minor*)

A sporadic rat-bite fever caused by *Spirillum minor (S. minus, Spirochaeta morsus muris)* is the common form of rat-bite fever in Japan and Asia. Untreated, the case fatality rate is approximately 10%. Clinically, *Spirillum minor* disease differs from streptobacillary fever in the rarity of arthritic symptoms, and the distinctive rash of reddish or purplish plaques. The incubation period is 1 to 3 weeks and the previously healed bite wound reactivates when symptoms appear. Laboratory methods are essential for differentiation; animal inoculation is used for isolation of the spirillum.

RELAPSING FEVER

ICD-9 087

1. **Identification**—A systemic spirochetal disease in which periods of fever lasting 2–9 days alternate with afebrile periods of 2–4 days; the number of relapses varies from 1–10 or more. Each pyrexial period terminates by crisis. The total duration of the louse-borne disease averages 13–16 days; the tick-borne disease usually lasts longer. Transitory petechial rashes are common during the initial period of fever. The overall case fatality rate in untreated cases is between 2–10%; it has exceeded 50% in epidemic louse-borne disease.

Diagnosis is made by demonstration of the infectious agent in darkfield preparations of fresh blood or stained thick or thin blood films, or by intraperitoneal inoculation of laboratory rats or mice with blood taken during the pyrexial period.

2. **Infectious agent**—In louse-borne disease—*Borrelia recurrentis,* a spirochete. In tick-borne disease—many different strains have been described by area of first isolation and/or vector rather than inherent biologic differences. Strains isolated during a relapse often show antigenic differences from those obtained during the immediately preceding paroxysm.

3. **Occurrence**—Characteristically epidemic where it is spread by lice, and endemic where it is spread by ticks. Louse-borne relapsing fever occurs in limited areas in Asia, eastern Africa (Ethiopia and the Sudan), northern and central Africa, and S America. The endemic tick-borne disease is widespread throughout tropical Africa; foci exist in Spain, northern Africa, Saudi Arabia, Iran, India, and parts of central Asia, as well as in N and S America. Epidemic louse-borne relapsing fever has not been reported in the USA for many years; human cases and occasional outbreaks of tick-borne disease occur in limited areas of several western states.

4. **Reservoir**—For louse-borne disease, man; for tick-borne relapsing fevers, wild rodents and ticks through transovarian transmission.

5. **Mode of transmission**—Not directly transmitted from person to person. Epidemic relapsing fever is acquired by crushing an infective louse, *Pediculus humanus,* over the bite wound or an abrasion of the skin. Man also is infected by the bite or coxal fluid of an argasid tick, principally *Ornithodoros turicata* and *O. hermsi* in the USA, *O. rudis* and *O. talaje* in Central and S America, *O. moubata* in tropical Africa, and *O. tholozani* in the Near and Middle East. These ticks usually feed at night, rapidly engorge and leave the host.

6. **Incubation period**—Five to 15 days; usually 8 days.

7. **Period of communicability**—The louse becomes infective 4–5 days after ingestion of blood from an infected person and remains so for life

(20–40 days). Infected ticks can live without feeding for several years, remain infective during this period and pass the infection transovarially to their progeny.

8. Susceptibility and resistance—Susceptibility is general. Duration of immunity after clinical attack is unknown; probably under 2 years.

9. Methods of control—

A. *Preventive measures:*

1) Louse control by measures prescribed for louse-borne typhus fever (see Typhus Fever, Epidemic Louse-Borne).
2) Tick control by measures prescribed for Rocky Mountain spotted fever. Tick-infested human habitations present difficult problems and eradication is difficult or impossible. Spraying with benzene hexachloride or an isomer may be tried.

B. *Control of patient, contacts and the immediate environment:*

1) Report to local health authority: Report of louse-borne relapsing fever required as a Disease under Surveillance by WHO, Class 1A (see Preface). Tick-borne disease, in selected areas, Class 3B.
2) Isolation: Blood/body fluid precautions. The patient, his clothing, all household contacts and the immediate environment should be deloused or freed of ticks.
3) Concurrent disinfection: None, if proper disinfestation has been carried out.
4) Quarantine: None.
5) Immunization of contacts: None.
6) Investigation of contacts and source of infection: For the individual tick-borne case, search for sources of infection; for louse-borne disease, application of appropriate lousicidal preparation (see Pediculosis).
7) Specific treatment: Tetracyclines.

C. *Epidemic measures:* When reporting has been good and cases are localized, apply insecticides with residual effect to contacts of all reported cases. Where infection is known to be widespread, systematic application of an effective residual insecticide to all persons in the community.

D. *Disaster implications:* A serious potential hazard among louse-infested populations. Epidemics are common in wars, in famine, or in other situations where malnourished, overcrowded populations with poor personal hygiene enhance the prevalence of pediculosis.

E. *International measures:*

1) Telegraphic notification by governments to WHO and to adjacent countries of the occurrence of an outbreak of louse-borne relapsing fever in an area previously free of the disease.

2) Louse-borne relapsing fever is not a disease subject to the International Health Regulations, but the measures outlined in 9E1, above, should be followed since it is a Disease under Surveillance by WHO.

RESPIRATORY DISEASE, ACUTE VIRAL (EXCLUDING INFLUENZA)
(Acute viral rhinitis*, A.v. pharyngitis*, A.v. laryngitis*, etc.)

Numerous acute respiratory illnesses of known and presumed viral etiology are grouped here under the general title of Respiratory Disease, Acute Viral. Clinically, and by CIOMS taxonomy, infections of the upper respiratory tract can be designated as acute viral rhinitis (upper respiratory infections, URI), acute viral pharyngitis, and acute viral laryngitis; and infections involving the lower respiratory tract can be designated as acute viral tracheobronchitis, bronchitis, bronchiolitis or acute viral pneumonia. These respiratory syndromes are associated with a large number of viruses, each of which is capable of producing a wide spectrum of acute respiratory illnesses. The illnesses caused by known agents have important epidemiological attributes in common, such as reservoir and mode of transmission. Many of the viruses invade any part of the respiratory tract; others show a predilection for certain anatomical sites. Some predispose to bacterial complications. Morbidity and mortality from acute respiratory diseases are especially significant in pediatric practice; in adults the relatively high incidence and resulting disability, with consequent economic loss, make diseases of this group a major health problem worldwide.

Several other nonbacterial infections of the respiratory tract are recognized as disease entities and are presented as separate diseases because they are sufficiently uniform in their clinical and epidemiological manifestations and occur in such regular association with specific infectious agents: ornithosis, influenza, enteroviral vesicular pharyngitis (herpangina) and epidemic myalgia (pleurodynia) are examples.

Symptoms of upper respiratory tract infection, mainly pharyngotonsillitis can be produced by bacterial agents, of which group A streptococcus is the most common. Practical management of acute respiratory disease depends on the differentiation of viral infections from disease entities for which specific antimicrobial measures are available; thus, it is important to rule out group A streptococcal infection by appropriate culture even though more illnesses are caused by viruses. In addition, in outbreaks or epidemics of continuing high incidence not due to the streptococcus, it is important to identify the cause in a representative sample of typical cases by appropriate clinical and laboratory methods to rule out other diseases, e.g., mycoplasmal or chlamydial pneumonia and Q fever, for which specific treatment may be effective.

I. ACUTE FEBRILE RESPIRATORY DISEASE

ICD-9 461-466; 480

1. **Identification**—Viral diseases of the respiratory tract may be characterized by fever and one or more constitutional reactions such as chills or chilliness, headache, general aching, malaise and anorexia; in infants by occasional gastrointestinal disturbances. Localizing signs also occur at various sites in the respiratory tract, either alone or in combination, such as rhinitis, pharyngitis or tonsillitis, laryngitis, laryngotracheitis, bronchitis, bronchiolitis, pneumonitis or pneumonia. There may be associated conjunctivitis. Symptoms and signs usually subside in 2 to 5 days without complications; infection may, however, extend or be complicated by bacterial sinusitis, otitis media, pneumonitis, or persistent bronchitis. WBC counts and respiratory bacterial flora are within normal limits unless modified by complications.

Specific diagnosis depends on isolation of the etiologic agent from respiratory secretions in appropriate cell or organ cultures, identification of viral antigen in nasopharyngeal cells by FA, ELISA and RIA tests and/or antibody studies of paired sera.

2. **Infectious agents**—Parainfluenza virus, types 1, 2, 3 and rarely type 4; respiratory syncytial virus (RSV); adenovirus, especially types 1–5, 7, 14, and 21; rhinoviruses; certain coronaviruses; certain types of coxsackievirus groups A and B; and echoviruses are considered etiologic agents of acute febrile respiratory illnesses. Some of these agents have a greater tendency to cause more severe illnesses; others have a predilection for certain age groups and populations. RSV, the major viral respiratory tract pathogen of early infancy, produces illness with greatest frequency during the first 2 years of life; it is the major known etiologic agent of bronchiolitis, and is a cause of pneumonia, croup, bronchitis, otitis media and febrile upper respiratory illness. The parainfluenza viruses are the major known etiologic agents of croup and also cause bronchitis, pneumonia, bronchiolitis and febrile upper respiratory illness in pediatric populations. Adenoviruses are associated with several forms of respiratory disease; types 4, 7 and 21 are common causes of acute respiratory disease (ARD) in unimmunized military recruits.

3. **Occurrence**—Worldwide. Seasonal in temperate zones, with greatest incidence during fall and winter and occasionally spring. In tropical zones, respiratory infections tend to be more frequent in wet and colder weather. In large communities, some viral illnesses are constantly present, usually with little seasonal pattern (e.g., adenovirus type 1); others tend to occur in sharp outbreaks (e.g., RSV).

Annual incidence is high, particularly in infants and children, and depends upon the number of susceptibles and the virulence of the agent. During autumn, winter and spring, attack rates for preschool children may average 2% per week as compared to 1% for school children and 0.5% for adults. Under special host and environmental conditions, certain viral infections may disable more than half of a closed community within a few weeks, e.g., outbreaks of adenovirus types 4 or 7 in military recruits.

4. **Reservoir**—Man. Many known viruses produce inapparent infections; adenoviruses may remain latent in tonsils and adenoids.

5. **Mode of transmission**—Directly by oral contact or by droplet spread; indirectly by hands, handkerchiefs, eating utensils or other articles freshly soiled by respiratory discharges of an infected person. Viruses discharged in the feces, including enteroviruses and adenoviruses, may be involved. Outbreaks of illness due to adenovirus type 3, 4 and 23 have been related to swimming pools.

6. **Incubation period**—From 1 to 10 days.

7. **Period of communicability**—Shortly prior to and for the duration of active disease; little is known about subclinical or latent infections. Especially in infants, RSV shedding may very rarely persist for several weeks or longer after clinical symptoms subside.

8. **Susceptibility and resistance**—Susceptibility is universal. Illness is more frequent and more severe in infants, children and the elderly. Infection induces specific antibodies which are usually short-lived. Reinfection with RSV and parainfluenza viruses is common, but generally milder.

9. **Methods of control**—

    A. *Preventive measures:*

        1)   When possible, avoid crowding in living and sleeping quarters, especially in institutions, in barracks and on shipboard.

        2)   Educate the public in personal hygiene, as in covering the mouth when coughing and sneezing, in sanitary disposal of discharges from mouth and nose and in frequent handwashing.

        3)   Oral live adenovirus vaccines have proven effective against

certain type-specific infections in military recruits, but are not indicated in civilian populations because of the low incidence of specific disease.

B. *Control of patient, contacts and the immediate environment:*

1) Report to local health authority: Obligatory report of epidemics; no individual case report, Class 4 (see Preface).
2) Isolation: Contact isolation is desirable in childrens' hospital wards. Outside of hospitals, ill persons should avoid direct and indirect exposure of young children, debilitated or aged persons or patients with other illnesses.
3) Concurrent disinfection: Of eating and drinking utensils; sanitary disposal of oral and nasal discharges.
4) Quarantine: None.
5) Immunization of contacts: None.
6) Investigation of contacts: Not generally indicated.
7) Specific treatment: None. Indiscriminate use of antibiotics is to be discouraged; they should be reserved for identified bacterial complications such as pneumonia, tracheobronchitis, otitis, tonsillitis and sinusitis. Aerosolized ribavarin has given promise of effectiveness in treatment of RSV.

C. *Epidemic measures:* No effective measures known. Isolation may be helpful in institutions; procedures such as ultraviolet irradiation, aerosols and dust control have not proved useful. Avoid crowding. (See 9A2, above.)

D. *Disaster implications:* None.

E. *International measures:* WHO Collaborating Centres (see Preface).

II. THE COMMON COLD   ICD-9 460
(Acute viral rhinitis*, Acute coryza)

1. Identification—Acute catarrhal infections of the upper respiratory tract characterized by coryza, sneezing, lacrimation, irritated nasopharynx, chilliness and malaise lasting 2 to 7 days. Fever is uncommon in children and rare in adults. No fatalities reported, but disability is important because it affects work performance, industrial and school absenteeism, and predisposes to more serious complications such as sinusitis, otitis media, laryngitis, tracheitis and bronchitis. WBC counts are usually normal and bacterial flora of the respiratory tract are within normal limits in the absence of complications.

Cell or organ culture studies of nasal secretions may demonstrate a known virus in 20–35% of cases. Specific clinical, epidemiologic and other manifestations aid differentiation from similar diseases due to toxic, allergic, physical or psychologic stimuli.

2. Infectious agents—Rhinoviruses, of which there are more than 100 recognized serotypes, are the major known etiologic agents of the common cold in adults, especially in the fall season. Coronaviruses such as 229E, OC43, and B814 are also responsible for common colds in adults; they appear to be especially important in the winter and early spring when the prevalence of rhinoviruses is low. Other known respiratory viruses account for a small proportion of common colds in adults. In infants and children parainfluenza viruses, RSV, adenoviruses, certain enteroviruses, and coronaviruses cause common cold-like illnesses. The etiology of over half of common colds has not been identified.

3. Occurrence—Worldwide, both endemic and epidemic. In temperate zones, incidence rises in fall, winter and spring. Many persons, except in small isolated communities, have 1 to 6 colds yearly. Incidence is highest in children under 5 years; gradual decline with increasing age.

4. Reservoir—Man.

5. Mode of transmission—Presumably by direct contact or by inhalation of airborne droplets; indirectly by hands and articles freshly soiled by discharges of nose and throat of an infected person. Rhinovirus is transmitted effectively by contaminated hands carrying virus to the conjunctivae.

6. Incubation period—Between 12 and 72 hours, usually 48 hours.

7. Period of communicability—Nasal washings taken 24 hours before onset and for 5 days after onset have produced symptoms in experimentally infected volunteers.

8. Susceptibility and resistance—Susceptibility is universal. Inapparent and abortive infections occur; frequency of healthy carriers is undetermined, but known to be rare with some viral agents, notably rhinoviruses. The frequently repeated attacks may be due to short duration of homologous immunity, to the multiplicity of agents or to other causes.

9. Methods of control—

A. *Preventive measures:* See I, 9A, above.

B. *Control of patient, contacts and the immediate environment:*

   1) Report to local health authority: Official report not ordinarily justifiable, Class 5 (see Preface).
   2) through 7): See I, 9B, above.

C., D., and E.: See I, 9C, 9D, and 9E, above.

RICKETTSIOSES, TICK-BORNE ICD-9 082
(Spotted Fever Group)

A group of clinically similar diseases caused by closely related rickettsiae. They are transmitted by *Ixodid* (hard) ticks which are widely distributed throughout the world; species differ markedly by geographical area. For all of these rickettsial fevers similar control measures are applicable and the tetracyclines and chloramphenicol are effective therapeutically.

CF tests, using group-specific spotted fever antigens, and the sensitive specific micro-IFA tests become positive in the 2nd week of illness. The Weil-Felix reactions with *Proteus* OX-19 and *Proteus* OX-2 become positive with less regularity.

I. ROCKY MOUNTAIN SPOTTED FEVER ICD-9 082.0
(New World spotted fever, Tick-borne typhus fever, São Paulo fever)

1. **Identification**—This prototype disease of the spotted fever group is characterized by sudden onset with moderate to high fever which ordinarily persists for 2–3 wks, significant malaise, deep muscle pain, severe headache, chills and conjunctival injection. A maculopapular rash, appearing on the extremities about the 3rd day, soon includes the palms and soles and spreads rapidly to most of the body; petechiae and hemorrhages are common. The case fatality rate is about 15–20% in the absence of specific therapy; with prompt recognition and treatment death is uncommon, yet 4–6% of cases reported in the USA during recent years have died. Absence or delayed appearance of the typical rash contributes to delay in diagnosis and increased fatality.

This clinical syndrome, especially early RMSF, may be confused with atypical measles (see Measles), with meningococcemia (see Meningitis), and with enteroviral infection.

Presumptive diagnosis is based on serologic response. The rickettsiae have been identified in skin biopsies using IF antisera. Positive identification requires isolation of the agent from the blood of patients but this may be hazardous to inexperienced laboratory workers.

2. **Infectious agent**—*Rickettsia rickettsii.*

3. **Occurrence**—Throughout the USA during spring, summer and fall. Two-thirds of cases reported in recent years have been in N and S Carolina,

Virginia, Maryland, Georgia, Tennessee and Oklahoma. Few cases have been reported from the Rocky Mountain region. In western USA adult males are infected most frequently, while in the East the incidence is higher in children; the difference relates to conditions of exposure to infected ticks. The case fatality rate increases with age. Infection also occurs in Canada, western and central Mexico, Panamá, Costa Rica, Colombia and Brazil.

4. Reservoir—Maintained in nature in ticks by transovarian and transstadial passage. The rickettsiae can be transmitted to dogs, various rodents and other animals.

5. Mode of transmission—Ordinarily by bite of an infected tick. Several hours (4–6) of attachment of the tick are required before the rickettsiae become reactivated to infect man. Contamination of skin with crushed tissues or feces of the tick may also cause infection. In eastern and southern USA the common vector is the dog tick, *Dermacentor variabilis;* in northwestern USA the wood tick, *D. andersoni;* in southwestern USA, occasionally the Lone Star tick, *Amblyomma americanum.* The principal vector in Latin America is *A. cajennense.*

6. Incubation period—From 3 to about 14 days.

7. Period of communicability—Not directly transmitted from person to person. The tick remains infective for life, commonly as long as 18 months.

8. Susceptibility and resistance—Susceptibility is general. One attack probably confers lasting immunity.

9. Methods of control—

A. Preventive measures:

1) Avoid tick-infested areas when feasible; search total body area every 3–4 hours for attached ticks if working or playing in infested area. Remove any ticks promptly and carefully without crushing, using gentle steady traction to avoid leaving mouth parts in the skin; protect hands when removing ticks from man or animals. Deticking dogs minimizes the tick population near residences. Tick repellents may be of value.

2) Measures designed to reduce tick populations are generally impractical.

3) Educate the public in mode of transmission by ticks and the means for personal protection.

4) No vaccine is presently licensed in the USA for public use.

B. Control of patient, contacts and the immediate environment:

1) Report to local health authority: In selected areas (USA); in many countries not a reportable disease, Class 3B (see Preface).
2) Isolation: None.
3) Concurrent disinfection: Carefully remove all ticks from patients.
4) Quarantine: None.
5) Immunization of contacts: Unnecessary.
6) Investigation of contacts and source of infection: Not profitable except as a community measure; see I, 9C, below.
7) Specific treatment: Tetracyclines or chloramphenicol (the latter is preferred for children under 8 and pregnant women) in daily oral doses until the patient is afebrile (usually 3 days) and for 1–2 additional days. Treatment should be initiated on clinical and epidemiologic considerations without waiting for laboratory confirmation of the diagnosis.

C. *Epidemic measures:* In hyperendemic areas particular attention should be paid to identification of the tick species involved and of the areas infested, and to recommendations in 9A1, 2, and 3, above.

D. *Disaster implications:* None.

E. *International measures:* WHO Collaborating Centres (see Preface).

II. BOUTONNEUSE FEVER   ICD-9 082.1
(Marseilles fever, African tick typhus, Kenya tick typhus, India tick typhus, Mediterranean tick fever)

1. Identification—A mild to moderately severe febrile illness of a few days to 2 wks, usually characterized by a primary lesion at the site of a tick bite. The lesion (tâche noire), usually present at the onset of fever, is a small ulcer 2–5 mm in diameter with a black center and red areola; regional lymph nodes are enlarged. However, in some areas, such as the Negev in Israel, primary lesions are rarely seen in serologically confirmed cases. A generalized maculopapular erythematous rash usually involving palms and soles appears about the 4th-5th day and persists 6–7 days; with antibiotic treatment, fever lasts no more than 2 days. The case fatality rate is <3%, even without specific therapy.

2. Infectious agent—*Rickettsia conorii.*

3. Occurrence—Widely distributed throughout the African Continent,

in India and in those parts of Europe and the Middle East adjacent to the Mediterranean, Black and Caspian Seas, and possibly in Mexico. Expansion of the European endemic zone to the north is occurring because tourists often carry their dogs with them; they acquire infected ticks which establish tick colonies when they return home and transmission occurs. In more temperate areas, highest incidence is during warmer months when ticks are numerous; in tropical areas throughout the year. Outbreaks may occur when groups of susceptibles are brought into an endemic area; a disease of travelers.

4. **Reservoir**—As in Rocky Mountain spotted fever, above.

5. **Mode of transmission**—In the Mediterranean area, by bite of infected *Rhipicephalus sanguineus,* a dog tick. In S Africa, ticks infected in nature and presumed to be vectors include *Haemaphysalis leachi, Amblyomma hebraeum, R. appendiculatus, Boophilus decoloratus,* and *Hyalomma aegyptium.*

6. **Incubation period**—Usually 5–7 days.

7. **Period of communicability; 8. Susceptibility and resistance;** and 9. **Methods of Control**—As in Rocky Mountain spotted fever, above.

III. QUEENSLAND TICK TYPHUS ICD-9 082.3

1. **Identification**—Clinically similar to Boutonneuse fever.

2. **Infectious agent**—*Rickettsia australis.*

3. **Occurrence**—Queensland, Australia.

4. **Reservoir**—As in Rocky Mountain spotted fever.

5. **Mode of transmission**—As in Rocky Mountain spotted fever. *Ixodes holocyclus,* infesting small marsupials and wild rodents, is probably the major vector.

6. **Incubation period**—About 7–10 days.

7. **Period of communicability; 8. Susceptibility and resistance;** and 9. **Methods of Control**—As in Rocky Mountain spotted fever.

IV. NORTH ASIAN TICK FEVER ICD-9 082.2
(Siberian tick typhus)

1. **Identification**—Clinically similar to Boutonneuse fever.

2. **Infectious agent**—*Rickettsia siberica.*

3. **Occurrence**—Asiatic USSR and the Mongolian People's Republic.

4. **Reservoir**—As in Rocky Mountain spotted fever.

5. Mode of transmission—By the bite of ticks in the genera *Dermacentor* and *Haemaphysalis,* which infest certain wild rodents.

6. Incubation period—Two to 7 days.

7. Period of communicability; 8. Susceptibility and resistance; and 9. Methods of control—As in Rocky Mountain spotted fever.

RICKETTSIALPOX   ICD-9 083.2
(Vesicular rickettsiosis)

An infection manifested by an initial skin lesion at the site of a mite bite, associated with lymphadenopathy. Followed by fever; then a disseminated skin rash appears, generally not involving the palms and soles and lasting only a few days. It may be confused with chickenpox. Death is uncommon and the infection is responsive to broad-spectrum antibiotics. Diagnosis is made by CF or IFA testing. The disease is caused by *Rickettsia akari,* a member of the spotted fever group of rickettsiae, transmitted to man from mice *(Mus musculus)* by a mite *(Liponyssoides sanguineus).* It has occurred in urban areas of the eastern USA, primarily in New York, and in the USSR. The incidence has been markedly reduced by changes in management of garbage in tenement housing, so that only 6 cases have been diagnosed in New York since 1971. In the USSR, commensal rats are reported to be sources of infection. Rickettsial isolations have been made in Africa and Korea. Prevention is by rodent elimination followed by mite control.

RUBELLA   ICD-9 056
(German measles)
CONGENITAL RUBELLA   ICD-9 771.0
(Congenital rubella syndrome)

1. Identification—Rubella is a mild febrile infectious disease with a diffuse punctate and macular rash sometimes resembling that of measles or scarlet fever. Children may present few or no constitutional symptoms but adults may experience a 1–5 days prodrome of low-grade fever, headache, malaise, mild coryza, and conjunctivitis. Postauricular, suboccipital or posterior cervical lymphadenopathy is common but not pathognomonic; occasionally adenopathy is generalized. As many as half of infections may occur without evident rash. Leukopenia is common and thrombocytopenia occurs but hemorrhagic manifestations are rare. Arthralgia or arthritis complicates a substantial proportion of infections, particularly among adult females. Encephalitis is a rare complication, occurring more frequently in adults than in children.

Rubella is important because of its ability to produce anomalies in the developing fetus. Congenital rubella syndrome occurs among 25% or more of infants born to women who acquired rubella during the 1st trimester of pregnancy; the risk of a single congenital defect falls to approximately 10% by the 16th week and defects are rare when the maternal infection occurs after the 20th week of gestation. Fetuses infected early are at greatest risk of intrauterine death, spontaneous abortion and congenital malformations of major organ systems. These include single or combinations of defects: deafness, cataracts, microphthalmia, microcephaly, mental retardation, patent ductus arteriosus, atrial or ventricular septal defects, congenital glaucoma, purpura, hepatospleno-megaly, jaundice, radiolucent bone disease or meningoencephalitis. Mod-erate and severe cases of congenital rubella are recognizable at birth; mild cases with only slight cardiac involvement or partial deafness may not be detected for months or even years after birth. Insulin-dependant diabetes mellitus is recognized as a frequent late manifestation of congenital rubella in certain geographic areas. These congenital malformations and even fetal death may occur following inapparent maternal rubella.

Differentiation of rubella from measles (q.v.), scarlet fever (see Streptococcal Diseases), and other infections of similar nature is often necessary (see erythema infectiosum and exanthem subitum, below). Macular and maculopapular rashes occur in 1–5% of patients with infectious mononucleosis (especially if given ampicillin) and also in infections with certain enteroviruses and after certain drugs.

Diagnosis of rubella, especially in pregnant women, can be confirmed by a fourfold rise in specific antibody titer between acute and convalescent phase serum specimens by HI, passive hemagglutination, latex agglutina-tion or ELISA testing, or by the presence of rubella-specific IgM which indicates a recent infection. Sera should be collected as early as possible (within 7–10 days) after onset of illness and again at least 7–14 days, and preferably 2–3 weeks, later. Virus may be isolated from the pharynx 1 week before until 2 weeks after onset of rash. Blood, urine or stool specimens may yield virus. The diagnosis of congenital rubella in the newborn is confirmed by the presence of specific IgM antibodies in a single specimen, or the persistence of an HI titer beyond the time expected from passive transfer of maternal IgG antibody or isolation of the virus.

2. **Infectious agent**—Rubella virus (family Togaviridae; genus *Rubivirus*).

3. **Occurrence**—Worldwide; universally endemic except in remote and isolated communities, especially certain island groups which have epidem-ics every 10–15 yrs. Prevalent in winter and spring. Extensive epidemics have occurred in the USA in 1935, 1943 and 1964 and in Australia in 1940.

Before vaccine was licensed in 1969, peaks of rubella incidence occurred in the USA every 6–9 yrs. In unvaccinated populations, rubella is primarily a disease of childhood but occurs more often in adolescents and adults than does measles or chickenpox. Where children are well immunized, adolescent and young adult infections become more important, with epidemics in institutions, colleges and military populations. Congenital rubella incidence has declined in the USA since 1979.

4. Reservoir—Man.

5. Mode of transmission—Contact with nasopharyngeal secretions of infected persons. Infection is by droplet spread or direct contact with patients, or presumably by indirect contact with articles freshly soiled with discharges from nose and throat, and with blood, urine, or feces. In closed environments such as among military recruits, all susceptibles may be infected. Infants with congenital rubella may shed large quantities of virus in their pharyngeal secretions and in urine, and serve as source of infection to their contacts.

6. Incubation period—Sixteen to 18 days with a range of 14–23 days.

7. Period of communicability—For about 1 wk before and at least 4 days after onset of rash. Highly communicable. Infants with congenital rubella may shed virus for months after birth.

8. Susceptibility and resistance—Susceptibility is general after loss of transplacentally acquired maternal antibody. Active immunity is acquired by natural infection or by vaccination and is usually permanent after natural infection and is expected to be long-term, probably lifelong, after vaccination. In the USA, 15–25% of young adults remain susceptible. Infants born to immune mothers are ordinarily protected for 6–9 months, depending on the amount of maternal antibody acquired transplacentally.

9. Methods of control—Rubella control is needed primarily to prevent defects in the offspring of women who acquire the disease during pregnancy.

    A. Preventive measures:

        1) A single dose of live attenuated rubella virus vaccine (Rubella Virus Vaccine, Live) elicits a significant antibody response in approximately 95% of susceptibles. The vaccine in dried form and after reconstitution must be kept at 2° to 8°C (35.6°-46.4°F) or colder and protected from light to retain potency; frozen vaccine must be kept at −10° to −30°C·(14° to −22°F) to retain potency. Vaccine virus may be recovered from the nasopharynx of some recipients for several wks but is not communicable. In the USA, immunization of all children over 12 months of age

is recommended; as a part of a combined vaccine containing measles vaccine, it should be given at 15 months or later. The continuing occurrence of rubella among women of childbearing age indicates that emphasis should continue to be placed on vaccinating susceptible adolescent and adult females of childbearing age. Vaccine is especially recommended for susceptible premarital or postpartum women and for teachers, nurses, doctors and other staff likely to come into contact with individuals who have rubella, and into contact with patients in prenatal clinics; and for those in situations where young adults congregate, such as colleges and other types of institutions.

Vaccine should not be given to anyone with an immunodeficiency or on immunosuppressive therapy. Because vaccine virus theoretically might harm the fetus if given to a susceptible woman early in pregnancy, women known to be pregnant should not be vaccinated. However, no defects attributable to vaccine virus have been detected in about 300 offspring of susceptible women vaccinated shortly before conception or during the 1st trimester of pregnancy, including over 150 who had received the RA 27/3 vaccine which is now used in the USA.

Reasonable precautions in a rubella immunization program include asking postpubertal females if they are pregnant, excluding those who say they are, and explaining the theoretical risks to the others and the need to prevent pregnancy for the next 3 months. The immune status of an individual can be determined reliably only by serological testing, but this is not necessary before vaccination since vaccine can be given safely to an immune person. In some countries, e.g., UK and Australia, routine immunization is given to girls between 11–13 years with or without prior antibody testing. For greater general detail, see Measles, 9A1.

2) In case of natural infection early in pregnancy, abortion should be considered because of risk of damage to the fetus. Although vaccine virus has been isolated from products of conception, congenital defects in live-born infants have not been seen; therefore, vaccination of a woman subsequently discovered to be pregnant need not be considered an indication for an abortion, but the potential risks should be explained; the final decision rests with the individual woman and her physician.

3) IG given after exposure early in pregnancy may not prevent infection or viremia but it may modify or suppress

symptoms. It is sometimes given in huge doses (20 ml) to a susceptible pregnant woman exposed to the disease who would not consider abortion under any circumstances, but its value has not been established.

B. *Control of patient, contacts and the immediate environment:*

1) Report to local health authority: All cases of rubella and of congenital rubella should be reported. In the USA, report is obligatory; Class 3B (see Preface). Early reporting of suspected cases will permit early establishment of control measures.

2) Isolation: In hospitals and institutions, patients suspected of having rubella should be managed under contact isolation precautions and placed in a private room; attempts should be made to prevent exposure of nonimmune pregnant women (see 9B5, below). Exclude children from school and adults from work for 7 days after onset of rash.

3) Concurrent disinfection: None.

4) Quarantine: None.

5) Immunization of contacts: Immunization, while not contraindicated (except during pregnancy), will not necessarily prevent infection or illness. Passive immunization with IG is not indicated (except possibly as in 9A3, above).

6) Investigation of contacts: Identify pregnant female contacts, especially those in the 1st trimester. Such contacts should be tested serologically for susceptibility or early infection (IgM antibody) and advised accordingly.

7) Specific treatment: None.

C. *Epidemic measures:* An outbreak of rubella in a school or comparable population may justify mass immunization. The medical community and general public should be informed about rubella epidemics in order to identify and protect susceptible pregnant women.

D. *Disaster implications:* None.

E. *International measures:* None.

ERYTHEMA INFECTIOSUM
(Fifth disease)

ICD-9 057.0

A mild, usually nonfebrile erythematous eruption occurring as epidemics among children, characterized by a striking erythema of the cheeks (slapped-face appearance) and reddening of the skin which fades and recurs. The body may show a lace-like serpigenous rash; exaggerated by exposure to sunlight or heat (i.e., bathing); accompanied by only mild constitutional symptoms. Nonfatal. The human parvovirus has been implicated in one outbreak.

EXANTHEM SUBITUM
(Roseola infantum)

ICD-9 057.8

An acute illness of probable viral etiology, usually in children under 4 years, commonly at about 1 year. A fever, sometimes as high as 41°C (106°F), suddenly appears and lasts 3–5 days. A maculopapular rash on the trunk and later on the rest of the body ordinarily follows lysis of the fever and rash fades rapidly. Incidence is greatest in the spring. The incubation period is about 10 days. Unrecognized infections occur.

SALMONELLOSIS

ICD-9 003

1. **Identification**—A bacterial disease commonly manifested by an acute enterocolitis, with sudden onset of headache, abdominal pain, diarrhea, nausea and sometimes vomiting. Dehydration, especially among infants, may be severe. Fever is nearly always present. Anorexia and loose bowels often persist for several days. Infection may begin as acute enterocolitis and develop into enteric fever with septicemia or focal infection. The infectious agent may rarely localize in any tissue of the body, producing abscesses and causing arthritis, cholecystitis, endocarditis, meningitis, pericarditis, pneumonia, pyoderma or pyelonephritis. Ordinarily deaths are uncommon except in the very young, the very old, or the debilitated. However, morbidity and associated costs of salmonellosis may be high.

In cases of enteric fever and septicemia, *Salmonella* may be isolated on enteric media from feces and from blood during the acute stages of illness. In cases of enterocolitis, fecal excretion usually persists for several days or weeks beyond the acute phase of illness; administration of antibiotics may increase the duration of excretion of organisms. For detection of asymptomatic infections, 3–10 g of fecal material is preferred to rectal swabs. Serologic tests are not useful in diagnosis.

2. Infectious agents—Numerous serotypes of *Salmonella* are pathogenic for both animals and man (strains of human origin causing typhoid and paratyphoid fevers are presented separately). There is much variation in the relative prevalence of the different serotypes isolated from country to country; in most countries which maintain *Salmonella* surveillance, *S. typhimurium* is most commonly reported. Of approximately 2000 known serotypes, only about 200 are detected in the USA in any given year. In most areas, a small number of serotypes account for the majority of confirmed cases.

3. Occurrence—Worldwide, more extensively reported in N America and Europe; classified as a foodborne disease (see Foodborne Intoxication) because food is the predominant vehicle of infection. Only a small proportion of cases are recognized clinically and as few as 1% of clinical cases are reported. The incidence rate for infection is highest for infants and young children. Epidemiologically, *Salmonella* enterocolitis may occur in small outbreaks in the general population. Large outbreaks in hospitals, institutions for children, restaurants and nursing homes are common, and usually arise from food contaminated at its source, or, less often, during handling by an ill patient or a carrier, but may be due to person-to-person spread. There are estimated to be 2 to 3 million *Salmonella* infections in the USA annually.

4. Reservoir—Domestic and wild animals, including poultry, swine, cattle, rodents and pets such as tortoises, turtles, chicks, dogs and cats; also man, i.e., patients and convalescent carriers and especially mild and unrecognized cases. Chronic carriers are rare.

5. Mode of transmission—By ingestion of the organisms in food derived from infected food animals or contaminated by feces of an infected animal or person. This includes raw (especially cracked) eggs and egg products; raw milk and raw milk products; meat and meat products; poultry; pet turtles and chicks; and unsterilized pharmaceuticals of animal origin. Infection is also disseminated by animal feeds and fertilizers prepared from contaminated meat scraps, tankage, fish meal and bones. Fecal-oral transmission from person to person is important especially when diarrhea is present; infants and stool-incontinent adults pose a greater risk of transmission than do asymptomatic carriers. The ingestion of a few organisms can cause infection in highly susceptible persons, but usually $>10^{2-3}$ organisms are required.

Epidemics of *Salmonella* infection are usually traced to foods such as commercially processed meat products, inadequately cooked poultry or poultry products, raw sausages, lightly cooked foods containing eggs or egg products, unpasteurized milk or dairy products including dried milk, foods contaminated with feces by a rodent or by an infected foodhandler. They are also traced to foods such as meat and poultry products which have been processed or prepared with contaminated utensils or to work surfaces or tables contaminated in previous use. The organisms can multiply in a variety of foods, especially milk, to attain a very high infective level. Hospital epidemics tend to be protracted, with organisms persisting in the environment; they often start with contaminated food and continue by person-to-person transmission via the hands of personnel or contaminated instruments. Maternity units with sometimes asymptomatic infection of the infants are sources of further spread. Fecal contamination of unchlorinated public water supplies has been involved in some extensive outbreaks.

6. Incubation period—Six to 72 hours, usually about 12–36 hours.

7. Period of communicability—Throughout the course of infection. Extremely variable, usually several days to several wks; a temporary carrier state occasionally continues for months, especially in infants. About 1% of infected adults and 5% of children under 5 yrs excrete the organism for over 1 year. The administration of antibiotics, even those to which the organisms are sensitive in laboratory tests, can prolong the period of communicability.

8. Susceptibility and resistance—Susceptibility is general and is usually increased by achlorhydria, antacid therapy, gastrointestinal surgery, prior broad-spectrum antibiotic therapy, neoplastic disease, immunosuppressive therapy or other debilitating conditions including malnutrition. Severity of the disease is related to the serotype, the number of organisms ingested and host factors.

9. Methods of control—

A. Preventive measures:

1) Thorough cooking of all foodstuffs derived from animal sources, particularly poultry (especially frozen), egg products and meat dishes. Avoid recontamination within the kitchen after cooking is completed. Avoid consuming raw eggs, as in egg-nogs or homemade ice cream, and using dirty or cracked eggs. All milk and egg products should be pasteurized.

2) Educate foodhandlers and food-preparers in the importance of handwashing before, during and after food preparation; in the importance of refrigerating food, maintaining a sanitary kitchen, and protecting prepared foods against rodent or insect contamination.

3) Exclude individuals with diarrhea from foodhandling and from care of hospitalized patients.

4) Recognize, control and prevent *Salmonella* infections in domestic animals and pets. Chicks, ducklings and turtles are particularly dangerous as pets for small children.

5) Meat and poultry inspection, with adequate supervision of abattoirs, food-processing plants, feed-blending mills, egg-grading stations and butcher shops.

6) Adequately cook or heat-treat (followed by measures to avoid recontamination) foods prepared for animals (meat meal, bone meal, fish meal, pet food).

7) Thoroughly indoctrinate known carriers in the need for very careful postdefecatory handwashing (and before handling food), and discourage from handling food as long as they shed the organisms.

B. *Control of patient, contacts and the immediate environment:*

1) Report to local health authority: Obligatory case report, Class 2B (see Preface).

2) Isolation: For hospitalized patients, enteric precautions in the handling of feces and contaminated clothing and bed linen. Exclude symptomatic individuals from foodhandling and from direct care of hospitalized and institutionalized patients; exclusion of asymptomatic infected individuals is indicated for those with questionable hygienic habits and where required by local or state regulations. Release to return to work in a sensitive occupation, when exclusion is mandated, generally requires 2 consecutive negative stool cultures for *Salmonella,* collected not less than 24 hours apart; if antibiotics have been given, the initial culture should be taken at least 48 hours after the last dose. Proper handwashing should be stressed.

3) Concurrent disinfection: Of feces and articles soiled therewith. In communities with a modern and adequate sewage disposal system, feces can be discharged directly into sewers without preliminary disinfection. Terminal cleaning.

4) Quarantine: None.

5) Management of contacts: No immunization available.

6) Investigation of contacts: Culture stools of any household contacts who are involved in direct patient care or care of young children or elderly persons in institutional settings.

7) Specific treatment: For uncomplicated enterocolitis, none generally indicated except rehydration and electrolyte replacement with oral glucose-electrolyte solution (see Cholera, 9B7); antibiotics may prolong the carrier state and lead to resistant strains. However, in infants under 2 months, the elderly and the debilitated, or with continued or high fever or manifestations of extra-intestinal infection, antibiotic therapy should be given. Antimicrobial

resistance of nontyphoidal *Salmonellae* is variable; ampicillin or amoxicillin is usually recommended, with TMP-SMX or chloramphenicol when antimicrobial-resistant strains are involved.

C. *Epidemic measures:* See Foodborne Intoxication, Staphylococcal Food Poisoning, 9C1 and 9C2. Search for a history of diarrhea among foodhandlers and collect stool specimens for culture if indicated.

D. *Disaster implications:* A danger in a situation with mass feeding and poor sanitation.

E. *International measures:* WHO Collaborating Centres (see Preface).

SCABIES
(Sarcoptic itch, Acariasis)

ICD-9 133.0

1. **Identification**—An infectious disease of the skin caused by a mite whose penetration is visible as papules or vesicles, or as tiny linear burrows containing the mites and their eggs. Lesions are prominent around finger webs, anterior surfaces of wrists and elbows, anterior axillary folds, belt line, thighs and external genitalia in men; nipples, abdomen, and lower portion of buttocks are frequently affected in women. In infants, the head, neck, palms and soles may be involved; these areas are usually spared in older individuals. Itching is intense, especially at night, but complications are limited to lesions secondarily infected from scratching. In immunodeficient individuals and in senile patients, infestation often appears as a generalized dermatitis more widely distributed than the burrows, with extensive scaling and sometimes vesiculation and crusting (Norwegian scabies); the usual severe itching may be reduced or absent. When scabies is complicated by β-hemolytic streptococci, risk of acute glomerulonephritis is increased.

Diagnosis may be established by recovering the mite from its burrow and identifying it microscopically. Care should be taken to choose lesions for scraping or biopsy which have not been excoriated by repeated scratching. Prior application of mineral oil facilitates collecting the scrapings and examining them under a cover slip. Applying ink to the skin and then washing it off will disclose the burrows.

2. **Infectious agent**—*Sarcoptes scabiei,* a mite.

3. **Occurrence**—Widespread. Past epidemics were attributed to pov-

erty, poor hygiene, and crowding due to war and economic crises. The recent wave of infestation in the USA and Europe has evolved in the absence of major social disturbances and has affected people from all socioeconomic levels without regard to age, sex, race, or standards of personal hygiene. It is endemic in many developing countries.

4. **Reservoir**—Man; *Sarcoptes* and other mites of animals can live on man but do not reproduce in the skin.

5. **Mode of transmission**—Transfer of parasites is by direct skin-to-skin contact; transfer from undergarments or bedclothes occurs only if these have been contaminated by infected persons immediately beforehand; can be acquired during sexual contact. Mites can burrow beneath the skin surface in 2.5 minutes. Norwegian scabies is highly infectious because of the large number of mites in the exfoliating scales.

6. **Incubation period**—Two to 6 wks before onset of itching in persons without previous exposure. Persons who have been previously infested develop symptoms 1–4 days after reexposure.

7. **Period of communicability**—Until mites and eggs are destroyed by treatment, ordinarily after 1 or occasionally 2 courses of treatment a week apart.

8. **Susceptibility and resistance**—Some resistance is suggested since immunologically compromised persons are susceptible to hyperinfestation; fewer mites succeed in establishing themselves on persons previously infected than on those with no prior exposure.

9. **Methods of control**—

A. *Preventive measures:* Educate the public and medical community on mode of transmission. Early diagnosis and treatment of infested patients and contacts.

B. *Control of patient, contacts and the immediate environment:*

1) Report to local health authority: Official report not ordinarily justifiable, Class 5 (see Preface).

2) Isolation: Exclude infested individuals from school or work until the day after treatment. For hospitalized patients, contact isolation for 24 hours after start of effective treatment.

3) Concurrent disinfection: Laundering underwear, clothing and bed sheets worn or used by patient in the 48 hours prior to treatment using hot cycles of washer and dryer has been suggested but is of questionable value.

4) Quarantine: None.

5) Immunization of contacts: None.

6) Investigation of contacts: Search for unreported or unrecognized cases among companions or household members; single infestations in a family are uncommon. Treat persons prophylactically who have had skin-to-skin contact with infested persons (including family members, sexual contacts, others).

7) Specific treatment: Application of 1% gamma benzene hexachloride (lindane, Kwell®), crotamiton (Eurax®), tetraethylthiuram monosulfide (Tetmosol®) in 5% solution twice daily (not available in USA), or an emulsion of benzyl benzoate to the whole body except the head and neck; treatment details vary with the drug. On the next day, a cleansing bath is taken and a change made to fresh clothing and bedclothes. Itching may persist for 1–2 wks and during this period should not be regarded as a sign of drug failure or reinfestation; overtreatment is common and should be avoided because of toxicity of some of these agents, especially gamma benzene hexachloride. In about 5% of cases a second course of treatment may be necessary after an interval of 7–10 days if eggs survived the 1st treatment. Close supervision of treatment, including bathing, is necessary.

C. *Epidemic measures:*

1) Treatment is undertaken on a coordinated mass basis.
2) Case-finding efforts are extended to screen whole families, military units or institutions, with segregation of infested individuals if possible.
3) Soap and facilities for mass bathing and laundering are essential. Tetmosol soap, where available, helps to prevent infection.
4) Health education of infested individuals and others at risk, as well as treatment. Cooperation of civilian or military authorities, often both, is needed.

D. *Disaster implications:* A potential nuisance in situations of overcrowding.

E. *International measures:* None.

SCHISTOSOMIASIS
(Bilharziasis, Snail fever)

ICD-9 120

1. **Identification**—A blood fluke (trematode) infection with adult male and female worms living in mesenteric or vesical veins of the host over a life span of many years. Eggs produce minute granulomata and scars in organs where they lodge or are deposited. Symptomatology is related to the number and location of the parasites in the human host; *Schistosoma mansoni* and *S. japonicum* give rise primarily to hepatic and intestinal symptoms, including diarrhea, abdominal pain and hepatosplenomegaly; and *S. haematobium,* to urinary manifestations, including dysuria, frequency and terminal hematuria. The most important pathological effects are the complications that arise from chronic infection; liver fibrosis and portal hypertension in the intestinal form, while obstructive uropathy, super-imposed bacterial infection and possibly bladder cancer occur in the urinary form of schistosomiasis. CNS manifestations may occur during the acute or chronic stages of infection from deposition of eggs in ectopic sites.

The larvae of certain schistosomes of birds and mammals may penetrate the human skin and cause a dermatitis, sometimes known as "swimmer's itch"; these schistosomes do not mature in man. Such infections may be prevalent among bathers in lakes in many parts of the world, including the Great Lakes region of N America and certain coastal beaches.

Definitive diagnosis depends on the demonstration of eggs in the stool, urine or biopsy specimen. Useful immunological tests include the circumoval precipitin test, IFA and ELISA with adult worm antigen, and RIA with purified egg or adult antigens; positive results in serologic tests do not constitute proof of current infection.

2. **Infectious agents**—*Schistosoma mansoni, S. haematobium* and *S. japonicum* are the major species causing human disease. *S. mekongi* and *S. intercalatum* are of importance only in limited areas.

3. **Occurrence**—*S. mansoni* is found in Africa and the Arabian Peninsula, Brazil, Surinam and Venezuela in S America and in some Caribbean islands. *S. haematobium* is found in Africa and the Middle East. *S. japonicum* is found in China, Japan, Philippines and Sulawesi. *S. mekongi* is found in the Mekong River area of Laos and Kampuchea and in Thailand. *S. intercalatum* occurs in parts of west Africa, including Cameroon, Central African Republic, Chad, Gabon and Zaire. None of these species is indigenous to N America.

4. **Reservoir**—Man is the principal reservoir of *S. haematobium, S. intercalatum,* and *S. mansoni.* Man, dogs, cats, pigs, cattle, water buffalo, horses and wild rodents are potential hosts of *S. japonicum;* their relative epidemiologic importance varies in different regions. Persistence of the parasite depends on the presence of an appropriate snail as intermediate

host, i.e., species of the genera *Biomphalaria* for *S. mansoni, Bulimus* for *S. haematobium* and *S. intercalatum, Oncomelania* for *S. japonicum* and *Tricula* for *S. mekongi.*

5. **Mode of transmission**—Infection is acquired from water containing free-swimming larval forms (cercariae) which have developed in snails. The eggs of *S. haematobium* leave the mammalian body mainly in the urine, those of the other species in the feces. The eggs hatch in water and the liberated larvae (miracidia) penetrate into suitable freshwater snail hosts. After several weeks, the cercariae emerge from the snail and penetrate human skin, usually while the person is working, swimming or wading in water; they enter the bloodstream, are carried to blood vessels of the lung, migrate to the liver, develop to maturity, and then migrate to veins of the abdominal cavity. Adult forms of *S. mansoni, S. japonicum, S. mekongi* and *S. intercalatum* usually remain in mesenteric veins; those of *S. haematobium* usually migrate through anastomoses into the vesical plexus of the urinary bladder. Eggs are deposited in venules and escape into the lumen of the bowel or urinary bladder, or lodge in other organs, including the liver and the lungs.

6. **Incubation period**—Severe acute systemic manifestations (Katayama fever) may occur in primary infections 2–6 weeks after exposure, immediately preceding and during initial egg deposition. Acute manifestations are rare with *S. haematobium* infections.

7. **Period of communicability**—Not communicable from person to person, but the infected person may spread the infection by discharging eggs in urine for approximately 5 years with *S. haematobium,* and in feces for ≧20 years with *S. mansoni.* Infected snails may release cercariae for several weeks.

8. **Susceptibility and resistance**—Susceptibility is universal; any resistance developing as a result of infection is variable and poorly defined.

9. **Methods of control**—

   A. *Preventive measures:*

   1) Dispose of feces and urine so that viable eggs will not reach bodies of fresh water containing snail intermediate hosts. Control of animals infected with *S. japonicum* is desirable but usually not practical.
   2) Improve irrigation and agricultural practices; reduce snail habitats by removing vegetation or by drainage and filling.
   3) Treat snail breeding places with molluscicides.
   4) Prevent exposure to contaminated water (e.g., rubber boots). To minimize cercarial penetration towel dry vigorously and completely skin surfaces wet with suspected

water. Apply 70% alcohol immediately to the skin to kill surface cercariae.

5) Provide water for drinking, bathing and washing clothes from sources free from cercariae or treated to kill them.

6) Educate people in endemic areas regarding mode of transmission and methods of protection.

7) Treatment in endemic areas to prevent disease progression and to reduce transmission through reduction in egg passage.

B. *Control of patient, contacts and the immediate environment:*

1) Report to local health authority: In selected endemic areas; in many countries not a reportable disease, Class 3C (see Preface).

2) Isolation: None.

3) Concurrent disinfection: Sanitary disposal of feces and urine.

4) Quarantine: None.

5) Immunization of contacts: None.

6) Investigation of contacts: Examine contacts for infection from a common source. Search for source is a community effort, see 9C, below.

7) Specific treatment: Praziquantel (Biltricide®) is the drug of choice against all three species. Alternative drugs are oxamniquine for *S. mansoni,* and metrifonate for *S. haematobium.*

C. *Epidemic measures:* Examine the people for schistosomiasis and treat all who are infected, but especially those with moderate to heavy intensities of egg passage, with particular attention to children. Provide clean water, warn people against contact with waters potentially containing cercariae, and prohibit contamination of water. Treat areas with high snail densities with molluscicides.

D. *Disaster implications:* None.

E. *International measures:* WHO Collaborating Centres (see Preface).

SHIGELLOSIS
(Bacillary dysentery)

ICD-9 004

1. **Identification**—An acute bacterial disease involving the large and small intestine, characterized by diarrhea accompanied by fever, nausea and sometimes toxemia, vomiting, cramps and tenesmus. Convulsions may be an important complication in young children. In typical cases the stools contain blood, mucus and pus (dysentery) resulting from the confluent microabscesses caused by the invasive organisms; watery diarrhea with vomiting may also occur, attributable to an enterotoxin elaborated by the organisms. Bacteremia is uncommon. Mild and asymptomatic infections occur. Illness is usually self-limited, lasting several days to weeks, with an average of 4–7 days. The severity of illness and the case fatality rate are functions of the host (age and preexisting state of nutrition), the size of the infecting dose and the serotype of the organism. *Shigella dysenteriae* (Shiga's bacillus) is often associated with serious disease; case fatality rates have been as high as 20% among hospitalized cases even in recent years. In contrast, many infections with *Shigella sonnei* result in a short clinical course and an almost negligible case fatality rate, except in compromised hosts.

Bacteriologic diagnosis is made by isolation of *Shigella* from feces or rectal swabs. Prompt laboratory processing of specimens and use of several media increase the likelihood of *Shigella* isolation. Infection is usually associated with the presence of pus cells in the stool exudate.

2. **Infectious agents**—The genus *Shigella* is comprised of 4 species or sub-genera: Group A, *S. dysenteriae;* Group B, *S. flexneri;* Group C, *S. boydii;* and Group D, *S. sonnei*. Groups A, B and C are further divided into some 40 serotypes, designated by arabic numbers. A specific plasmid has been associated with virulence.

3. **Occurrence**—Worldwide; two-thirds of the cases, and most of the deaths, are in children under 10 years; common during the weaning period. Illness in infants under 6 months is unusual. Secondary attack rates in households are high, ranging from 10–40%. Outbreaks commonly occur under conditions of crowding and poor sanitation, such as in jails, institutions for children, day-care centers, mental hospitals, crowded camps and aboard ships. Shigellosis is endemic in both tropical and temperate climates; reported cases represent only a small proportion of cases, even in developed areas.

More than one serotype commonly is present in a community; mixed infections with other intestinal pathogens also occur. In general at this time, *S. boydii, S. dysenteriae,* and *S. flexneri* account for most isolates from developing countries. In contrast, *S. sonnei* is most common and *S. dysenteriae* is uncommon in developed countries. Multi-antibiotic-resistant *Shigella* (including *S. dysenteriae*) have appeared in many areas of the world, possibly related to widespread use of antimicrobial agents.

4. Reservoir—The only significant reservoir is man. However, outbreaks have occurred in primate colonies.

5. Mode of transmission—By direct or indirect fecal-oral transmission from a patient or carrier. Infection may occur after the ingestion of very few (10–100) organisms. Individuals primarily responsible for transmission are those who fail to clean hands and under fingernails thoroughly after defecation. They may then spread infection to others by direct physical contact or indirectly by contaminating food. Water, milk, cockroach and fly-borne transmission may occur as the result of direct fecal contamination.

6. Incubation period—One to 7 days, usually 1–3 days.

7. Period of communicability—During acute infection and until the infectious agent is no longer present in feces, usually within 4 weeks after illness. Asymptomatic carriers may transmit infection; rarely, the carrier state may persist for months, or longer.

8. Susceptibility and resistance—Susceptibility is general with infection following ingestion of a small number of organisms; the disease is more severe in children than in adults, among whom many infections may be asymptomatic. The elderly, debilitated individuals, and persons of all ages suffering from malnutrition, are particularly susceptible to severe disease and death. Studies with experimental serotype-specific live oral vaccines have shown protection of short duration against infection with the homologous strain.

9. Methods of control—Because of the diverse problems which may be involved in shigellosis, local health authorities must be prepared to evaluate the local situation and take appropriate steps to prevent the spread of infection. It is not possible to provide a specific set of guidelines applicable to all situations. The potentially high case fatality rate in infections with *S. dysenteriae* type 1, coupled with antibiotic resistance, calls for measures comparable to those for typhoid fever, including the need to identify source(s) of infection. In contrast, an infection with *S. sonnei* in a private home would not merit such an approach. Institutional outbreaks, without regard to the infecting species, may require special measures, including separate housing for cases and new admissions, and repeated cultures of patients and attendants. The most difficult epidemics to control are those involving young children (not yet toilet-trained), the mentally defective, and situations where there is an inadequate supply of water.

    A.   *Preventive measures:* Same as those listed under typhoid fever, 9A, 1–10, except that no commercial vaccines are yet available.

    B.   *Control of patient, contacts and the immediate environment:*

        1)   Report to local health authority: Case report is obligatory

in most states and countries, Class 2B (see Preface). Recognition and report of epidemics in schools and institutions is especially important.

2) Isolation: During acute illness, enteric precautions. Because of the extremely small infective dose, patients with known *Shigella* infections should not be employed to handle food or to provide child or patient care until 2 successive fecal samples or rectal swabs, (collected ≥ 24 hours apart, but not sooner than 48 hours following discontinuance of antimicrobials) are found to be free of *Shigella*.

3) Concurrent disinfection: Of feces and contaminated articles. In communities with a modern and adequate sewage disposal system, feces can be discharged directly into sewers without preliminary disinfection. Terminal cleaning.

4) Quarantine: None.

5) Management of contacts: Whenever feasible, ill contacts of shigellosis patients should be excluded from foodhandling and the care of children or patients until diarrhea ceases and 2 successive negative stool cultures are obtained. Thorough handwashing after defecation and before handling food or caring for children or patients must be stressed if such contacts are unavoidable.

6) Investigation of contacts: The search for unrecognized mild cases and convalescent carriers among contacts may be unproductive for sporadic cases and seldom contributes to the control of an outbreak. Cultures of contacts should generally be confined to foodhandlers, attendants and children in hospitals, and other situations where the spread of infection is particularly likely.

7) Specific treatment: Fluid and electrolyte replacement is the most important consideration (see Cholera, 9B7). Antibiotics (TMP-SMX, ampicillin, tetracyclines, nalidixic acid, and chloramphenicol) shorten the duration of illness and of positive cultures and should be used in individual cases if warranted by the severity of the illness or to protect contacts (i.e., in day-care centers or institutions) when epidemiologically indicated. Multi-resistance to antibiotics is common so the choice of specific agents will depend on the antibiogram of the isolated strain or on local antimicrobial susceptibility patterns. Antimotility agents are contraindicated.

C. *Epidemic measures:*

1)   Groups of cases of acute diarrheal disorder should be reported at once to the local health authority, even in the absence of specific identification of the causal agent.

2)   Investigation of food, water and milk supplies, and general sanitation.

3)   Prophylactic administration of antibiotics is generally not recommended.

D.   *Disaster implications:* A potential problem where personal and environmental sanitation are deficient (see Typhoid fever).

E.   *International measures:* WHO Collaborating Centres (see Preface).

SMALLPOX   ICD-9 050

The last naturally acquired case of smallpox in the world occurred in October 1977 and global eradication was certified 2 years later by the WHO and confirmed by the World Health Assembly in May 1980. Thus, the occurrence of even a single case anywhere in the world is an international epidemiological emergency. Because of the imperative need for rapid diagnosis and immediate institution of effective control measures should a case occur (in nature or from a laboratory accident), this disease, now extinct, warrants this full presentation.

1. Identification—A systemic viral disease with an exanthem which is usually characteristic. Onset is sudden, with fever, malaise, headache, severe backache, prostration and occasionally abdominal pain. After 2–4 days the temperature falls and a rash appears. This rash passes through successive stages of macules, papules, vesicles, pustules and finally scabs which fall off at the end of the 3rd-4th week; fever frequently rises as the rash progresses to the pustular stage. The lesions become evident first on the face and subsequently on the body and extremities, are more abundant on the face and extremities than on the trunk (centrifugal distribution), and are abundant over prominences and extensor surfaces. In previously vaccinated persons, the rash may be significantly modified to the extent that systemic symptoms are mild to nil and only a few highly atypical lesions are seen which sometimes do not pass through the usual successive stages of rash.

Two principal clinico-epidemiologic varieties of smallpox were recognized: variola minor (alastrim) and variola major (classical smallpox). In variola major, the case fatality rate among the unvaccinated was 15–40%; death occurred as early as the 3rd-4th day but more usually during the 2nd week. Approximately 3% of hospitalized variola major cases experienced a fulminating disease characterized by a severe prodrome, prostration and bleeding into the skin and mucous membranes, uterus and genital tract, especially in pregnant women; such hemorrhagic cases were rapidly fatal. When the usual rash did not appear, disease was confused with severe acute leukemia, meningococcemia or idiopathic thrombocytopenic purpura. In the highly lethal "flat" variety, observed in about 5% of cases, the focal lesions were slow to develop, and the vesicles containing very little fluid tended to project only slightly above the surrounding skin and were soft and velvety to the touch. In the few patients with this type who survived, the lesions sometimes resolved without the usual pustulation and crusting.

Outbreaks of variola minor were associated with a case fatality rate of $\leqq 1\%$. Although the rash was similar to that observed in variola major, the patient generally experienced less severe systemic reactions, and "hemorrhagic" and "flat" types were rarely observed.

Most frequently confused with varicella (chickenpox), smallpox was usually distinguished by the clear-cut prodromal illness, by the centrifugal distribution of the rash, by the appearance of all lesions more or less simultaneously, by the similarity in appearance of all lesions in a given area, and by its more deeply seated lesions.

Laboratory confirmation is made by isolation of the virus on chorioallantoic membrane or tissue culture from scrapings of lesions, vesicular or pustular fluid or crusts and by a rise in titer in serological tests. A rapid provisional diagnosis is often possible by EM or, if not available, by the precipitation-in-gel technique. These last two procedures cannot distinguish smallpox from vaccinia or from monkeypox.

2. Infectious agent—Variola virus.

3. Occurrence—Formerly a worldwide disease, the WHO global program culminated in the eradication of smallpox. The last known case of naturally acquired variola major occurred in Bangladesh on 16 October 1975. Variola minor persisted in the Horn of Africa until 26 October 1977. Since that date, 2 cases occurred in 1978 in Birmingham, England, related to a research laboratory.

4. Reservoir—Prior to eradication, man was the reservoir; now it is held only in stocks of virus in a few restricted laboratories.

5. Mode of transmission—By close contact with respiratory discharges and skin lesions of patients, or material which they had recently contaminated; infrequently airborne spread. Household, hospital and school contacts were especially at risk. Spread to laundry workers by bedding and other linens was frequently observed. Inapparent infections have not been implicated, but unrecognized cases sometimes led to extensive secondary spread.

6. Incubation period—From 7–17 days; commonly 10–12 days to onset of illness and 2–4 days more to onset of rash.

7. Period of communicability—From the time of the development of the earliest lesions to disappearance of all scabs; about 3 weeks. Most communicable during first week.

8. Susceptibility and resistance—Susceptibility is universal; long-term immunity usually followed recovery; second attacks were rare.

9. Methods of control—

   A. *Preventive measures:*

     1) Since smallpox has now been eradicated, routine vaccination is no longer justified. International Certificates of Vaccination against smallpox are no longer required of any travelers.

     2) Vaccination is recommended only for those few research workers in laboratories still conducting research on variola virus or related orthopox viruses; in the USA, vaccine for this purpose can be obtained from the CDC, Division of Host Factors, Clinical Medicine Branch, Atlanta GA 30333; telephone (404) 329-3356.

     3) Military forces in some countries continue to be vaccinated to protect against the remote possibility of biological warfare, even though international convention precludes such warfare. Appropriate measures should be taken by such services to minimize risk to unvaccinated contacts. (See 9A4, below).

     4) Vaccination, should it ever be required, is accomplished by inserting potent vaccinia virus into the superficial layers of the skin. Freeze-dried vaccine, now stockpiled by WHO and many countries, retains adequate potency. The preferred site for vaccination is the outer aspect of the upper arm over the insertion of the deltoid muscle. No cleansing of the skin is needed unless the vaccination site is obviously dirty, in which case it should be gently cleansed with water, and permitted to dry.

       Two different vaccination techniques may be used—multiple puncture and jet injection with the Ped-o-jet. In the **multiple puncture technique**, a forked (bifurcated) needle is used. The needle is dipped into the vaccine and then, holding the needle perpendicular to the skin, punctures are made in an up-and-down manner within an area about 3 mm (1/8 inch) in diameter. Five punctures are made for previously unvaccinated and 15 for revaccinations. A trace of blood should be observed at the vaccination site. For jet injection, a special bacteria-free vaccine is required. Any vaccine on the surface should be removed.

To minimize risk of infection of unvaccinated contacts, a loose dressing should be applied over any lesion which might develop; the individual should avoid physical contact with others, especially those with a history of eczema. Vaccination is repeated as above 1 wk later unless a "major reaction" is present, indicating that an immunizing vaccinal infection has occurred. A "major reaction" is one which, 1 wk after vaccination, presents a vesicular or pustular lesion, or an area of definite induration or erythema surrounding a scab or ulcer remaining at the point of vaccine insertion. All other responses are "equivocal reactions" and the individual should be vaccinated again, using a more vigorous technique. All primary vaccinations should elicit a major reaction; revaccinations, except in highly immune groups, should produce major reactions in 80–90% of subjects. Persons with a high level of cellular immunity may exhibit an allergic reaction in the first 2–3 days after vaccination, even with a vaccine which has lost its infectivity, with erythema and papules or vesicles resulting in a scab which may still be present at the end of 1 week.

Major complications and undesirable sequelae of vaccination are: (1) encephalitis, very rare with current vaccine strains; (2) progressive vaccinia (vaccinia necrosum), exceptionally rare, occurring in individuals with immunological defects or in those who are receiving immunosuppressive drugs, corticosteroids or radiation; (3) eczema vaccinatum occurring in those with past or present eczema, which may occur in eczematous siblings of vaccinees.

More frequent but minor complications include (1) generalized vaccinia with multiple vaccinial lesions appearing in 5–10 days on various parts of the body; (2) autoinoculation of mucous membranes or abraded skin; (3) benign erythema multiforme type rash, usually generalized and symmetrical which may frequently occur at the height of the vaccinia, and (4) secondary infections, caused by tetanus, staphylococci or other organisms, from contamination of the vaccination site. Vaccinia immune globulin (VIG), 0.3–0.6 ml/kg, is indicated in the treatment of eczema vaccinatum and progressive vaccinia. It may be obtained in the USA on an emergency basis by contacting the CDC, Atlanta (see Preface). Methisazone (Marboran) may be of benefit in treatment of these conditions.

5) Vaccination of those at special risk of experiencing complications. These are: (1) persons with eczema, leukemia, lymphoma or other reticuloendothelial malignancies and dysgammaglobulinemia; (2) patients receiving immunosuppressive drugs such as steroids or antimetabolites or ionizing radiation; (3) pregnant women. If such an individual should require vaccination, VIG, 0.3 ml/kg, should be given concurrently with vaccination. If there has been possible exposure to a case of smallpox, vaccination is indicated even if VIG is not available.

6) The past policy of immediate widespread vaccination when a suspected case of smallpox was detected is no longer justified. Vaccination should not be performed unless a presumptive diagnosis of smallpox is established on examination by a physician with extensive experience in the clinical and epidemiologic diagnosis of smallpox and on a laboratory report confirming that poxvirus particles have been demonstrated by electron microscopy. In any case, initial vaccination should be limited to household and other close contacts.

B. *Control of patient, contacts and the immediate environment:*

1) Report to local health authority: AN INTERNATIONAL EPIDEMIOLOGICAL EMERGENCY. REPORT BY TELEPHONE OR TELEGRAPH TO HEALTH AUTHORITIES. All suspected cases should be investigated immediately by clinical and laboratory study by state, national and, appropriately, international authorities. The occurrence of even one laboratory-confirmed case of smallpox would be an international emergency as it would call into question the status of eradication or indicate that virus had escaped from a research laboratory. Occurrence of cases only clinically suspected to be smallpox constitute a public health emergency.

2) Isolation: Strict isolation precautions until all scabs have separated. Infection can be transmitted by air currents and virus can be carried outside the hospital by various materials contaminated by the patient, especially on clothing and linen.

3) Concurrent disinfection: Deposit oral and nasal discharges in a paper container and burn. Bedclothes and other fabrics should be sterilized by boiling or autoclaving. Terminal disinfection: The floors, walls and other hard surfaces

should be fumigated, or sprayed or mopped with disinfecting agents known to kill poxviruses and allowed to remain for 4 hours before washing with water. Compounds found to be of value include phenolic and quaternary ammonium compounds, formalin and chlorine preparations. When fumigation is practiced, spaces can be disinfected by exposure to moist formalin vapor for 6 hours, or to ethylene oxide. Exposure to ultraviolet light or sunlight for several hours is also effective if surfaces are fully exposed.

4) Quarantine: All persons living in the same house with the smallpox patient as well as face-to-face contacts should be vaccinated promptly with known potent vaccine (see 9B5, below) and placed under daily surveillance for 17 days after last contact with the smallpox patient. Quarantine should be substituted for surveillance of intimate contacts whose cooperation is uncertain. At the first sign of fever or other illness, the individual should be isolated. Any who refuse vaccination or have not been vaccinated (as determined by absence of vaccination scar) and who have been in intimate contact with the patient, should be placed under quarantine for the period when disease might appear, i.e., from 7 days after the first contact to 17 days after the last exposure to a case.

5) Immunization of contacts: All contacts of a laboratory-confirmed smallpox case, both intimate and casual, should be promptly vaccinated, employing a known potent vaccine. Previously vaccinated contacts exposed $\geqq 7$ days before, as well as all unvaccinated contacts, should receive VIG, if available, 0.3 ml/kg (see 9A4, above).

6) Investigation of contacts and source of infection: Prompt investigation to determine the source of infection is of the greatest importance. The diagnosis in some outbreaks was not made until the 3rd-4th generation of cases. Since inapparent cases of smallpox are rare and do not appear to transmit infection, the chain of infection can almost always be determined. Persons with supposed "chickenpox" or those who have recently experienced pustular or hemorrhagic disease (especially fatal cases) should be considered as possible sources of infection.

7) Specific treatment: None.

C. *Epidemic measures:*

1) Isolation of patients, laboratory confirmation of diagnosis, vaccination of contacts and investigation of source of infection (see 9B, above).

2) Immediate assistance should be obtained from national and international authorities for detailed investigation and for implementation of necessary control measures. Vaccine can be made available quickly from national stockpiles or the WHO emergency reserve. The amount of vaccination which might be required would depend on circumstances, but in most outbreaks, vaccination of a few hundred to a few thousand persons has successfully stopped spread. Mass vaccination of entire communities was neither necessary nor desirable to control an outbreak.

D. *Disaster implications:* Introduction of variola virus into a nonimmune population could result in a major disaster unless controlled promptly.

E. *International measures:*

1) Telegraphic notification by governments to WHO and to adjacent countries if any case of smallpox is found or suspected.

2) In December 1979, the Global Commission for the Certification of Smallpox Eradication concluded that: (1) smallpox eradication had been achieved throughout the world; and (2) that there was no evidence that smallpox would return as an endemic disease. Recommendations were submitted to assure the permanence of the eradication; these were accepted by the World Health Assembly on 8 May 1980. These recommendations include (1) discontinuance of smallpox vaccination except for those at special risk of exposure and elimination of the international certificate of vaccination for travelers; (2) the establishment of a stockpile of freeze-dried vaccine sufficient to vaccinate 200 million people to be maintained by WHO in two independent refrigerated depots (presently Geneva and Lausanne); (3) investigate thoroughly all cases of suspected smallpox with WHO participation, under a WHO coordinated system, with full dissemination of all information; (4) stocks of variola virus to be held and handled at no more than 2 WHO Collaborating Centres with adequate containment facilities which will be inspected periodically by WHO; (5) a special surveillance program for human monkeypox which will continue until 1989; and (6) WHO to encourage and coordinate diagnostic work and research on orthopoxviruses. At the present time, 163 of WHO's 164 member states and associated members have officially discontinued routine

vaccination; vaccination is being continued only in Albania. The 2 laboratories known to retain stocks of variola virus are the CDC, Atlanta, GA, USA and the Research Institute for Viral Preparations, Moscow, USSR.

MONKEYPOX   ICD-9 051.9

Human monkeypox is a rare zoonosis that was not recognized until smallpox was eliminated from the area where monkeypox occurs. Between 1970 and June 1984, 195 cases had been reported from tropical rain forest areas of west and central Africa; 180 of these cases occurred in Zaire. Clinically the disease resembles smallpox. The case fatality rate is 12–16%, comparable to that of smallpox when it was in that area. Cases have occurred in close contacts of earlier cases, suggesting a secondary attack rate of about 10%, much lower than that for smallpox (usually 40–80%). The virus is a member of the orthopoxviruses, but distinct from variola virus; smallpox vaccination protects against disease. Monkeypox virus has been isolated from outbreaks in captive animals, but no strains have been isolated from wild animals. With elimination of vaccination and waning immunity against these viruses, an increase in human cases may occur but is not considered a threat to the permanence of smallpox eradication.

SPOROTRICHOSIS   ICD-9 117.1

1. **Identification**—A fungal disease, usually of the skin, often of an extremity, which begins as a nodule. As the nodule grows, lymphatics draining the area become firm and cordlike and form a series of nodules, which in turn may soften and ulcerate. Arthritis, pneumonitis and other visceral infections are rare. A fatal result is uncommon.

Laboratory confirmation is made by culture of the pus or exudate, preferably aspirated from an unopened lesion; organisms rarely visualized by direct smear. Biopsied tissue should be examined with fungal stains.

2. **Infectious agent**—*Sporothrix schenckii,* a dimorphic fungus.

3. **Occurrence**—Reported from all parts of the world, in males more frequently than in females, and in adults more than in children; often an occupational disease of farmers, gardeners and horticulturists. No differences in racial susceptibility. The disease is characteristically sporadic, and relatively uncommon. An epidemic among gold miners in S Africa involved some 3,000 persons; fungus was growing on mine timbers.

4. **Reservoir**—Soil, vegetation, wood.

5. Mode of transmission—Introduction of fungus through the skin by pricks of thorns or barbs, the handling of sphagnum moss or by slivers from wood or lumber. Outbreaks have occurred among children playing and adults working with baled hay. Pulmonary sporotrichosis is assumed to arise by inhalation of conidia.

6. Incubation period—The lymphatic form may develop 1 wk to 3 months after injury.

7. Period of communicability—Not transmitted from person to person.

8. Susceptibility and resistance—Man probably is highly susceptible.

9. Methods of control—

A. *Preventive measures:* Treat lumber with fungicides in industries where disease occurs.

B. *Control of patient, contacts and the immediate environment:*

1) Report to local health authority: Official report not ordinarily justifiable, Class 5 (see Preface).
2) Isolation: None.
3) Concurrent disinfection: Of discharges and dressings. Terminal cleaning.
4) Quarantine: None.
5) Immunization of contacts: None.
6) Investigation of contacts and source of infection: To seek undiagnosed and untreated cases.
7) Specific treatment: Orally administered iodides are effective in lymphocutaneous infection; in other forms, amphotericin B (Fungizone®) is effective.

C. *Epidemic measures:* In the S African epidemic, mine timbers were sprayed with a mixture of zinc sulfate and triolith. This and other sanitary measures controlled the epidemic.

D. *Disaster implications:* None.

E. *International measures:* None.

STAPHYLOCOCCAL DISEASE

Staphylococci produce a variety of syndromes with clinical manifestations that range from a single pustule to impetigo to septicemia and death. A lesion or lesions containing pus is the primary clinical finding, abscess formation the typical pathology. Virulence of bacterial strains varies greatly. The most useful index of pathogenicity is an ability to coagulate plasma (coagulase); almost all virulent strains are coagulase-positive.

Staphylococcal disease has distinctly different clinical and epidemiological patterns in the general community, in newborns, in menstruating women, or among hospitalized patients. Therefore, each will be presented separately. Staphylococcal food poisoning, an intoxication and not an infection, is discussed separately (see Foodborne Intoxication, Staphylococcal); attention here is to local and general staphylococcal infections.

I. STAPHYLOCOCCAL DISEASE IN THE COMMUNITY

BOILS, CARBUNCLES, FURUNCLES	ICD-9 680, 041.1
IMPETIGO	ICD-9 684, 041.1
CELLULITIS, ABSCESSES	ICD-9 682.9, 041.1
STAPHYLOCOCCAL SEPTICEMIA	ICD-9 038.1
STAPHYLOCOCCAL PNEUMONIA	ICD-9 482.4
OSTEOMYELITIS	ICD-9 730, 041.1
ENDOCARDITIS	ICD-9 421.0, 041.1

1. **Identification**—The common skin lesions are impetigo, boils, carbuncles, abscesses and infected lacerations. The basic lesion of impetigo is described in II, below; in addition, a distinctive scalded skin syndrome is associated with certain strains of *Staphylococcus aureus,* most often those of phage group II which elaborate an exfoliative toxin. The other skin lesions are localized and discrete. Constitutional symptoms are unusual; if lesions extend or are widespread, fever, malaise, headache or anorexia may develop. Usually, lesions are uncomplicated but seeding of the bloodstream may lead to pneumonia, lung abscess, osteomyelitis, septicemia, endocarditis, pyarthrosis, meningitis, or brain abscess. In addition to primary lesions of the skin, staphylococcal conjunctivitis and osteomyelitis are relatively frequent. Staphylococcal pneumonia is a well recognized complication of influenza. Staphylococcal endocarditis and other complications of staphylococcal bacteremia may result from parenteral use of illicit drugs. It is a frequent cause of secondary infection of skin lesions.

2. **Infectious agents**—Various coagulase-positive strains of *Staphylococcus aureus* which may be characterized by phage type, antibiotic resistance or serological agglutination; epidemics are caused by relatively few specific strains and these are usually resistant to penicillin G. Coagulase-negative *S. epidermidis* may also cause septicemia, endocarditis and urinary infections and are increasingly involved in the etiology of disease.

3. **Occurrence**—Worldwide. Maximal incidence is in areas where

personal hygiene (especially the use of soap and water) is suboptimal and people are crowded. Common among children, especially in warm weather. Occurs sporadically and as small epidemics in families and summer camps, with various members developing recurrent illness due to the same staphylococcal strain.

4. Reservoir—Man.

5. Mode of transmission—The major site of colonization is the anterior nares; 30–40% of the general population carry coagulase-positive staphylococci there. Auto-infection is responsible for at least one-third of infections. Persons with a draining lesion or any purulent discharge are the most common source of epidemic spread. Transmission is by contact with a person who either has a purulent lesion or is an asymptomatic (usually nasal) carrier of a pathogenic strain. Some carriers are more effective disseminators of infection than others. The rôle of contaminated objects has been overstressed; the hands are the most important instrument for transmitting infection. Airborne spread is rare but has been demonstrated in infants with associated viral respiratory disease.

6. Incubation period—Variable and indefinite. Commonly 4–10 days.

7. Period of communicability—As long as purulent lesions continue to drain or the carrier state persists. Auto-infection may continue for the period of nasal colonization or duration of active lesions.

8. Susceptibility and resistance—Immune mechanisms are not well understood. Susceptibility is greatest among the newborn and the chronically ill. Elderly and debilitated persons, as well as those with diabetes mellitus, cystic fibrosis, agammaglobulinemia, agranulocytosis, neoplastic disease and burns are particularly susceptible. Use of steroids and antimetabolites also increases susceptibility.

9. Methods of control—

   A. *Preventive measures:*

      1) Educate in personal hygiene, especially handwashing and the importance of avoiding common use of toilet articles.

      2) Prompt treatment of initial cases in children and families.

   B. *Control of patient, contacts and the immediate environment:*

      1) Report to local health authority: Obligatory report of outbreaks in schools, summer camps or other population groups; also any recognized concentration of cases in the community. No individual case report, Class 4 (see Preface).

      2) Isolation: Not practical in most communities; infected

persons should avoid contact with infants and debilitated persons.

3) Concurrent disinfection: Place dressings from open lesions and discharges in disposable bag and burn, or dispose in other practical and safe manner. Terminal cleaning.

4) Quarantine: None.

5) Immunization of contacts: None.

6) Investigation of contacts: Search for draining lesions; occasionally, determination of nasal carrier status of the pathogenic strain among family members is useful.

7) Specific treatment: In localized skin infections, systemic antibiotics are not indicated unless infection spreads significantly or complications ensue. Abscesses should be incised to permit drainage of pus. For severe staphylococcal infections employ a penicillinase-resistant penicillin or, when hypersensitivity to penicillins is present, use a cephalosporin (unless there is a history of immediate hypersensitivity to penicillin), clindamycin or vancomycin. In severe systemic infections the selection of antibiotics should be governed by results of susceptibility tests on isolates. Vancomycin is the treatment of choice for severe infections with methicillin-resistant *S. aureus*. Prompt parenteral treatment is important. Staphylococci are generally insensitive to sulfonamides unless they are used in combination with trimethoprim (e.g., in TMP-SMX).

C. *Epidemic measures:*

1) Search for and treat persons with clinical disease, especially those with draining lesions, with local application of an appropriate antibiotic (such as bacitracin, 4 times/d). Institute strict personal hygiene with emphasis on handwashing. Culture for nasal carriers of the epidemic strain, and treat locally (see II, 9C3, below).

2) An unusual or abrupt increase in prevalence of staphylococcal infections in the community should be investigated for a possible common source such as an unrecognized hospital epidemic.

D. *Disaster implications:* None.

E. *International measures:* WHO Collaborating Centres (see Preface).

II. STAPHYLOCOCCAL DISEASE IN HOSPITAL NURSERIES
IMPETIGO
ABSCESS OF BREAST

ICD-9 684, 041.1
ICD-9 675.1, 041.1

1. **Identification**—Impetigo of the newborn (pemphigus neonatorum) and other purulent skin manifestations are the most frequent nursery-acquired staphylococcal diseases; the characteristic skin lesions develop secondary to colonization of nose or umbilicus, conjunctiva, circumcision site or rectum of infants with a pathogenic strain. (Colonization of these sites with nonpathogenic strains of staphylococci is a normal occurrence in infants and does not imply disease.) Lesions most commonly are in diaper and intertriginous areas but may be distributed anywhere on the body; they are initially vesicular, rapidly turning seropurulent, surrounded by an erythematous base. Rupture of pustules favors peripheral spread. Though less common, scalded skin syndrome or Ritter's disease may occur with clinical manifestations ranging from diffuse scarlatiniform erythema to scattered bullous impetigo to generalized disease (Ritter's). Complications are unusual although furunculosis, breast abscess, staphylococcal pneumonia, septicemia, meningitis, osteomyelitis, brain abscess or other serious disease has been reported.

2. **Infectious agents**—Same as for staphylococcal disease in the community (I., above).

3. **Occurrence**—Worldwide. Problems occur mainly in hospitals, are promoted by laxity in aseptic techniques and are exaggerated by development of antibiotic-resistant strains of the infectious agent, i.e., hospital strains.

4. **Reservoir**—Same as for staphylococcal disease in the community (I., above).

5. **Mode of transmission**—Primary mode is spread by hands of hospital personnel; rarely airborne.

6. **Incubation period**—Commonly 4–10 days but disease may not occur until several months after colonization.

7. **Period of communicability**—Same as for staphylococcal disease in the community (I., above).

8. **Susceptibility and resistance**—Susceptibility in the newborn appears to be general. Infants remain at risk of disease for duration of colonization with pathogenic strains.

9. **Methods of control**—

   A. *Preventive measures:*

1)   Use aseptic techniques and adequate handwashing before each infant contact in nurseries.
2)   A rotational system ("cohorting") in the nursery whereby one unit (A) is filled and subsequent babies are admitted to a second nursery (B), while the initial unit (A) discharges infants and is cleaned before new admissions. If facilities are present for rooming-in of baby with mother, this may reduce risk. Colonized or infected infants should be isolated.
3)   Surveillance and supervision through an active hospital Infection Control Committee, including a regular system of reporting, investigating and reviewing all hospital-acquired infections. Illness developing after discharge from hospital should also be investigated and recorded.
4)   Some advocate routine application of antibacterial substances such as triple dye (brilliant green, crystal violet, acriflavine), chlorhexidine, or bacitracin ointment to the umbilical cord stump while the baby is in the hospital.

B. *Control of patient, contacts and the immediate environment:*

1)   Report to local health authority: Obligatory report of epidemics; no individual case report, Class 4 (see Preface).
2)   Isolation: Without delay place all known or suspect cases in the nursery on isolation precautions. Do not permit hospital personnel with minor staphylococcal lesions (pustules, boils, abscesses, paronychia, conjunctivitis, severe acne, otitis externa or infected lacerations) to work in the nursery.
3)   through 5) Same as for staphylococcal disease in the community. (I9B3–5, above.)
6)   Investigation of contacts and source of infection: See epidemic measures in 9C, below.
7)   Specific treatment: For localized impetiginous lesions: remove crusts, cleanse skin, treat with bacitracin ointment or wash with an iodophor solution 4–6 times/d. Systemic antibiotics are not indicated unless disease is progressive with fever, malaise or secondary complications. For serious infections, treat as in I, 9B7, above.

C. *Epidemic measures:*

1)   The occurrence of 2 or more concurrent cases of staphylococcal disease related to a nursery or a maternity ward is presumptive evidence of an epidemic and warrants investigation. Culture all lesions to determine antibiotic resistance pattern of epidemic strain. Clinically important

isolates should be kept by the laboratory for 2–4 wks before discarding. This makes possible epidemiologic investigation using antibiotic sensitivity patterns and phage typing.

2) In a nursery outbreak, institute isolation precautions for cases and contacts until all have been discharged. Before admitting new patients, wash cribs, beds, isolettes and other furniture with an approved disinfectant. Autoclave instruments and basins, wipe mattresses and sterilize bedding and diapers.

3) Examine all patient-care personnel, including physicians, nurses' aides and attendants, for draining lesions anywhere on the body. Culture nasal specimens from all persons in contact with infants. Under circumstances of continuing disease it may become necessary to exclude and treat all carriers of the epidemic strain until cultures are negative. Treatment of asymptomatic carriers is directed at suppression of the nasal carrier state, usually accomplished by the local application of appropriate antibiotic ointments to the nasal vestibule, rather than by systemic treatment.

4) Investigate adequacy of nursing procedures; emphasize strict aseptic technique. Personnel assigned to isolation and quarantine nurseries should not work with normal newborns.

5) Although prohibited for routine use in the USA because CNS damage may result from systemic absorption, preparations containing 3% hexachlorophene may be employed during an outbreak. Full-term infants may be bathed in the diaper area only as soon after birth as possible and daily until they are discharged. After bathing is completed, the hexachlorophene should be washed off thoroughly.

III. STAPHYLOCOCCAL DISEASE IN MEDICAL AND SURGICAL WARDS OF HOSPITALS

1. Identification—Lesions vary from simple furuncles or stitch abscesses to extensively infected bedsores or surgical wounds, septic phlebitis, chronic osteomyelitis, fulminating pneumonia, endocarditis or septicemia. Postoperative staphylococcal disease is a constant threat to the convalescence of the hospitalized surgical patient. The increasing complexity of surgical operations, with greater organ exposure and more prolonged anesthesia, promotes entry of staphylococci. Frequent and sometimes injudicious use of antibiotic therapy has increased the prevalence of

antibiotic-resistant staphylococci. Staphylococcal enteritis is a serious complication which occasionally occurs in antibiotic-treated patients.

Verification depends on isolation of *Staphylococcus aureus,* associated with a clinical illness compatible with the bacteriologic findings.

2. Infectious agent—*Staphylococcus aureus;* see I, section 2, above. Predominantly antibiotic resistant with 85–90% resistant to penicillin and increasing proportions resistant to semi-synthetic penicillins (e.g., methicillin) and the aminoglycosides (e.g., gentamicin).

3. Occurrence—Worldwide. Staphylococcal infection is a major form of acquired sepsis in the general wards of hospitals. At times, attack rates assume epidemic proportions. Spread to the community may occur when persons infected in the hospital are discharged.

4. Reservoir; 5. Mode of transmission; 6. Incubation period; 7. Period of communicability—Same as for staphylococcal disease in the community. (I, above.)

8. Susceptibility and resistance—Susceptibility is general, but greatest in chronically ill or debilitated patients, those receiving systemic steroid or antimetabolite therapy and those undergoing major and prolonged surgical operation and convalescence. The widespread use of continuous i.v. therapy with in-dwelling plastic catheters and parenteral injections have opened new portals of entry for infectious agents.

9. Methods of control—

    A. Preventive measures:

        1) Strictly enforced aseptic techniques and programs of monitoring nosocomial infections coordinated through a hospital Infection Control Committee.

        2) Educate hospital medical staff to use common antibiotics for simple infections and reserve certain antibiotics (e.g., vancomycin, cephalosporins) for penicillin-resistant staphylococcal infections.

        3) Replace all in-dwelling peripheral venous catheters at least every 72 hours; sites of i.v. infusions every 48 hours.

    B. Control of patient, contacts and the immediate environment:

        1) Report to local health authority: Obligatory report of epidemics; no individual case report, Class 4 (see Preface).

        2) Isolation: Whenever a moderate or heavy abundance of staphylococci is known or suspected to be present in draining pus or the sputum of a patient with pneumonia, the patient should be placed on the appropriate isolation precautions promptly. Isolation is not required when

wound drainage is scanty provided that an occlusive dressing is employed and care is taken in changing dressings to prevent contamination of the environment.

3) Concurrent disinfection: As in staphylococcal disease in the community (I, 9B3, above).

4) Quarantine: None.

5) Immunization of contacts: None.

6) Investigation of contacts and source of infection: Not practical for sporadic cases (see 9C, below).

7) Specific treatment: Appropriate antibiotics as determined by antibiotic sensitivity tests.

C. *Epidemic measures:*

1) The occurrence of 2 or more cases with epidemiologic association is sufficient to suspect epidemic spread and to initiate investigation.

2) Same as II, 9C3, above.

3) Review and enforce rigid aseptic techniques.

D. *Disaster implications:* None.

E. *International measures:* WHO Collaborating Centres (see Preface).

TOXIC SHOCK SYNDROME   ICD-9 785.59

Toxic Shock Syndrome (TSS) is a severe illness characterized by sudden onset of high fever, vomiting, profuse watery diarrhea and myalgia, followed by hypotension, and in severe cases, shock. An erythematous, "sunburn-like" rash is present during the acute phase; about 10 days after onset there is desquamation of the skin, especially of palms and soles. Fever is usually higher than 38.9°C (102°F), the systolic blood pressure <90 mm mercury and three or more organ systems are involved. Those involved include the gastrointestinal; muscular (severe myalgia and/or creatine phosphokinase level greater than twice the normal upper limit); mucous membranes (hyperemia of vaginal, pharyngeal or conjunctival); renal (blood urea nitrogen or creatinine more than twice normal and/or sterile pyuria); hepatic (SGOT or SGPT greater than twice normal); hematological (platelets <100,000); and the CNS (disorientation or alterations in consciousness without focal neurological signs). Blood, throat and CSF are negative for other pathogens on culture although the recovery of *S. aureus* from any of these sites does not invalidate a case; serological tests for Rocky Mountain spotted fever, leptospirosis and measles are negative.

During 1980, almost 900 cases were reported within the USA, 97.1% in women, with a case fatality rate of 5%; 324 cases were reported in 1983. Approximately 95% of the reported female cases occurred during the menstrual period. Epidemiological studies indicated that toxin-producing strains of *S. aureus* were responsible; that virtually all isolated strains have been penicillin-resistant, and that most cases with onset during menstruation have been associated with the use of vaginal tampons; a few cases have been associated with the use of vaginal contraceptive sponges. The incidence of severe cases was estimated to be 3–6/100,000 women of menstrual age/year. In the male cases and the female cases not associated with menstruation, *S. aureus* has been isolated from focal lesions of the skin, bone and lung.

Menstrual TSS can be almost entirely avoided by not using vaginal tampons; the risk may be reduced by using tampons intermittently during each menstrual cycle (that is, not used all day and all night during the period) and possibly by using less absorbant tampons. Instructions for sponge use indicating that they should not be left in place for more than 30 hours should be heeded. Women who develop a high fever and vomiting or diarrhea during the menstrual period should immediately discontinue tampon use and consult a physician. It is not known when those who have had an episode of menstrual TSS can safely resume tampon use.

STREPTOCOCCAL DISEASES CAUSED BY GROUP A (BETA HEMOLYTIC) STREPTOCOCCI

ICD-9 034, 035, 670

(Streptococcal sore throat, Scarlet fever, Impetigo, Erysipelas, Puerperal fever)

1. **Identification**—Group A streptococci cause a variety of diseases. The more frequently encountered conditions are streptococcal sore throat and streptococcal skin infections (impetigo or pyoderma). Other diseases include scarlet fever, puerperal fever, septicemia, erysipelas, cellulitis, mastoiditis, otitis media, pneumonia, peritonitis and wound infections. In outbreaks, one form of clinical disease often predominates.

Streptococcal sore throat patients frequently exhibit fever, sore throat, exudative tonsillitis or pharyngitis and tender anterior cervical lymph nodes. The pharynx, the tonsillar pillars and soft palate may be injected and edematous; petechiae may be present against a background of diffuse redness. There may be a minimum of symptoms. Coincident or subsequent otitis media or peritonsillar abscess may occur; acute rheumatic fever or acute glomerulonephritis or chorea may appear in 1-5 weeks; rheumatic heart disease is a later complication.

Streptococcal skin infection (pyoderma, impetigo) is usually superficial and may proceed through vesicular, pustular, and encrusted stages.

Scarlatiniform rash is unusual and rheumatic fever is not a sequel. Glomerulonephritis, however, may occur later.

Scarlet fever is a form of streptococcal disease characterized by a skin rash; it occurs when the infecting strain of streptococcus is a toxin-producer and the patient is sensitized but not immune to the toxin. Clinical characteristics may include all those symptoms occurring with a streptococcal sore throat (or it may be associated with a wound, skin or puerperal infection) as well as enanthem, strawberry tongue, and exanthem. The rash is usually a fine erythema, commonly punctate, blanching on pressure, often felt (like sandpaper) better than seen and appearing most often on the neck, chest, in folds of the axilla, elbow and groin, and on inner surfaces of the thighs. Typically, the rash does not involve the face, but there is flushing of the cheeks and circumoral pallor. High fever, nausea and vomiting often accompany severe infections. During convalescence, desquamation of the skin occurs at the tips of fingers and toes, less often over wide areas of trunk and limbs, including palms and soles. Incidence and severity of the disease have declined in the USA in recent years. The case fatality rate in some parts of the world, however, has occasionally been as high as 3%. Scarlet fever may be followed by the same sequelae as follow streptococcal sore throat.

Erysipelas is an acute cellulitis characterized by fever, constitutional symptoms, leukocytosis and a red, tender, edematous, spreading lesion of the skin, often with a definite raised border. The central point of origin tends to clear as the periphery extends. Face and legs are common sites. Recurrences are frequent. The disease is more common in women and may be especially severe, with bacteremia, in patients suffering from debilitating disease. Case fatality rates vary greatly depending on the part of the body affected and whether there is an associated disease. Erysipelas due to group A streptococci is to be distinguished from erysipeloid, caused by *Erysipelothrix rhusiopathiae (insidiosa),* a localized cutaneous infection seen primarily as an occupational disease of persons handling animals, meat, poultry and fish.

Streptococcal puerperal fever is an acute disease, usually febrile, accompanied by local and general symptoms and signs of bacterial invasion of the genital tract and sometimes the bloodstream in the postpartum or postabortion patient. Case fatality rate from streptococcal puerperal fever is low when adequately treated. Many puerperal infections are caused by organisms other than hemolytic streptococci; while clinically similar, they differ bacteriologically and epidemiologically. Epidemiologic characteristics and other methods of control are generally the same as those for group A streptococcal infections.

Streptococci of other groups can produce human disease. β-hemolytic organisms of group B are frequently found in the human vagina and may cause neonatal sepsis and suppurative meningitis (q.v.). Group D organisms (including enterococci), hemolytic or nonhemolytic, are involved in subacute bacterial endocarditis and urinary tract infections. α-hemolytic streptococci are also a common cause of subacute bacterial endocarditis.

Provisional laboratory findings which support group A streptococcal disease are based on the isolation of organisms from the affected tissues on blood agar or other appropriate media, identified by the morphology of colonies, production of clear (β-) or α-hemolysis on blood agar, and inhibition by special antibiotic discs containing 0.02–0.04 units of bacitracin. Definitive identification depends upon specific grouping procedures. However, a few group A strains produce little or no β-hemolysis (these may be nephritogenic or rheumatogenic). Latex agglutination, IF techniques, and coagglutination tests are also available for rapid identification. A rise in serum antibody titer (antistreptolysin O, antihyaluronidase, anti-DNA-ase B) may be demonstrated between acute and convalescent stages of illness.

2. **Infectious agent**—*Streptococcus pyogenes,* group A streptococci of approximately 75 serologically distinct types which may vary greatly in geographic and time distributions. Group A streptococci producing skin infections are usually of different serologic types from those associated with throat infections. In scarlet fever, 3 immunologically different types of erythrogenic toxin (A, B and C) have been demonstrated. While β-hemolysis is characteristic of group A streptococci, strains of groups B, C and G are often β-hemolytic. On occasion, groups C and G have produced pharyngitis and group B is the leading cause of neonatal disease (see Group B Streptococcal Disease of the Newborn, below).

3. **Occurrence**—Streptococcal sore throat and scarlet fever are common in temperate zones, well recognized in semitropical areas and less frequently recognized in tropical climates. Inapparent infections are at least as common in tropic as in temperate zones. In the USA, streptococcal diseases may be endemic, epidemic or sporadic in character. Group A streptococcal infections due to a limited number of specific M-types, especially type 12, have frequently been associated with the development of acute glomerulonephritis. Acute rheumatic fever may occur as a nonsuppurative complication following infection with almost any group A serotype with capacity to produce clinical infection of the upper respiratory tract; this complication has virtually disappeared from the industrialized countries but remains a great problem in the developing world. Apart from foodborne epidemics which may occur in any season, the highest incidence is during late winter and spring. The 3–15 year age group is most often affected; no sex or racial differences in incidence have been defined; military and school populations are frequently affected.

The highest incidence of streptococcal impetigo occurs in young children in late summer and fall in hot climates. Nephritis following skin infections is associated with a limited number of M-types of streptococci, e.g., type 49, which generally differ from those associated with nephritis following infections of the upper respiratory tract.

Geographic and seasonal distributions of erysipelas are similar to those for scarlet fever and streptococcal sore throat; most common after 20 years of age and also frequent in infants. Occurrence is sporadic, even during epidemics of streptococcal infection.

Reliable morbidity data do not exist for puerperal fever. In developed countries morbidity and mortality have generally declined precipitously since the advent of antibiotics. It is now chiefly a sporadic disease, although epidemics may occur in institutions where aseptic techniques are faulty.

4. Reservoir—Man.

5. Mode of transmission—Results from direct or intimate contact with patient or carrier, rarely by indirect contact through objects or hands. Nasal carriers are particularly likely to transmit disease. Casual contact rarely leads to infection. In populations where impetigo is prevalent, group A streptococci may be recovered from the normal skin for 1–2 weeks before skin lesions develop; the same strain may appear in the throat (without clinical evidence of throat infection) usually late in the course of the skin infection. Anal carriers have been responsible for nosocomial outbreaks of wound infections. Dried streptococci reaching the air via contaminated floor dust, lint from bedclothing, handkerchiefs, etc., are viable but apparently noninfectious for mucous membranes or intact skin.

Explosive outbreaks of streptococcal sore throat may follow ingestion of contaminated foods. Milk and milk products have been associated most frequently with foodborne outbreaks; egg salad and deviled hard-boiled eggs have recently been implicated with increasing frequency.

6. Incubation period—Short, usually 1–3 days, rarely longer.

7. Period of communicability—In untreated uncomplicated cases 10–21 days; in untreated conditions with purulent discharges, weeks or months. With adequate penicillin therapy, transmissibility generally is terminated within 24–48 hours.

8. Susceptibility and resistance—Susceptibility to streptococcal sore throat and to scarlet fever is general, although many persons develop either antitoxic or type-specific antibacterial immunity, or both, through inapparent infection. Antibacterial immunity develops only against the specific M-type of group A streptococcus that induced infection and may last for years. Antibiotic therapy may interfere with the development of type-specific immunity. Repeated attacks of sore throat or other streptococcal disease due to different types of streptococci are relatively frequent. Immunity against erythrogenic toxin, and hence to rash, develops within a week after onset of scarlet fever and is usually permanent; second attacks of scarlet fever are rare but may occur because of the 3 immunological forms of toxin. Both active and passive immunization against erythrogenic toxin are possible but not practical. Passive immunity to group A streptococcal disease occurs in newborns with transplacental maternal type-specific antibodies.

One attack of erysipelas appears to predispose individuals to subsequent attacks.

9. Methods of control—

A. *Preventive measures:*

1) Provide easily accessible laboratory facilities for recognition of group A hemolytic streptococci.

2) Educate the public in modes of transmission, in the relationship of streptococcal infection to acute rheumatic fever, Sydenham's chorea, rheumatic heart disease and glomerulonephritis, and the necessity for completing the full course of antibiotic therapy prescribed for streptococcal infections.

3) Boil or pasteurize milk and exclude infected persons from handling milk likely to become contaminated. Milk from any cow with evidence of mastitis should be excluded from sale or use.

4) Other foods such as deviled eggs should be prepared just prior to serving or be adequately refrigerated in small quantities at $\leq 5°C$ (41°F).

5) Exclude foodhandlers with respiratory illness or skin lesions from their usual work.

6) Strict asepsis in obstetrical procedures, with special attention to avoid contamination from mouths and noses of attendants, as well as by hands and instruments. Protect patients during labor and the postpartum period from attendants, visitors and other patients with respiratory or skin infection.

7) Long-term antimicrobial prophylaxis: Monthly injections of long-acting benzathine penicillin G or daily penicillin or sulfadiazine orally for persons to whom recurrent streptococcal infection constitutes a special risk, such as individuals who have had rheumatic fever, chorea, or recurrent erysipelas. Those who do not tolerate penicillin or sulfonamides may be given erythromycin.

B. *Control of patient, contacts and the immediate environment:*

1) Report to local health authority: Obligatory report of epidemics; no individual case report, Class 4 (see Preface).

2) Isolation: Drainage/secretion precautions; may be termi-

nated after 24 hours' treatment with penicillin or other effective antibiotics; therapy should be continued for 10 days to avoid development of rheumatic heart disease.

3) Concurrent disinfection: Of purulent discharges and all articles soiled therewith. Terminal cleaning.

4) Quarantine: None.

5) Immunization of contacts: None.

6) Investigation of contacts: In well-documented epidemics of streptococcal infection and in high-risk situations (e.g., evidence of streptococcal infection in a rheumatic family, occurrence of cases of rheumatic fever or acute nephritis in a population group), search for and treat carriers.

7) Specific treatment: Penicillin. Several forms are acceptable for treatment, i.e., i.m. benzathine penicillin G (treatment of choice), i.m. procaine penicillin G, oral penicillin G, or oral penicillin V. Therapy should provide adequate penicillin levels for 10 days. Such treatment initiated within the first 24–48 hours may ameliorate the acute illness, reduce the frequency of suppurative complications and prevent the development of most cases of acute rheumatic fever. Therapy may also reduce the risk of acute glomerulonephritis and prevent further spread of the organism. Erythromycin is the preferred treatment for penicillin-sensitive patients. Sulfonamides are not effective in eliminating the streptococcus from the throat and in preventing nonsuppurative complications. Many strains are resistant to the tetracyclines.

C. *Epidemic measures:*

1) Determine the source and manner of spread, person-to-person, by milk or by food. Outbreaks can often be traced to an individual with an acute or persistent streptococcal infection or carrier state (nose, throat or perianal area) through identification of the serologic type of the streptococcus.

2) Prompt investigation of any unusual grouping of cases for the possibility of contaminated milk or foods.

3) Under special circumstances, penicillin prophylaxis may be given to limited population groups, especially household or other intimate contacts, or those known to have been exposed to contaminated milk or food, or even to an entire population group.

D. *Disaster implications:* Patients with thermal burns or wounds are highly susceptible to streptococcal infections of the affected area.

E. *International measures:* WHO Collaborating Centres (see Preface).

GROUP B STREPTOCOCCAL DISEASE OF THE NEWBORN

ICD-9 038.0

Group B streptococci *(S. agalactiae)* of human subtypes produce important diseases of newborn children; about 90% of cases have septicemia, about 40% have evidence of pulmonary involvement, and about 30% have meningeal involvement. In approximately two-thirds of cases, age at onset is under 1 week of age; these infections are acquired within the amniotic sac or during passage through the birth canal, and have a case fatality rate of 50% with higher rates in very premature infants. The remaining cases, with onset from 1 week–3 months after birth and a case fatality rate of 20%, are probably acquired from the environment. Half of the survivors of meningitis cases are left with hearing loss, blindness, cerebral palsy, mental retardation and/or epilepsy.

While the manner of acquisition is unclear, approximately 10–30% of pregnant women harbor Group B streptococci in the genital tract. Approximately 1% of their offspring develop symptomatic infection; risk of serious disease is greatest in premature infants.

Attempts to eradicate genital tract group B streptococci in women during pregnancy with oral antibiotics have been only partially successful. There are high relapse rates when antibiotics have been discontinued, possibly due to reinfection from rectal carriage of the organism or by possible reacquisition from culture-positive sexual partners.

The administration of i.v. penicillin or ampicillin at the onset and throughout labor to women who are colonized with group B streptococci and who are at high risk of delivering an infected infant (premature gestational age or premature rupture of membranes or intrapartum fever) may be considered. Preliminary studies suggest that this interrupts transmission of group B streptococci to newborn infants and may decrease actual infection and mortality. However, some strains of the organism are moderately resistant to penicillin and require treatment with ampicillin or penicillin plus an aminoglycoside.

STRONGYLOIDIASIS   ICD-9 127.2

1. **Identification**—A helminthic infection of the duodenum and upper jejunum, asymptomatic in the majority of cases. Clinical manifestations include transient dermatitis when larvae of the parasite penetrate the skin on initial infection; cough, râles and sometimes a demonstrable pneumonitis when they pass through the lungs; or abdominal symptoms caused by the adult female in the mucosa of the intestine. Symptoms of chronic infection may be mild or severe, depending upon intensity of infection. Classic symptoms are abdominal pain (usually epigastric and often suggesting peptic ulcer), diarrhea and urticaria; they may also include nausea, weight loss, vomiting, weakness and constipation. Intensely pruritic dermatitis radiating from the anus may occur; stationary wheals lasting 1–2 days may occur as well as a migrating serpigenous rash moving several cm/hour. Rarely, intestinal autoinfection with increasing worm burden may lead to disseminated strongyloidiasis with wasting, pulmonary involvement and death, particularly but not exclusively in the immunocompromised host. In these cases secondary gram-negative sepsis is common. Eosinophilia is usually moderate in the chronic stage but may be absent with overwhelming autoinfection.

Diagnosis is made by identifying larvae in stool specimens (motile in freshly passed feces), in duodenal aspirates or in sputum in disseminated infections. Held at room temperature for ≧24 hours, feces may show developing stages of the parasite including filariform (infective) larvae and free-living adults (which must be distinguished from larvae of hookworm species).

2. **Infectious agent**—*Strongyloides stercoralis,* a nematode.

3. **Occurrence**—Throughout the tropical and temperate areas, more common in warm, wet regions. Prevalence in endemic areas is not accurately known. May be prevalent in institutions where personal hygiene is poor.

4. **Reservoir**—Man and possibly dogs.

5. **Mode of transmission**—Infective (filariform) larvae, which develop in feces or moist soil contaminated with feces, penetrate the skin, enter the venous circulation and are carried to the lungs. They penetrate capillary walls, enter alveoli, ascend the trachea to the epiglottis, and descend the digestive tract to reach the upper part of the small intestine where development of the adult parasitic female is completed. The adult worm, a parthenogenetic female, lives embedded in the mucosal epithelium of the intestine, especially the duodenum, where eggs are deposited. They hatch and liberate noninfective rhabditiform larvae which migrate into the lumen of the intestine, leave the host in the feces and develop into either infective filariform larvae (which may infect the same or a new host) or into

free-living adults after reaching the soil. The free-living, fertilized females produce eggs which soon hatch, liberating rhabditiform larvae, which may become filariform larvae within 24–36 hours. In some individuals, particularly those with compromised immune status, liberated rhabditiform larvae may develop to the infective stage before leaving the body and passing through the intestinal mucosa or perianal skin; the resulting autoinfection can cause overwhelming worm burdens and persistent infection for many years.

6. **Incubation period**—From penetration of the skin by filariform larvae until rhabditiform larvae appear in the feces is about 2 weeks; the period until symptoms appear is indefinite and variable.

7. **Period of communicability**—As long as living worms remain in the intestine; up to 35 years with autoinfection.

8. **Susceptibility and resistance**—Susceptibility to infection is universal. Acquired immunity has been demonstrated in laboratory animals but not in man. Patients with malignant disease or on immunosuppressive medication may experience massive hyperinfection.

9. **Methods of control**—

   A. *Preventive measures:*

       1) Sanitary disposal of human feces.
       2) Rigid attention to hygienic habits.
       3) Rule out strongyloidiasis before initiating immunosuppressive therapy.

   B. *Control of patient, contacts and the immediate environment:*

       1) Report to local health authority: Official report not ordinarily justifiable, Class 5 (see Preface).
       2) Isolation: None.
       3) Concurrent disinfection: Sanitary disposal of feces.
       4) Quarantine: None.
       5) Immunization of contacts: None.
       6) Investigation of contacts: Members of the same household or institution should be examined for evidence of infection.
       7) Specific treatment: Because of the potential for autoinfection, all infections, regardless of worm burden, should be treated preferably with thiabendazole (Mintezol®) or alternatively, mebendazole (Vermox®) or albendazole (Zentel®). Repeated courses of treatment may be required.

   C. *Epidemic measures:* Not applicable; a sporadic disease.

D. Disaster implications: None.

E. International measures: None.

SYPHILIS
I. VENEREAL SYPHILIS   ICD-9 090-097
(Lues)

1. Identification—An acute and chronic treponemal disease characterized clinically by a primary lesion, a secondary eruption involving skin and mucous membranes, long periods of latency, and late lesions of skin, bone, viscera, the CNS and the cardiovascular system. The primary lesion usually appears about 3 weeks after exposure as a papule at the site of the initial invasion; after erosion, it presents a variety of forms, the most distinctive, although not the most frequent, is an indurated painless chancre with a serous exudate. Invasion of the bloodstream precedes the initial lesion, and a firm, nonfluctuant, painless satellite lymph node (bubo) commonly follows. Infection may occur without chancre. After 4–6 weeks, even without specific treatment, the chancre begins to involute and a generalized secondary eruption may appear, often accompanied by mild constitutional symptoms. Secondary manifestations disappear spontaneously within weeks up to 12 months, with subsequent clinical latency of weeks to years. In the early years there may be recurrence of infectious lesions of the skin and mucous membrane or developing lesions of the eye and the CNS. Latency sometimes continues through life and spontaneous recovery may occur. In other instances, and unpredictably, late (5–20 years after initial infection) disabling lesions occur in the cardiovascular system and CNS. Destructive noninfectious lesions of the skin, viscera, bone, and mucosal surface may occur. Death or serious disability does not occur during early stages; late manifestations shorten life, impair health and limit occupational efficiency.

Fetal infection occurs in high frequency with untreated primary and secondary infections of pregnant women and in lower frequency with latency; transplacental infection is uncommon before the 4th month of gestation. It frequently causes abortion or stillbirth or may cause infant deaths due to preterm delivery of low birth weight infants or from generalized systemic disease. Congenital infection may result in late manifestations occasionally causing such stigmata as Hutchinson's teeth, saddlenose, saber shins, interstitial keratitis and deafness.

Primary and secondary syphilis are confirmed by darkfield or phase-contrast examination of exudates of lesions or aspirates from lymph nodes (if no antibiotic has been administered), and by serologic tests of blood and

CSF. Positive tests with nontreponemal antigens should be confirmed by tests employing treponemal antigens, i.e., FA or treponemal hemagglutination, to aid in excluding biologic false-positive reactions. A darkfield examination of all genital ulcerative lesions is indicated and is indispensable in suspected early seronegative primary syphilis.

2. Infectious agent—*Treponema pallidum,* a spirochete.

3. Occurrence—A widespread communicable disease, involving primarily young persons between 15–30 years old. Differences in racial incidence are related more to social than to biologic factors; more prevalent in urban than rural areas and in males than in females; high prevalence among male homosexuals. Since 1957, early venereal syphilis has increased significantly throughout much of the world.

4. Reservoir—Man.

5. Mode of transmission—By direct contact with infectious exudates from obvious or concealed moist early lesions of skin and mucous membrane, body fluids and secretions (saliva, semen, blood, vaginal discharges) of infected persons during sexual contact; rarely by kissing or by fondling children with congenital disease. Transmission can occur through blood transfusion if the donor were in the early stage of disease. Infection by indirect contact with contaminated articles is possible, but rarely occurs. Health professionals have developed primary lesions on the hands following clinical examination of infectious lesions. Fetal infection may occur through placental transfer.

6. Incubation period—Ten days to 10 wks, usually 3 wks.

7. Period of communicability—Variable and indefinite. During primary and secondary stages and also in mucocutaneous recurrences; some cases may be communicable intermittently for 2–4 yrs. Extent of communicability through sexual activity during the latent period (2–4 yrs) is not established; possible inapparent lesions make this stage potentially infectious. Congenital transmission is most probable during early maternal syphilis but can occur throughout the latent period. Adequate penicillin treatment usually ends infectivity within 24–48 hours.

8. Susceptibility and resistance—Susceptibility is universal, though only approximately 10% of exposures result in infection. There is no natural immunity. Infection leads to gradually developing resistance against *Treponema pallidum* and to some extent against heterologous treponemes; immunity may fail to develop because of early treatment in the primary or secondary stage. In late latency, superinfection may cause destructive lesions of the skin, bone and mucous membranes.

9. Methods of control—

A. Preventive measures: For syphilis, emphasis on control of patients with disease in a transmissible stage should not preclude search for persons with latent syphilis to prevent relapse and disability due to late manifestations. Congenital syphilis is prevented by serologic examination in both early and late pregnancy and treatment of positive reactors.

In general, the following are applicable to all sexually transmitted diseases (STD): syphilis, chancroid, lymphogranuloma venereum, granuloma inguinale, gonorrhea, herpes simplex type 2 virus infection, trichomonal vaginitis, bacterial vaginosis, sexually transmitted hepatitis B, and diseases caused by *Chlamydia* and the genital mycoplasms.

1) General health promotion measures, health and sex education and preparation for marriage. Syphilis serology should be included in the workup of all cases of STD and as part of all prenatal examinations, preferably performed both early and late in pregnancy.

2) Protection of the community by control of prostitution and, in cooperation with social agencies, discouragement of sexual promiscuity; by teaching methods of personal prophylaxis applicable before, during and after exposure, especially the use of a condom in high-risk sex contacts.

3) Provision of facilities for early diagnosis and treatment; encouragement of their use through education of the public about symptoms of the STD and modes of spread, and through making these services readily accessible and acceptable, irrespective of economic status. Intensive case-finding programs, to include interview of patients and tracing of contacts; for syphilis, repeated mass serologic examination of special groups with known high incidence of STD.

B. Control of patient, contacts and the immediate environment:

1) Report to local health authority: Case report of early infectious syphilis and congenital syphilis is required in all states, and variously in other countries, Class 2A (see Preface); report of positive serology and darkfield examinations by laboratories is required in most states. Privacy of the individual must be safeguarded.

2) Isolation: For hospitalized patients, drainage/secretion precautions; blood/body fluid precautions are appropriate for patients with primary or secondary syphilis. Precautions are unnecessary for latent or tertiary disease. Patients should refrain from sexual intercourse until

lesions clear and with untreated previous partners to avoid reinfection.

3) Concurrent disinfection: None in adequately treated cases; care to avoid contact with discharges from open lesions and articles soiled therewith.

4) Quarantine: None.

5) Immunization of contacts: Not applicable.

6) Investigation of contacts: The fundamental feature of programs for syphilis control is interview of patients to identify contacts. Trained interviewers obtain best results. The stage of disease determines the criteria for contact-tracing: (1) for primary syphilis, all sexual contacts during the 3 months preceding onset of symptoms; (2) for secondary syphilis, those of the preceding 6 months; (3) for early latent syphilis, those of the preceding year, if time of primary and secondary lesions cannot be established; (4) for late and late latent syphilis, marital partners and children of infected mothers; (5) for congenital syphilis, all members of the immediate family. **All identified contacts of confirmed cases of early syphilis should receive therapy.**

7) Specific treatment: Long-acting penicillin G (benzathine penicillin) given in a single dose of 2.4 million units on the day of diagnosis assures effective therapy even if the patient fails to return; this or 10 daily i.m. doses of aqueous procaine penicillin G 600,000 units, or amoxicillin 3.0 g plus probenicid 1.0 g orally for 15 days, is usually effective for both primary, secondary and recently acquired (<2 years duration) latent syphilis. Increased dosages and longer periods of therapy are indicated for the late stages of syphilis; i.e., benzathine penicillin 2.4 million units weekly for 3 wks; *Or* aqueous procaine penicillin 600,000 units/d for 15 days. For cardiovascular and neurosyphilis, aqueous procaine penicillin 600,000 units/d for 20 days is recommended. Success in therapy should be checked by following serologic titers and appropriate CSF examinations. Tetracycline 2.0 g/d (in 4 doses) for 15–30 days may be used in penicillin-sensitive persons. Erythromycin 2.0 g/d for 15–30 days may be used for penicillin-sensitive pregnant women. These patients and their babies require extended posttreatment observation and follow-up checks of serologic reactions to assure that cure has been achieved; compliance with a regimen of four doses/d for 2–4 wks is a frequent problem.

C. *Epidemic measures:* Intensification of measures outlined under 9A and 9B, above.

D. **Disaster implications:** None.

E. *International measures:*

1) Appropriate examination of groups of adolescents and young adults moving from areas of high prevalence of treponemal infections.

2) Adherence to agreements among nations (e.g., Brussels Agreement) as to records, provision of diagnostic and treatment facilities and contact interviews at seaports for foreign merchant seamen.

3) Provision for rapid international exchange of information on contacts.

4) WHO Collaborating Centres (see Preface).

II. NONVENEREAL ENDEMIC SYPHILIS   ICD-9 104.0
(Bejel, Njovera)

1. Identification—An acute disease of limited geographical distribution, characterized clinically by an eruption of skin and mucous membrane, usually without an evident primary sore. Mucous patches of the mouth are often the first lesions, soon followed by moist papules in skin folds and by drier lesions of the trunk and extremities. Other early skin lesions are macular or papular, often hypertrophic, and frequently circinate resembling those of venereal syphilis. Plantar and palmar hyperkeratoses occur frequently, often with painful fissuring; patchy depigmentation and hyperpigmentation of the skin and alopecia are common. Inflammatory or destructive lesions of skin, long bones, and nasopharynx are late manifestations. Unlike venereal syphilis, the nervous and cardiovascular systems are rarely involved. The case fatality rate is low.

Organisms are demonstrable in lesions by darkfield examination. Serologic tests for syphilis are reactive in the early stages and remain so for many years of latency, gradually tending toward reversal; response to treatment as in venereal syphilis.

2. Infectious agent—*Treponema pallidum,* a spirochete indistinguishable from that of syphilis.

3. Occurrence—A common disease of childhood in localized areas where poor socioeconomic conditions and primitive sanitary and dwelling arrangements prevail. Present in eastern Mediterranean and Asian countries; numerous foci in Africa, particularly in arid regions.

4. Reservoir—Man.

5. Mode of transmission—Direct or indirect contact with infectious early lesions of skin and mucous membranes; the latter favored by common use of eating and drinking utensils and generally unsatisfactory hygienic conditions; congenital transmission does not occur.

6. Incubation period—Two weeks to 3 months.

7. Period of communicability—Until moist eruptions of skin and mucous patches disappear; sometimes several weeks or months.

8. Susceptibility and resistance—Similar to venereal syphilis.

9. Methods of control—

A. *Preventive measures:* Those of the nonvenereal treponematoses. See Yaws, 9A.

B. *Control of patient, contacts and the immediate environment:*

1) Report to local health authority: In selected endemic areas; in most countries not a reportable disease; Class 3B (see Preface).
2) through 7): See Yaws 9B applicable to all nonvenereal treponematoses.

C. *Epidemic measures:* Intensification of preventive and control activities.

D. *Disaster implications:* None.

E. *International measures:* See Yaws 9E. WHO Collaborating Centres, (see Preface).

TAENIASIS

TAENIASIS DUE TO *TAENIA SOLIUM*	ICD-9 123
INTESTINAL FORM	ICD-9 123.0
(Pork tapeworm)	
CYSTICERCOSIS	ICD-9 123.1
(Cysticerciasis, Infection by *Taenia solium cysticercus*)	
***TAENIA SAGINATA* INFECTION**	ICD-9 123.2
(Beef tapeworm) `	

1. Identification—Taeniasis is an intestinal infection with the adult stage of large tapeworms; cysticercosis is a tissue infection with the larval stage of one species, *Taenia solium*. Clinical manifestations of infection with the adult worm are variable and may include nervousness, insomnia, anorexia, loss of weight, abdominal pain and digestive disturbances. Except for the annoyance of having segments of worms emerging from the anus, many infections are asymptomatic. Taeniasis is usually a nonfatal infection but *T. solium* may cause fatal cysticercosis.

The larval infection, cysticercosis, is a serious somatic disease that may involve many different organs. When eggs of the pork tapeworm are swallowed by man they hatch in the small intestine and the larvae migrate to the subcutaneous tissues, striated muscles, and other tissues or vital organs of the body and form cysts (cysticerci). Consequences may be grave when larvae localize in the eye, CNS or heart. In the presence of somatic cysticercosis, epileptiform seizures, signs of intracranial hypertension or psychiatric disturbances strongly suggest cerebral involvement. Neurocysticercosis may cause serious disability with a relatively high case fatality rate.

Infection with an adult tapeworm is diagnosed by identification of proglottids (segments) of the worm, of eggs in the feces or on anal swabs. Eggs of *T. solium* and *T. saginata* cannot be differentiated from each other. Specific diagnosis is based on the morphology of the scolex (head) or gravid proglottids. Obtaining the scolex or head following treatment confirms the identification and assures elimination of the worm (usually only one worm is present). Subcutaneous cysticerci are visible or palpable; microscopic examination of an excised cysticercus confirms the diagnosis. Visceral cysticercosis may be recognized by CAT, or by x-ray when the cysticercus are calcified.

2. Infectious agents—*Taenia saginata,* the beef tapeworm, causes only intestinal infection with the adult worm in man; *T. solium,* the pork tapeworm, causes both intestinal infection with the adult worm and somatic infection with the larva (cysticercus).

3. Occurrence—Worldwide distribution; particularly frequent wherever beef or pork is eaten raw or insufficiently cooked. Prevalence is highest in parts of Latin America, Africa, SE Asia and eastern Europe. Infection with *T. solium* is rare in the USA and Canada, and exceedingly rare in UK and Scandinavia but frequently found in immigrants from endemic areas.

4. Reservoir—Man is the definitive host of both species of *Taenia;* cattle are the intermediate host for *T. saginata,* and pigs for *T. solium.*

5. Mode of transmission—Eggs of *T. saginata* passed in the stool of an infected person are infectious only to cattle, in the flesh of which the parasites develop into "Cysticercus bovis," the larval stage of *T. saginata.* Infection in man follows ingestion of raw or undercooked beef containing the cysticerci; in the intestine the adult worm develops attached to the jejunal mucosa. Human cysticercosis may occur by direct transfer of *T. solium* eggs from the feces of a person harboring an adult worm to his own or another's mouth, or indirectly by ingestion of food or water contaminated with eggs. When the eggs of *T. solium* are ingested by either man or pigs, the embryo escapes from the shell, penetrates the intestinal wall into lymphatics or blood vessels and is carried to the various tissues in which they develop to produce the human disease of cysticercosis, or into the larvae ("Cysticercus cellulosae") in the pig. Intestinal infection in man (taeniasis due to *T. solium*) follows ingestion of raw or undercooked infected pork ("measly pork") with subsequent development of the adult worm in the intestine.

6. **Incubation period**—For the adult *T. solium* tapeworm, from 8–12 wks; for *T. saginata,* 10–14 wks.

7. **Period of communicability**—*T. saginata* is not directly transmitted from person to person but *T. solium* may be; eggs of both species are disseminated into the environment as long as the worm remains in the intestine, sometimes more than 30 yrs; eggs may remain viable in the environment for months.

8. **Susceptibility and resistance**—Susceptibility is general. No apparent resistance follows infection.

9. **Methods of control**—

    A. Preventive measures:

        1) Identification and immediate treatment or institution of enteric precautions for persons harboring adult *T. solium* is essential to prevent human cysticercosis. *T. solium* eggs are infective immediately upon leaving the host and are capable of producing a severe human illness. Appropriate measures to protect the patient from himself and his contacts are necessary.

        2) Education of the public to prevent contamination of soil, water, human and animal food with human feces; to avoid use of sewage effluents for pasture irrigation; and to cook beef and pork thoroughly.

        3) Adequate inspection of the carcasses of cattle and swine will detect a proportion of infected carcasses and these should be condemned or processed.

        4) Deny swine access to human feces.

    B. Control of patient, contacts and the immediate environment:

        1) Report to local health authority: Selectively reportable, Class 3C (see Preface).

        2) Isolation: None recommended. Stools of patients with untreated taeniasis due to *T. solium* may be infective. (See 9A4, above.)

3) Concurrent disinfection: Sanitary disposal of feces; emphasize rigid sanitation, with handwashing after defecating and before eating, especially for *T. solium*.
4) Quarantine: None.
5) Immunization of contacts: None.
6) Investigation of contacts: Evaluate symptomatic contacts.
7) Specific treatment: Niclosamide (Niclocide®, Yomesan®) and praziquantel (Biltricide®) are effective in the treatment of *T. saginata* and *T. solium* intestinal infections. For cysticercosis: surgical intervention may relieve some symptoms; some patients with CNS involvement may benefit from praziquantel therapy under hospital conditions, since reactions to dying cysticerci can be severe.

C. *Epidemic measures:* None.

D. *Disaster implications:* None.

E. *International measures:* None.

TETANUS
(Lockjaw)

ICD-9 037

1. **Identification**—An acute disease induced by an exotoxin of the tetanus bacillus, which grows anaerobically at the site of an injury. The disease is characterized by painful muscular contractions, primarily of the masseter and neck muscles, secondarily of trunk muscles. A common first sign suggestive of tetanus is abdominal rigidity, though rigidity is sometimes confined to the region of injury. Generalized spasms occur, frequently induced by sensory stimuli; typical features of the tetanic spasm are the position of opisthotonus and the facial expression known as "risus sardonicus." History of an injury or apparent portal of entry may be lacking. The case fatality rate varies from 30–90%, according to age, length of incubation and therapy.

Laboratory confirmation is of little help. The organism is rarely recovered from the site of infection and usually there is no detectable antibody response.

2. **Infectious agent**—*Clostridium tetani,* the tetanus bacillus.

3. **Occurrence**—Worldwide. Occurs sporadically in the USA and most industrial countries; it is relatively uncommon (attack rate in the USA is <0.5 cases/ million) and usually occurs in older persons. It is more common in agricultural regions and in underdeveloped areas where contact with

animal excreta is more likely and immunization is inadequate. An important cause of death in many countries of Asia, Africa and S America, especially in rural and tropical areas where tetanus neonatorum is common. Parenteral use of drugs by addicts, particularly intramuscular or subcutaneous use, can result in individual cases or occasional circumscribed outbreaks.

4. Reservoir—Intestine of animals, including man, in which the organism is a harmless normal inhabitant. Soil contaminated with animal and rarely human feces.

5. Mode of transmission—Tetanus spores introduced into the body, usually through a puncture wound contaminated with soil, street dust or animal or human feces, or injected contaminated street drugs, but also through lacerations, burns and trivial or unnoticed wounds. The presence of necrotic tissue and/or foreign bodies favors growth of the anaerobic pathogen. Cases have followed injuries considered too trivial for medical consultation.

6. Incubation period—Usually 3–21 days, although it may range from 1 day to several months; dependent on character, extent and location of wound; average 10 days. Most cases occur within 14 days. Shorter incubation periods, in general, are associated with more heavily contaminated wounds, more severe disease and a worse prognosis.

7. Period of communicability—Not directly transmitted from person to person.

8. Susceptibility and resistance—Susceptibility is general. Active immunity is induced by tetanus toxoid and persists for at least 10 years after full immunization; transient passive immunity follows injection of tetanus immune globulin (TIG) or, tetanus antitoxin (equine origin). Recovery from tetanus may not result in immunity; second attacks can occur. Immunization is indicated after recovery.

9. Methods of control—

A. Preventive measures:

1) Active immunization with adsorbed tetanus toxoid gives durable protection for at least 10 yrs; after the initial basic series has been completed, single booster doses elicit high levels of immunity. The toxoid is generally administered together with diphtheria toxoid and pertussis vaccine as a triple antigen (DTP) or as a double antigen (DT) for children under 7, or Td, for adults; in some countries, DTP, DT and T are available combined with inactivated polio vaccine. There is no advantage to nonadsorbed ("plain") preparations, whether for primary immunization

or booster shots. Reactions following tetanus toxoid injections are infrequent but do occur after excessive numbers of prior doses have been given.

a) The schedule recommended for tetanus immunization is the same as for diphtheria (q.v.).

b) While tetanus toxoid is recommended for universal use regardless of age, it is especially important for workers in contact with soil, sewage or domestic animals, members of the military forces, policemen and others with greater than usual risk of traumatic injury.

c) Active protection should be maintained by administering booster doses of Td every 10 years. In UK, routine reinforcing doses are given only at school entry and school leaving; in New Zealand, booster doses are given every 20 yrs.

d) Where logistics or costs make the standard schedule impractical, there is evidence that a single dose of some toxoids may immunize 50–90% of children or adults; a booster 1 yr later usually brings all subjects above the immune threshold.

2) Prophylaxis in wound management: Tetanus prophylaxis in patients with wounds is based on careful determination and assessment of whether the wound is clean or contaminated, the immune status of the patient, proper use of tetanus toxoid and/or tetanus immune globulin (see Table 1, below), wound cleansing and, where required, surgical debridement and the proper use of antibiotics.

a) Those who have been completely immunized who sustain minor and uncontaminated wounds would require a booster dose of toxoid only if more than 10 yrs (5 yrs in UK) have elapsed since the last dose was given. For major and/or contaminated wounds, a single booster injection of tetanus toxoid should be administered promptly on the day of injury if the patient has not received tetanus toxoid within the preceding 5 yrs (1 yr in UK).

b) Persons who have not completed a full primary series of tetanus toxoid will require a dose of toxoid and may require passive immunization with human tetanus immune globulin (TIG) as soon as possible following the wound. DTP, DT or Td, as determined by the age of the patient and previous immunization history, should be used at the time of the wound and ultimately to complete the primary series. Passive immunization with at least 250 units of TIG i.m. (or 1,500 to 5,000 units of antitoxin of animal origin if TIG is not available) is indicated for patients with (1) other than clean, minor wounds and a history of no or only one previous tetanus toxoid dose; (2) an unknown or uncertain history of previous tetanus immunization; or (3) a history of only 2 previous toxoid doses and a wound >24 hours old. When tetanus toxoid and TIG or antitoxin are given concurrently, separate syringes and separate sites must be used. Penicillin given for 7 days may kill *C. tetani* in the wound but this does not obviate the need for prompt treatment of the wound together with appropriate immunization.

3) Education on the necessity of complete immunization with tetanus toxoid, the kinds of injury particularly liable to be complicated by tetanus, and the potential need after injury for active and/or passive prophylaxis.

B. *Control of patient, contacts and the immediate environment:*

1) Report to local health authority: Case report required in most states and countries, Class 2A (see Preface).
2) Isolation: None.
3) Concurrent disinfection: None.
4) Quarantine: None.
5) Immunization of contacts: None.
6) Investigation of contacts and source of infection: Case investigation to determine circumstances of injury.
7) Specific treatment: TIG i.m. (or i.v. if a preparation safe for i.v. administration is available) in doses of 500–6000 units. If TIG is not available, tetanus antitoxin (equine origin) in a single large dose should be given i.v. following appropriate testing for hypersensitivity; parenteral penicillin in large doses should be given daily for 10–14 days. Intrathecal administration of TIG 250–500 IU or antitoxin (free of phenolic preservatives) has given promising results. The wound should be debrided widely and excised if possible. Maintain an adequate airway; employ sedation as indicated; muscle relaxant drugs together with tracheotomy and mechanically assisted respiration may be life-saving. Active immunization should be initiated concurrently with therapy.

C. *Epidemic measures:* In the rare outbreak make a thorough search for inadequacies in detoxification in preparation of toxoid.

D. *Disaster implications:* Social upheavals (wars, riots) and nat-

TABLE 1.

Summary guide to tetanus prophylaxis in routine wound management[1]

History of tetanus immunization (doses)	Clean, minor wounds		All other wounds	
	Td*	TIG	Td*	TIG
Uncertain	Yes	No	Yes	Yes
0–1	Yes	No	Yes	Yes
2	Yes	No	Yes	No[2]
3 or more	No[3]	No	No[4]	No

[1]Important details in the text.

*For children <7 years old, DPT (DT, if pertussis vaccine is contraindicated) is preferred to tetanus toxoid alone. For persons ≧7 yrs, Td is preferred to tetanus toxoid alone.

[2]Yes, if wound >24 hours old.

[3]Yes, if >10 yrs since last dose.

[4]Yes, if >5 yrs since last dose. (More frequent boosters are not needed and can accentuate side effects).

ural disasters (floods, hurricanes, earthquakes) which cause many traumatic injuries in unimmunized populations will result in an increased need for TIG or tetanus antitoxin and toxoid for injured patients.

E. *International measures:* Up-to-date immunization against tetanus is advised for international travelers.

TETANUS NEONATORUM   ICD-9 771.3

Tetanus neonatorum is a serious health problem in many developing countries where maternity care services are limited and immunization against tetanus is inadequate. The mortality rates due to tetanus neonatorum range from 10 to 60/1000 live births in rural areas of some of these countries. Most newborn infants with tetanus have been delivered outside of a hospital to unimmunized mothers delivered by a traditional birth attendant.

The disease usually occurs through the infection of the umbilicus with tetanus spores during delivery by cutting the cord with an unclean instrument, or after delivery by "dressing" the umbilical stump with substances heavily contaminated with tetanus spores.

Tetanus neonatorum is typified by a newborn infant who sucks and cries well for the first few days after birth and subsequently develops progressive difficulty and then inability to feed because of trismus, generalized stiffness with spasms or convulsions and opisthotonus. The average incubation period is about 6 days, with a range from 3 to 28 days. Overall, neonatal tetanus case fatality rates are very high; among cases with short incubation periods, these exceed 80%.

Prevention of tetanus neonatorum can be achieved by two approaches; improving maternity care with emphasis on increasing the proportion of deliveries attended by trained attendants, and by increasing the immunization coverage of women of childbearing age, and especially pregnant women, with tetanus toxoid.

Important control measures include licensing of midwives, with provision of professional supervision and education as to methods, equipment and techniques of asepsis in childbirth; and education of mothers, relatives and attendants in the practice of strict asepsis of the umbilical stump of newborn infants. The latter is especially important in many less developed areas where ashes, cow dung poultices or other contaminated substances are traditionally applied to the umbilicus.

Unimmunized pregnant women in circumstances where risk of neonatal tetanus exists should receive at least 2 doses of tetanus toxoid at least 4 weeks apart, the second at least 2 weeks before delivery. A third dose of toxoid should be given during the next pregnancy. Inadequately immunized pregnant women should complete the primary series; those immunized more than 10 years previously should receive a booster dose.

TOXOCARIASIS ICD-9 128.0
(Visceral larva migrans, Larva migrans visceralis, *Toxocara (canis) (cati)* infection)

1. **Identification**—A chronic and usually mild disease of young children due to migration of certain nematode larvae in the organs and tissues. It is characterized by eosinophilia of variable duration, hepatomegaly, hyperglobulinemia, pulmonary symptoms and fever. In severe cases the WBC count may reach $\geqq 100,000/mm^3$, with 80–90% eosinophils. Symptoms may persist for a year or longer. Pneumonitis or neurological disturbances may occur. Rarely fatal. Endophthalmitis, caused by larvae entering the eye, may occur with some frequency in older children, with

loss of vision in the affected eye; a retinal lesion resembling retinoblastoma may lead to unnecessary enucleation of the eye.

Demonstration of larvae of *Toxocara* by liver biopsy confirms the clinical diagnosis but is rarely justified. ELISA testing with larval stage antigens after absorbing the serum with *Ascaris suum* may be of value.

2. Infectious agents—*Toxocara canis* and *T. cati*, predominantly the former.

3. Occurrence—Probably worldwide. Has had most attention in the USA and UK but prevalence is probably no greater in these countries than in some others. The severe form occurs sporadically as isolated cases in a family, affecting mainly children 14–40 months, but also occurs at older ages. The next older or younger sibling often shows eosinophilia or other evidence of light or residual infection. Adults are infrequently infected.

4. Reservoir—Dogs and cats respectively. Nearly all puppies are infected by transplacental and transmammary migration of larvae. Puppies start to pass eggs in their stools by the time they are 3–4 weeks old.

5. Mode of transmission—By direct or indirect transmission of infective *Toxocara* eggs from contaminated soil to the mouth; directly related to dirt-eating by young children. Eggs reach the soil in feces of infected cats or dogs; 24% of soil samples from certain parks in the UK contained eggs. They require 1–3 weeks incubation to become infective, but remain viable and infective in soil for many months; they are adversely affected by desiccation. After ingestion, embryonated eggs hatch in the intestine, larvae penetrate the wall and migrate to the liver and lungs by the lymphatic and circulatory systems. From the lungs, larvae spread to various organs, causing damage by migration and induction of granulomatous lesions.

6. Incubation period—Weeks or months, depending upon intensity of infection, reinfection and sensitivity of the patient.

7. Period of communicability—Not directly transmitted from person to person.

8. Susceptibility and resistance—The lower incidence in older children and adults relates mainly to less exposure. Dogs usually acquire infection as puppies; infection in the female dog may end or become dormant with sexual maturity; with pregnancy, however, *T. canis* larvae become active and infect the fetuses and the newborn pups through the milk. Sex and age differences are less marked for cats; older animals are somewhat less susceptible than young.

9. Methods of control—

 A. Preventive measures:

1) Prevent contamination of soil by cat and dog feces in areas immediately adjacent to houses and childrens' play areas, especially in urban areas and multiple housing projects.

2) Require removal of canine and feline feces passed in play areas. Children's sandboxes offer an attractive site for defecating cats; cover when not in use.

3) Deworm dogs and cats beginning at 3 weeks of age, repeated at 2–week intervals for 3 treatments and thereafter every 6 months. Also treat lactating and especially pregnant bitches. Dispose of feces passed as a result of treatment, as well as other stools, in a sanitary manner.

4) Educate the public and especially pet owners concerning sources and origin of the infection, particularly the danger of eating dirt and of exposure to areas contaminated with the feces of untreated puppies.

5) Hands should always be washed after handling soil and before eating.

6) Prevent pica in children.

B. *Control of patient, contacts and the immediate environment:*

1) Report to local health authority: Official report not ordinarily justifiable, Class 5 (see Preface).

2) Isolation: None.

3) Concurrent disinfection: None.

4) Quarantine: None.

5) Immunization of contacts: None.

6) Investigation of contacts and source of infection: (See 9A3, above.) Observed dirt-eating at area of known canine fecal contamination is presumptive evidence of infection. Disinfection of soil is not feasible.

7) Specific treatment: Diethylcarbamazine and thiabendazole have been used; effectiveness is at best questionable.

C. *Epidemic measures:* Not applicable.

D. *Disaster implications:* None.

E. *International measures:* None.

GNATHOSTOMIASIS   ICD-9 128.1

Another visceral larva migrans, common in Thailand and elsewhere in SE Asia, is caused by *Gnathostoma spinigerum,* a nematode parasite of cats and dogs. Following ingestion of undercooked fish containing third-stage larvae, the parasites migrate through the tissues of man or animals, forming transient inflammatory lesions or abscesses in various parts of the body.

Larvae may invade the brain, producing focal cerebral lesions associated with eosinophilic pleocytosis.

CUTANEOUS LARVA MIGRANS ICD-9 126
DUE TO *ANCYLOSTOMA*
BRAZILIENSE ICD-9 126.2
DUE TO *ANCYLOSTOMA CANINUM* ICD-9 126.9
(Creeping eruption)

Infective larvae of dog and cat hookworm *Ancylostoma braziliense* and *Ancylostoma caninum* cause a dermatitis in man, called "creeping eruption." This is a disease of utility men, gardeners, children, seabathers and others who come in contact with damp sandy soil contaminated with cat and dog feces; in the USA, most prevalent in the southeast. The larvae, which enter the skin, migrate intracutaneously for long periods, but eventually penetrate to deeper tissues. Each larva causes a serpiginous track, advancing several mm to a few cm a day, with intense itching more marked at night. The disease is self-limited with spontaneous cure after several weeks or months. Individual larva can be killed by freezing the area with ethyl chloride spray; thiabendazole is effective systemically or as a topical ointment.

TOXOPLASMOSIS ICD-9 130
CONGENITAL TOXOPLASMOSIS ICD-9 771.2

1. **Identification**—A systemic protozoal disease. Primary infection frequently is asymptomatic; acute disease may occur with fever, lymphadenopathy and lymphocytosis persisting for days or weeks. Rare manifestations include cerebral signs, pneumonia, generalized skeletal muscle involvement, myocarditis, a maculopapular rash and death. With development of antibodies the parasitemia decreases but *Toxoplasma* cysts remaining in the tissues contain viable organisms; these dormant infections can reactivate if the individual becomes immunologically incompetent as in AIDS patients, among whom cerebral toxoplasmosis occurs. A primary infection during early pregnancy may lead to fetal infection with death or chorioretinitis, brain damage with intracerebral calcification, hydrocephaly, microcephaly, fever, jaundice, rash, hepatosplenomegaly, xanthochromic CSF and convulsions evident at birth or shortly thereafter. Later in pregnancy, maternal infection results in mild or subclinical fetal disease with delayed manifestations, especially chronic chorioretinitis.

Diagnosis is based on clinical signs and supportive serologic results, demonstration of the agent in body tissues or fluids by biopsy or necropsy, or isolation in animals or tissue culture. Rising antibody levels are corroborative of active infection; specific IgM in infants and titer rises in sequential sera are conclusive evidence of congenital infection. High antibody levels may persist for years without relation to active disease.

2. **Infectious agent**—*Toxoplasma gondii,* an intracellular coccidian protozoan belonging to the Sporozoa.

3. **Occurrence**—Worldwide in mammals, birds and man. Infection in man is common.

4. **Reservoir**—Rodents, swine, cattle, sheep, goats, chickens, and birds are intermediate hosts of *T. gondii;* all may carry an infective stage (cystozoite or bradyzoite) of *T. gondii* encysted in tissue, especially muscle and brain. Cysts remain viable for long periods, perhaps the life of the animal. Cats acquire the infection as a feces-borne infection from other cats, or from eating infected mammals (especially rodents) or birds. Cats harbor the parasite in the intestinal tract where the sexual stage of the life cycle takes place. Only in felines can the sexual cycle of the parasite occur with excretion of the oocysts in feces for 10–20 days or, rarely, longer.

5. **Mode of transmission**—Transplacental infection in humans may occur only when a woman has a primary infection. Postnatal infections may be acquired by eating raw or undercooked infected meat (pork or mutton, more rarely beef) containing cysts or by the ingestion of infective oocysts in food, water or dust contaminated with feline feces. Children are at risk from ingesting infective oocysts in sandboxes in which cats have defecated. One outbreak was associated epidemiologically with consumption of raw goat's milk.

6. **Incubation period**—Ten to 23 days in one common source outbreak from ingestion of undercooked meat; 5–20 days in an outbreak associated with cats.

7. **Period of communicability**—Not directly transmitted from person to person except in utero. Cats shed oocysts for 7–20 days, possibly longer after ingestion of infected prey; the oocysts sporulate and become infective 2–5 days later and may remain infective in water or moist soil for months or years. Cysts in the flesh of an infected animal remain infective as long as the meat is edible and uncooked.

8. **Susceptibility and resistance**—Susceptibility is general. Duration and degree of immunity are unknown but assumed to be permanent; antibodies persist for years, probably for life. Patients undergoing immunosuppressive therapy or with complement defects are highly susceptible, and may display reactivated infection. A complication of AIDS.

9. **Methods of control**—

A. Preventive measures:

1) Cook meats thoroughly.
2) Feed cats dry, canned or boiled food and discourage from hunting or scavenging.
3) Dispose of cat feces and litter daily (before sporocysts become infective). Feces can be flushed down the toilet, burned or deeply buried. Disinfect litter pans daily by scalding; wear gloves when handling potentially infective material. Dried litter should be disposed of without shaking, to avoid dispersal of oocysts in the air.
4) Unless they are known to have antibodies to *T. gondii,* pregnant women should avoid cleaning litter pans or contact with cats of unknown feeding history. Wear gloves during gardening and thoroughly wash hands afterwards.
5) Control stray cats and prevent them from gaining access to sandboxes or sand piles used by children for play. Sandboxes should be covered when not in use.
6) Wash hands thoroughly after handling raw meat or contact with soil possibly contaminated with cat feces.

B. Control of patient, contacts and the immediate environment:

1) Report to local health authority: Not ordinarily required but desirable to facilitate further understanding of the epidemiology of the disease, Class 3C (see Preface).
2) Isolation: None.
3) Concurrent disinfection: None.
4) Quarantine: None.
5) Immunization of contacts: None.
6) Investigation of contacts: In congenital cases, determine antibodies in mother and members of the household; in acquired cases, determine contact with infected animals and common exposure to cat feces or raw meat.
7) Specific treatment: Pyrimethamine (Daraprim®) combined with sulfadiazine or triple sulfonamides and folinic acid for 4 weeks is the preferred treatment; accompanied by appropriate hematological control. In UK and France, spiramycin is the preferred treatment. Treatment is not indicated for mild disease.

C. Epidemic measures: None.

D. Disaster implications: None.

E. International measures: None.

TRACHOMA

ICD-9 076

1. **Identification**—A chlamydial keratoconjunctivitis of insidious or abrupt onset; the infection may persist for a few years if untreated but the characteristic lifetime duration of active disease in hyperendemic areas is the result of frequent reinfection. It is characterized by conjunctival inflammation with lymphoid follicles and papillary hyperplasia, associated with vascular invasion of the cornea (pannus) and, in its later stages, by conjunctival scarring which may lead to gross deformity of the eyelids, progressive visual disability and blindness. Associated bacterial infections are common in many areas and increase communicability, severity and modify clinical manifestations.

Acute infection may be indistinguishable from that of chlamydial conjunctivitis (q.v.) but the diseases are dissimilar in their distinct epidemiologic patterns and in the propensity to severe sequelae in trachoma. Other forms of chronic follicular conjunctivitis, occasionally with scarring and corneal pannus, include molluscum nodules of the lid margin, toxic reactions to chronically administered eye drops and chronic staphylococcal lid margin infection.

Laboratory diagnosis is made by demonstration of intracytoplasmic inclusion bodies in epithelial cells of conjunctival scrapings by Giemsa or IF staining; or by isolation of the agent in cell culture.

2. **Infectious agent**—*Chlamydia trachomatis* of immunotypes C, A and B. Some strains are indistinguishable from those of chlamydial conjunctivitis.

3. **Occurrence**—Worldwide, but with unequal and varying distributions, marked by differences in age of onset, clinical evolution, frequency of spontaneous cure and disabling sequelae and response to treatment. Widespread in the Middle East, in south Asia, in parts of north and sub-Saharan Africa and of S America; in the USA, it is rarely present, occurring among population groups with poor hygiene, poverty, and crowded living conditions, particularly in dry, dusty regions such as are found in some Indian reservations in the Southwest. There has been a high prevalence among Australian Aboriginees. Nomadic communities generally have a less severe form than stationary populations.

4. **Reservoir**—Man.

5. **Mode of transmission**—By direct contact with ocular discharges and possibly mucoid or purulent discharges of nasal mucous membranes from infected persons, or materials soiled therewith. Flies, especially *Musca sorbens,* may possibly contribute to spread of the disease but transmission occurs in their absence. Extraocular localization can take place with some

immunotypes and is mainly genital. Venereal transmission is possible and can result in symptomatic or asymptomatic infection of the cervix or urethra. Such localization can result in infection of the newborn taking the form of inclusion conjunctivitis and/or pneumonia.

6. **Incubation period**—Five to 12 days (based on volunteer studies).

7. **Period of communicability**—As long as active lesions are present in the conjunctivae and adnexal mucous membranes; this may last a few years. Concentration of the agent in the tissues is greatly reduced with cicatrization, but increases again with reactivation and recurrence of infective discharges.

8. **Susceptibility and resistance**—Susceptibility is general; there is no evidence that infection confers immunity nor that experimental vaccines are useful in preventing infection or in reducing the severity of established cases. In endemic areas children have active disease more frequently than adults. The severity of disease often is related to living conditions, particulary poor hygiene. Exposure to dry winds, dust and fine sand may contribute to the severity of the disease.

9. **Methods of control—**

   A. *Preventive measures:*

     1) Improved basic sanitation, including availability and use of soap and water; avoid common-use towels.

     2) Educate the public on the need for personal hygiene, especially the risk in common use of toilet articles.

     3) Provide adequate case-finding and treatment facilities, with emphasis on preschool children.

     4) Conduct epidemiological investigations to determine important factors in occurrence of the disease in each specific situation.

   B. *Control of patient, contacts and the immediate environment:*

     1) Report to local health authority: Case report required in some states and countries of low endemicity, Class 2B (see Preface).

     2) Isolation: Not practical in most areas where the disease occurs. For hospitalized patients: drainage/secretion precautions.

     3) Concurrent disinfection: Of eye discharges and contaminated articles.

     4) Quarantine: None.

     5) Immunization of contacts: None.

     6) Investigation of contacts: Members of family, playmates and schoolmates.

7) Specific treatment: In areas where the disease is severe and highly prevalent, mass treatment with topical tetracycline or erythromycin is frequently used. Oral tetracyclines and erythromycin are also effective in the active stages of the disease.

C. *Epidemic measures:* In regions of hyperendemic prevalence, mass treatment campaigns have been successful in reducing severity and frequency when associated with education of the people in personal hygiene and with improvement of the sanitary environment.

D. *Disaster implications:* None.

E. *International measures:* WHO Collaborating Centres (see Preface).

TRENCH FEVER
(Wolhynian fever, Quintana fever)

ICD-9 083.1

1. Identification—A nonfatal, febrile bacterial disease varying in manifestations and severity. It is characterized by headache, malaise, pain and tenderness, especially in the shins; onset either sudden or slow, with a fever which may be relapsing, typhoid-like, or limited to a single febrile episode lasting for several days. Splenomegaly is common and a transient macular rash may occur. Symptoms may continue to recur many years after the primary infection, which may be subclinical with organisms circulating in the blood for months with or without repeated recurrence of symptoms.

Laboratory diagnosis is made by culture of patient's blood on blood agar under 5% CO_2 tension in air. Microcolonies are visible after 2 weeks of incubation at 37°C (98.6°F). Infection evokes specific antibodies detectable by serological tests; ELISA tests are highly sensitive.

2. Infectious agent—*Rochalimaea quintana (Rickettsia quintana).*

3. Occurrence—Epidemics occurred in Europe during World Wars I and II among both troops and prisoners of war living under crowded, unhygienic conditions. Sporadic cases in areas of endemic foci are probably not recognized.

The organism probably can be found wherever the human body louse exists. Endemic foci of infection have been detected in Poland, USSR, Mexico, Bolivia, Burundi, Ethiopia and north Africa.

4. Reservoir—Man. The intermediate host is the body louse, *Pediculus humanus.* The organism multiplies extracellularly in the gut lumen for the duration of the insect's life, which is approximately 5 weeks after hatching. No transovarial transmission occurs.

5. Mode of transmission—Not directly transmitted from person to person. Man is infected by inoculation of the organism in louse feces through a break in the skin from either the bite of the louse or other means. Infected lice begin to excrete infectious feces 5–12 days after ingesting infective blood and continue for duration of life. Nymphal stages may become infected. The disease spreads when lice leave abnormally hot (febrile) or cold (dead) bodies in search of a normothermic clothed body.

6. Incubation period—Generally 7–30 days.

7. Period of communicability—Organisms may circulate in the blood (by which lice are infected) for weeks, months or years and may recur with or without symptoms. A history of trench fever is a permanent contraindication to blood donation. ·

8. Susceptibility and resistance—Susceptibility is general. After infection, the degree of protective immunity to either infection or disease is unknown.

9. Methods of control—

  A. *Preventive measures:* Delousing procedures will destroy the vector and prevent transmission to man. Dust clothing and body with an effective insecticide.

  B. *Control of patient, contacts and the immediate environment:*

      1) Report to local health authority: Cases should be reported so that an evaluation of louse infestation in the population may be made and appropriate measures taken, since lice also transmit epidemic typhus and relapsing fever; Class 3B (see Preface).
      2) Isolation: None after delousing.
      3) Concurrent disinfection: Louse-infested clothing should be treated to kill the lice.
      4) Quarantine: None.
      5) Immunization of contacts: None.
      6) Investigation of contacts and source of infection: Search the bodies and clothing of people at risk for the presence of lice; delouse if indicated.
      7) Specific treatment: Tetracyclines and chloramphenicol are probably effective, but have not yet been adequately tested in clinical cases.   ·

  C. *Epidemic measures:* Systematic application of residual insecticide to the clothing of all persons in the affected population (see 9A, above).

D. *Disaster implications:* Risk is increased when louse-infested people are forced to live in crowded, unhygienic shelters. (See 9B1, above.)

E. *International measures:* WHO Collaborating Centres (see Preface).

TRICHINOSIS
(Trichiniasis, Trichinellosis)

ICD-9 124

1. Identification—A disease caused by an intestinal roundworm whose larvae migrate to and become encapsulated in the muscles. Clinical disease in man is highly variable and can range from inapparent infection to a fulminating, fatal disease depending on the number of larvae ingested. Sudden appearance of muscle soreness and pain, and edema of upper eyelids is a common early and characteristic sign; it is sometimes followed by subconjunctival, subungual and retinal hemorrhages, pain and photophobia. Thirst, profuse sweating, chills, weakness, prostration and rapidly increasing eosinophilia may shortly follow ocular signs. Gastrointestinal symptoms, such as diarrhea, due to the intraintestinal activity of the adult worms, may precede the ocular manifestations. Remittent fever is usual, sometimes as high as 40°C (104°F); the fever terminates after 1–3 weeks. Respiratory and neurological complications may appear in the 3rd-6th week; death due to myocardial failure may occur in the 1st-2nd week and between the 4th-8th week.

Marked eosinophilia and serologic tests (most frequently bentonite flocculation) may aid in diagnosis. Biopsy of skeletal muscle, not earlier than about 10 days after exposure to infection, frequently provides conclusive evidence by demonstrating the parasite.

2. Infectious agent—*Trichinella spiralis,* an intestinal nematode. Separate taxonomic designations have been proposed for strains found in the Arctic *(T. spiralis nativa)* and in Africa *(T. s. nelsoni)*.

3. Occurrence—Worldwide but variable in incidence, depending in part on practices of eating and preparing pork, or wild animal meat, and the extent to which the disease is recognized and reported. Necropsy surveys reveal former wide prevalence in the USA; the age adjusted rate is now only ≤2%. Cases usually are sporadic and outbreaks localized, several from homemade sausage and other meat products using pork from noncommercial sources.

4. Reservoir—Swine, dogs, cats, rats and many wild animals, including fox, wolf, bear, polar bear and marine mammals in the Arctic, and hyena, jackal, lion and leopard in the tropics.

5. Mode of transmission—By eating raw or insufficiently cooked flesh of animals containing viable encysted larvae, chiefly pork and pork products, and "beef products" such as hamburger adulterated either intentionally or inadvertently with raw pork. In the mucosal epithelium of the small intestine, larvae develop into adults. Gravid female worms then produce larvae, which penetrate the lymphatics and are disseminated via the bloodstream throughout the body. The larvae become encapsulated in skeletal muscle.

6. Incubation period—Usually about 10–14 days after ingestion of infected meat; varies between 5–45 days.

7. Period of communicability—Not transmitted directly from person to person. Animal hosts remain infective for months and meat from such animals stays infected for appreciable periods unless cooked or frozen to kill the larvae. (See 9A4 and 9A5, below.)

8. Susceptibility and resistance—Susceptibility is universal. Infection results in partial immunity.

9. Methods of control—

   A. Preventive measures:

      1) Educate the public on the need to cook all fresh pork and pork products at a temperature and time sufficient to allow all parts to reach at least 65.6°C (150°F) or until meat changes from pink to grey, which allows a good margin of safety, unless it is established that these meat products have been processed either by heating, curing or freezing adequate to kill trichinae.

      2) Pork must be ground in a separate grinder or the grinder thoroughly cleaned before processing other meats.

      3) Regulations to assure adequate commercial processing of pork products. Testing carcasses for infection with a digestion technique is useful but is being replaced by immunodiagnosis with the ELISA test.

      4) Adopt suitable laws and regulations insuring cooking of garbage and offal before feeding to swine.

      5) Educate hunters to cook walrus, seal, wild boar, bear and meat of other wild animals thoroughly.

      6) Freezing temperatures maintained throughout infected meat are effective in killing trichinae, i.e., holding pieces of pork up to 15 cm thick at a temperature of −25°C (−13°F) or lower for 10 days will effectively destroy all

common types of *Trichinella* cysts. Thicker pieces should be frozen and held at this temperature for 20 days. These temperatures will not kill the cold-resistant Arctic strains (*T. s. nativa*) in walrus or bear meat.

B. *Control of patient, contacts and the immediate environment:*

1) Report to local health authority: Case report required in most states and countries, Class 2B (see Preface).
2) Isolation: None.
3) Concurrent disinfection: None.
4) Quarantine: None.
5) Immunization of contacts: None.
6) Investigation of contacts: Check other family members and persons who have eaten suspected meat for evidence of infection. Confiscate any remaining food.
7) Specific treatment: Mebendazole (Vermox®) is used in both the intestinal and muscular stage of infection. Corticosteroids are indicated in severe cases.

C. *Epidemic measures:* Institute epidemiologic study to determine the common food involved. Confiscate remainder of food and correct faulty practices.

D. *Disaster implications:* None.

E. *International measures:* None.

TRICHOMONIASIS   ICD-9 131
(Trichomoniasis due to *Trichomonas vaginalis*)

1. **Identification**—A common persistent disease of the genitourinary tract, characterized in women by vaginitis, with small petechial or sometimes punctate hemorrhagic lesions and a profuse, thin, foamy, yellowish discharge with foul odor; frequently asymptomatic. In men, the infectious agent invades and persists in the prostate, urethra, or seminal vesicles, but rarely produces symptoms or demonstrable lesions; it is thought to cause about 3% of nongonococcal urethritis and in these cases is associated with prostatitis.

Diagnosis is made through identification of the motile parasite either by microscopic examination of discharges or by culture, which is more sensitive.

2. **Infectious agent**—*Trichomonas vaginalis,* a flagellate protozoan.

3. Occurrence—Widespread; a frequent disease of all continents and people of all races, primarily of adults, with highest incidence among females 16–35 years. In sampled areas of the USA, the prevalence of infection among patients in gynecological clinics has been as high as 50%.

4. Reservoir—Humans.

5. Mode of transmission—By contact with vaginal and urethral discharges of infected persons during sexual intercourse and presumably by contact with contaminated articles.

6. Incubation period—Four to 20 days, average 7 days.

7. Period of communicability—For the duration of the persistent infection, which may last for years.

8. Susceptibility and resistance—Susceptibility to infection is general but clinical disease is mainly in females.

9. Methods of control—

A. *Preventive measures:* Educate the public as to the symptoms and mode of transmission; encourage women with symptoms to seek immediate treatment and to avoid sexual intercourse.

B. *Control of patient, contacts and the immediate environment:*

1) Report to local health authority: Official report not ordinarily justifiable, Class 5 (see Preface).
2) Isolation: None; avoid sexual relations during period of infection and treatment.
3) Concurrent disinfection: None, the organism cannot withstand drying.
4) Quarantine: None.
5) Immunization of contacts: None.
6) Investigation of contacts: Sexual partners should be treated concurrently.
7) Specific treatment: Metronidazole (Flagyl®) by mouth is effective in both male and female patients. It is contraindicated during the 1st trimester of pregnancy. Concurrent treatment of sexual partner(s) to prevent reinfection.

C. *Epidemic measures:* None.

D. *Disaster implications:* None.

E. *International measures:* None.

TRICHURIASIS
(Trichocephaliasis, Whipworm disease)

ICD-9 127.3

1. Identification—A nematode infection of the large intestine, usually asymptomatic. Heavy infections result in bloody mucoid stools and diarrhea. Rectal prolapse may occur in heavily infected children.

Diagnosis is made by demonstration of eggs in feces or by sigmoidoscopic observation of worms attached to the wall of the lower colon in heavy infections. Eggs must be differentiated from those of *Capillaria* spp.

2. Infectious agent—*Trichuris trichiura (Trichocephalus trichiurus),* a nematode; the human whipworm.

3. Occurrence—Worldwide, especially in warm, moist regions.

4. Reservoir—Man.

5. Mode of transmission—Indirect; not immediately transmissible from person to person. Eggs passed in feces require a minimum of 3 weeks in soil for embryonation. Ingestion of fully embryonated eggs from contaminated soil is followed by hatching the larvae, their attachment to the mucosa of the cecum and proximal colon and development into mature worms. Eggs appear in the feces about 90 days after ingestion of the embryonated eggs; symptoms may appear much earlier.

6. Incubation period—Indefinite.

7. Period of communicability—Several years in untreated carriers.

8. Susceptibility and resistance—Susceptibility is universal.

9. Methods of control—

    A. Preventive measures:

        1) Provide adequate facilities for feces disposal.
        2) Educate all members of the family, particularly children, in the use of toilet facilities.
        3) Encourage satisfactory hygienic habits, especially hand-washing before foodhandling; avoid ingestion of soil by washing vegetables and other soil-containing foods thoroughly.

    B. Control of patient, contacts and the immediate environment:

        1) Report to local health authority: Official report not ordinarily justifiable, Class 5 (see Preface). School health authorities should be advised of unusual frequency in school populations.
        2) Isolation: None.

3) Concurrent disinfection: None; sanitary disposal of feces.
4) Quarantine: None.
5) Immunization of contacts: None.
6) Investigation of contacts: Examine feces of all symptomatic members of the family group, especially children and playmates.
7) Specific treatment: Light infections (few eggs per microscopic field) require no treatment. Mebendazole (Vermox®) or albendazole (Zentel®) is the drug of choice; both are contraindicated in pregnancy. Oxantel is an alternative drug.

C. *Epidemic measures:* Not applicable.

D. *Disaster implications:* None.

E. *International measures:* None.

TRYPANOSOMIASIS
I. AFRICAN TRYPANOSOMIASIS   ICD-9 086.5
(African sleeping sickness)

1. Identification—A systemic protozoal disease. In the early stages a chancre may be observed at the primary tsetse fly bite site, with fever, intense headache, insomnia, lymph node enlargement (especially posterior cervical), anemia, local edema and rash. In the late stage, there is body wasting, somnolence and signs referable to the CNS. May run a protracted course of several years, or death may follow within a few months; frequently fatal.

Diagnosis in early stages is made by finding trypanosomes in lymph from punctured nodes and in slides prepared from capillary blood or the buffy coat. In advanced stages trypanosomes may also be found in the CSF. Inoculation of laboratory rats or mice is sometimes useful. Specific antibodies may be demonstrated by ELISA, FA and agglutination tests; high levels of immunoglobulins, especially IgM, are typical of African trypanosomiasis.

2. Infectious agents—*Trypanosoma brucei gambiense* and *T. b. rhodesiense,* hemoflagellates. Criteria for species differentiation are not absolute; isolates from cases of virulent, rapidly progressive disease are considered to be *T. b. rhodesiense,* especially if contracted in east Africa; west and central African cases are usually more chronic and considered to be due to *T. b. gambiense.*

3. Occurrence—The disease is confined to tropical Africa between 15°N and 20°S latitude, corresponding to the distribution of the tsetse fly. In some endemic regions, up to 30% of the population has been infected. Outbreaks can occur when, for any reason, man-fly contact is intensified or when trypanosomes are introduced into a tsetse-infected area by movement of infected flies or reservoir hosts. Where flies of the *Glossina palpalis* group are the principal vectors, as in west and central Africa, infection occurs mainly along streams; in east Africa and around Lake Victoria, where the main vector is *G. morsitans,* disease occurs over the broader dry savannas.

4. Reservoir—In *T. b. gambiense,* man is the major reservoir and domestic animals of minor importance. Wild game, especially bushbuck and antelopes, and domestic cattle are the chief animal reservoirs of *T. b. rhodesiense;* carnivores (lions and hyenas) also serve as reservoirs.

5. Mode of transmission—By bite of either sex of an infective *Glossina,* the tsetse fly. Six species are the principal vectors in nature: *Glossina palpalis, G. tachinoides, G. morsitans, G. pallidipes, G. swynnertoni,* and *G. fuscipes.* The tsetse fly is infected by ingesting blood of man or animal that carries trypanosomes. The parasite multiplies in the fly for 12–30 days, according to temperature and other factors, until infective forms develop in the salivary glands. Once infected, a tsetse fly remains infective for life (up to 3 months); infection is not passed from generation to generation in flies. Congenital transmission can occur in man. Direct mechanical transmission by blood on the proboscis of *Glossina* and other man-biting flies such as horseflies, or in laboratory accidents is possible.

6. Incubation period—In *T. b. rhodesiense* infection, usually 3 days to 3 wks; in *T. b. gambiense* infection, usually longer and extremely variable, i.e., it may be several months, or even years.

7. Period of communicability—To the tsetse fly, as long as the parasite is present in the blood of the infected person or animal. Parasitemia is extremely variable in untreated cases and occurs in late as well as early stages of the disease.

8. Susceptibility and resistance—Susceptibility is general. Occasional inapparent infections have been documented with both *T. b. gambiense* and *T. b. rhodesiense.* Spontaneous recovery in cases without CNS involvement is thought to occur but has not been confirmed.

9. Methods of control—

   A. Preventive measures:

       1)   Selection of appropriate methods of prevention must be based on knowledge of the local ecology of the vectors and

infectious agents. Thus, in a given geographic area, priority must be given to one or more of the following:

a) Reduction of parasite population by survey of human population for infection and treatment of those infected.

b) Destruction of vector tsetse fly habitats by selective and discriminatory brush clearing along water courses or around villages. If cleared areas can be reclaimed for agricultural use, a permanent solution to the vector problem may result.

c) Reduction of fly population by appropriate use of traps impregnated with decamethrin and by local use of residual insecticides (5% DDT or 3% dieldrin is effective), and in emergency situations, use of aerosol insecticides sprayed from aircraft.

d) Education on personal measures to protect against tsetse fly bites.

B. *Control of patient, contacts and the immediate environment:*

1) Report to local health authority: In selected endemic areas, establish records of prevalence and encourage control measures; not a reportable disease in most countries, Class 3B (see Preface).

2) Isolation: Not practicable. Prevent tsetse flies from feeding on patients with trypanosomes in their blood. In some countries legal restrictions are placed on movement of untreated patients.

3) Concurrent disinfection: None.

4) Quarantine: None.

5) Immunization of contacts: None.

6) Investigation of contacts: None.

7) Specific treatment: Early in the course of infection (prior to invasion of the CNS) suramin is the drug of choice for *T. b. rhodesiense* infections, and pentamidine for *T. b. gambiense* infections. Melarsoprol has been used effectively for treatment of patients with CNS infection of either parasite. These drugs are available from CDC Drug Service, Atlanta, on an investigational basis (see Preface).

C. *Epidemic measures:* Mass surveys, treatment for identified infections and tsetse fly control are urgent. If epidemics recur in an area despite control measures, it may be necessary to move whole villages to safer districts. Other measures as in 9A, above.

D. *Disaster implications:* None.

E. *International measures:* Promote cooperative efforts of governments in endemic areas. Disseminate information and increase the availability of simple diagnostic tests for screening and simple means of vector control, develop systems for effective distribution of reagents and drugs. Stimulate training at national and international levels. WHO Collaborating Centres (see Preface).

II. AMERICAN TRYPANOSOMIASIS   ICD-9 086.2
(Chagas' disease)

1. Identification—Acute disease generally occurs in children; chronic manifestations generally appear later in life. Many infected people have no clinical manifestations. The acute disease is characterized by variable fever, malaise, lymphadenopathy and hepatosplenomegaly. An inflammatory response at the site of infection (chagoma) may last up to 8 weeks. Unilateral bipalpebral edema (Romaña's sign) occurs in a significant percentage of acute cases. Life-threatening or fatal manifestations include myocarditis and rarely meningoencephalitis. Chronic sequelae include myocardial damage with cardiac dilatation and arrhythmias, and intestinal tract involvement with megaesophagus and megacolon. Late manifestations are rare in Panamanian infections and megaviscera do not occur.

Infection with *Trypanosoma rangeli* occurs in focal areas of endemic Chagas' disease extending from Central America to Peru and Venezuela; a prolonged parasitemia occurs, sometimes coexisting with *T. cruzi* flagellates (with which it shares reservoir hosts) but no clinical manifestations attributable to this infection have been noted.

Diagnosis of Chagas' disease in the acute phase is established by demonstration of the organism in blood (rarely, in a lymph node or in skeletal muscle) by direct examination, culture, intracerebral inoculation of suckling mice, or xenodiagnosis (feeding uninfected triatomid bugs on the patient and finding the parasite in the bug's feces several weeks later). Parasitemia is most intense during febrile episodes early in the course of infection. In the chronic phase xenodiagnosis and blood culture on diphasic media may be positive but other methods rarely reveal parasites. Parasites are differentiated from those of *T. rangeli* by their shorter length (20μ v. 36μ). Serologic tests are valuable for individual diagnosis as well as for screening purposes.

2. Infectious agents—*Trypanosoma cruzi (Schizotrypanum cruzi)*, a protozoan that occurs in man as a hemoflagellate and as an intracellular parasite without an external flagellum.

3. Occurrence—The disease is confined to the Western Hemisphere, with wide geographic distribution in rural Mexico and Central and S America; highly endemic in some areas. Three human infections acquired

within the USA have been reported (2 in Texas, 1 in California); serologic studies suggest the possible occurrence of other asymptomatic cases. *T. cruzi* has been found in small mammals in Alabama, Arizona, California, Florida, Georgia, Louisiana, Maryland, New Mexico, Texas, Arkansas and Utah.

4. **Reservoir**—Infected people and many domestic and wild animals including the dog, cat, pig, guinea pig, bat, house rat, wood rat, fox, opossum, raccoon and armadillo.

5. **Mode of transmission**—By trypanosomes in the feces of infected vectors, i.e., blood-sucking species of *Reduviidae* (cone-nosed bugs), especially from *Triatoma, Rhodnius* and *Panstrongylus* spp. while biting. Infection of humans and other mammals occurs when freshly excreted bug feces containing the parasite contaminates conjunctiva, mucous membranes, abrasions or skin wounds (including the bite wound); defecation occurs during feeding. The bugs become infected when they feed on a parasitemic animal; the organisms multiply in the gut. Transmission may occur by blood transfusion; organisms may cross the placenta to cause congenital infection and transmission by ingestion of milk from infected females has been reported for humans and other mammals. Accidental laboratory infections are not uncommon.

6. **Incubation period**—About 5–14 days after bite of the insect vector; 30–40 days if infected by blood transfusion.

7. **Period of communicability**—Organisms are present regularly in the blood during the acute period and may persist in very small numbers throughout life in symptomatic and asymptomatic people. The vector becomes infective in 10–30 days after biting an infected host and the gut infection in the bug persists for life (as long as 2 years).

8. **Susceptibility and resistance**—All ages are susceptible, but in younger persons the disease usually is more severe.

9. **Methods of control**—

   A. *Preventive measures:*
   1) Systematic attack on vectors infesting poorly constructed houses through use of effective insecticides with residual action.
   2) Construct or repair living areas to eliminate lodging places for the insect vector and shelter for domestic and wild reservoir animals.
   3) Use bed nets in houses infested by the vector.
   4) Educate the public on the mode of spread and methods of prevention.
   5) In endemic areas screen blood donors by appropriate

serologic tests to prevent infection by transfusion. Addition of gentian violet (25 ml of 0.5% solution/ 500 ml of blood 24 hours before use) may prevent transmission.

B. *Control of patient, contacts and the immediate environment:*

1) Report to local health authority: In selected endemic areas; not a reportable disease in most countries, Class 3B (see Preface).
2) Isolation: Not generally practical. Blood/body fluid precautions for hospitalized patients.
3) Concurrent disinfection: None.
4) Quarantine: None.
5) Immunization of contacts: None.
6) Investigation of contacts and source of infection: Search thatched roofs, bedding and rooms for the vector. All members of the family of a case should be examined.
7) Specific treatment: Nifurtimox (Bayer 2502), a nitrofurfurylidene derivative, is most useful in treatment of acute cases and is available from the CDC Drug Service, Atlanta, on an investigational basis (see Preface). Benznidazole, a 2–nitroimidazole derivative, has also proved to be effective in acute cases.

C. *Epidemic measures:* In areas of high incidence, field survey to determine distribution and density of vectors and animal hosts.

D. *Disaster implications:* None.

E. *International measures:* None.

TUBERCULOSIS
(TB, Phthisis)

ICD-9 010-018

1. **Identification**—A mycobacterial disease important as a cause of disability and death in many parts of the world. The initial infection usually goes unnoticed; tuberculin sensitivity appears within a few weeks; lesions commonly heal, leaving no residual changes except pulmonary or tracheobronchial lymph node calcifications. It may progress directly to pulmonary tuberculosis or, by lymphohematogenous dissemination of bacilli, to produce pulmonary, miliary, meningeal or other extrapulmonary involvement. Serious outcome of the initial infection is more frequent in infants, adolescents and young adults.

Extrapulmonary tuberculosis is less common than pulmonary. It includes tuberculous meningitis, acute hematogenous (miliary) tuberculosis and involvement of lymph nodes, pleura, pericardium, kidneys, bones and joints, larynx, skin, intestines, peritoneum or eyes.

Progressive pulmonary tuberculosis generally arises from a latent focus remaining from the initial infection. If untreated it has a variable course with exacerbations and remissions; appropriate chemotherapy nearly always results in a cure. Clinical status is based mainly on the presence or absence of tubercle bacilli in the sputum and also on the nature of chest x-ray changes. Abnormal x-ray densities indicative of pulmonary infiltration, cavitation or fibrosis can occur before clinical manifestations. Fatigue, fever and weight loss may occur early, while localizing symptoms of cough, chest pain, hemoptysis and hoarseness become prominent in advanced stages.

People who are or have been infected with *Mycobacterium tuberculosis* and *M. bovis* will almost always react to a low dose tuberculin skin test, i.e., bio-equivalent to 5 International Units (IU) (or 5 Tuberculin Units—5 TU) of the International Standard of Purified Protein Derivative-Standard (PPD). The reaction may be suppressed in critically ill tuberculosis patients; during certain acute infectious diseases, notably measles; and in persons who are immunosuppressed by disease or drugs. Positive reactions caused by other mycobacteria, including BCG, tend to be smaller; their relative frequency varies with the prevalence of these other mycobacteria in the environment and inversely with the frequency of tuberculous infections. A positive or significant reaction is usually defined as one with a diameter of ≥ 10 mm of actual induration; this must be recognized as an arbitrary cut-point and not suitable for all situations.

The cut-point for true positive reactions will vary and may be as high as an induration of 15 mm in diameter if the subjects are young children living in areas with little tuberculosis but a high frequency of other mycobacteria; on the other hand, among household contacts of infectious tuberculosis cases, as little as 5 mm of induration should be considered indicative of tuberculous infection. When periodic tuberculin testing of adults is done, if the reaction is less than that locally accepted as significant, a 2nd test should be done 1 week later; an increase in size of reaction indicates a boosted reaction unless there has been exposure to an infectious case within the previous few weeks. If the second test elicits a response considered significant, the person may be assumed to have been infected with mycobacteria at some time in the past; if this reaction too is less than that considered significant, the individual is considered not to have been infected. After such two-step testing, a subsequent reaction with an increase in size of ≥ 6 mm, and to a diameter of ≥ 10 mm is considered conversion, indicative of a recent tuberculous infection.

In general, a tuberculous infection may be inferred when the tuberculin test has converted or when a single test presents ≥ 10 mm of induration. A presumptive diagnosis of current disease is made by demonstration of acid-fast bacilli in stained smears from sputum or other body fluids; a positive smear justifies initiation of antituberculosis therapy. The diagnosis is confirmed by isolation of tubercle bacilli on culture; this also permits determination of the drug sensitivity of the infecting organism. In the absence of bacteriologic confirmation, current disease can be diagnosed if there is a significant reaction to the tuberculin test and clinical and/or x-ray evidence of an ongoing disease process.

2. **Infectious agents**—*Mycobacterium tuberculosis* and *M. africanum* primarily from humans, and *M. bovis* primarily from cattle. Other mycobacteria occasionally produce disease of the lymph nodes and lungs clinically indistinguishable from tuberculosis, identified only by culture of the organisms.

3. **Occurrence**—Worldwide; numerous countries have shown downward trends of mortality and morbidity for many years. Mortality rates in the 1970s ranged from 1–76/100,000 population/yr. Mortality and morbidity rates increase with age; in older persons, these are higher in males than in females; much higher among the poor than the rich; usually higher in cities than in rural areas. In 1983, the reported incidence of clinical disease in the USA was 10.2/100,000 population with rates for the individual states ranging from 1.3–23.1/100,000. In low incidence areas, most tuberculosis is endogenous, i.e., it is a reactivation from latent foci remaining from the initial infection. Although tuberculosis ranks low among communicable diseases in infectiousness per unit of time of exposure, the long exposure of some contacts, notably household associates, may lead to a 30% risk of becoming infected, and a 1–2% chance of the infection progressing to disease within a year. For infected infants, the lifetime risk of developing disease may approach 10%. Epidemics have been reported among persons congregated in enclosed spaces.

Prevalence of infection detected by tuberculin testing increases with age. The incidence of infection in developed countries has declined rapidly in recent decades; in the USA, the annual rate of new infections is estimated to average about 1:5000 persons or less. In areas where human infection with mycobacteria other than tubercle bacilli is prevalent, cross reactions complicate interpretation of the tuberculin reaction.

Infection with the bovine tubercle bacillus in man is rare in the USA but is still a problem in areas where the disease in cattle has not been controlled and raw milk is used.

4. **Reservoir**—Primarily man; in some areas, also diseased cattle.

5. **Mode of transmission**—Exposure to bacilli in airborne droplet nuclei from sputum of persons with infectious tuberculosis. Prolonged close exposure to an infectious case may lead to infection of contacts. Direct invasion through mucous membranes or breaks in the skin may occur, but is extremely rare. Bovine tuberculosis results from exposure to tubercu-

lous cattle, usually by ingestion of raw unpasteurized milk or dairy products and sometimes by airborne spread to farmers and animal handlers.

6. Incubation period—From infection to demonstrable primary lesion or significant tuberculin reaction, about 4–12 wks. While the subsequent risk of progressive pulmonary or extrapulmonary tuberculosis is greatest within the year or two after infection, it may persist for a lifetime as a latent infection.

7. Period of communicability—Theoretically, as long as infectious tubercle bacilli are being discharged in the sputum. Some untreated or inadequately treated patients may be sputum-positive intermittently for years. The degree of communicability depends on the number of bacilli discharged, the virulence of the bacilli and opportunities for their aerosolization by coughing, sneezing, talking or singing. Effective antimicrobial therapy reduces communicability promptly. Extrapulmonary tuberculosis is generally not communicable, even if there is a draining sinus.

8. Susceptibility and resistance—Susceptibility is general. The most hazardous period for development of clinical disease is the first 6–12 months after infection. The risk of developing disease is highest in children under 3 years old, lowest in later childhood and high again in adolescents and young adults. Relapses of long latent infections, particularly in older persons, account for a large proportion of cases of clinical disease. For those infected, susceptibility to disease is increased among underweight or undernourished persons; among persons with silicosis, diabetes, or gastrectomies; and among alcoholics and the immunosuppressed.

9. Methods of control—

    A. Preventive measures:

        1) Improve those social conditions which increase the risk of becoming infected, such as overcrowding; educate the public in mode of spread and methods of control.

        2) Make available medical, laboratory and x-ray facilities for examination of patients, contacts and suspects, and of facilities for early treatment of cases and high-risk infected persons; beds for those needing hospitalization.

        3) Public health nursing and outreach service for home supervision of patients to encourage compliance with the therapeutic regimen and arrange for examination and preventive treatment of contacts.

        4) Preventive treatment with isoniazid has been shown to be effective in preventing the progression of latent infection to clinical disease in a high proportion of individuals. It is indicated for infected persons under 35 years of age.

Because of the increased risk of isoniazid-associated hepatitis among older persons, isoniazid is not routinely advised for infected persons over 35 years of age unless one or more of the following is present: recent infection, close or household association with a current case, tuberculosis never effectively treated with antimicrobial drugs, diabetes, silicosis or prolonged therapy with corticosteroids or immunosuppressants. Persons started on preventive treatment should be informed of possible adverse effects such as hepatitis, drug fever or severe rash and advised to discontinue treatment and seek medical advice if any suggestive symptoms develop. No more than one month's supply of medication should be given at any time. Patients should be queried at each monthly return visit about adverse effects. Biochemical monitoring for hepatitis need not be done routinely, but is mandatory if symptoms or signs of hepatitis occur.

Isoniazid therapy is contraindicated where there is a history of a previous severe adverse reaction to the drug or when there is acute liver disease of any etiology. During pregnancy it may be wise to postpone preventive treatment until after delivery. Isoniazid should be given with added caution to persons who use alcohol regularly.

A policy of preventive treatment, even of special risk groups, is unrealistic and unsuitable for mass application in a community health program unless the treatment program for patients suffering from infectious tuberculosis is widespread and well organized, achieving a high rate of cure.

5) BCG vaccination of uninfected (tuberculin-negative) persons can induce tuberculin sensitivity in >90% of vaccinees. The protection conferred has varied markedly in different field trials, perhaps related to some special characteristics of the population or to the quality of the vaccine. Some controlled trials have provided evidence that protection may persist for as long as 20 years in high incidence situations, while others have shown no protection at all. Because the risk of infection is very low in the USA, BCG is not routinely used. It may be considered for persons at high and unavoidable risk of becoming infected, including health care personnel in high-risk areas where periodic tuberculin testing and preventive treatment of reactors are not feasible. In areas with a high risk of infection and minimal resources, BCG vaccine in infants and young children may be an important tuberculosis

control measure. BCG is contraindicated for persons with immunodeficiency diseases.

6) Eliminate tuberculosis among dairy cattle by tuberculin testing and slaughter of reactors; pasteurize or boil milk.

7) Measures to prevent silicosis in industrial plants and mines.

8) In high-incidence areas, examination of sputum by direct microscopy and by culture of persons who present themselves to health services because of chest symptoms may give a high yield of infectious tuberculosis. In many situations, direct microscopy may be the most cost-effective method of case finding and is the method of choice for developing countries.

9) In the USA and developed areas where BCG vaccination is not routinely carried out, selective tuberculin testing may be done on groups at high risk of becoming infected, e.g., contacts of infectious cases and immigrants from areas where tuberculosis is prevalent. In population groups where disease still occurs, tuberculin testing surveys, at school entry and at 14 yrs of age may help to identify foci of infection and to indicate trends in the incidence of infection. X-ray examination should be restricted to positive tuberculin reactors and is especially indicated whenever persistent chest symptoms are noted.

B. *Control of patient, contacts and the immediate environment:*

1) Report to local health authority: Obligatory case report in most states and countries, Class 2B (see Préface). Case report should indicate if bacteriologically positive or if based on significant tuberculin reaction and clinical and/or x-ray findings. Health departments should maintain a current register of cases needing treatment.

2) Isolation: Control of infectivity is best achieved by prompt specific drug therapy, which usually produces sputum conversion within a few weeks. Hospital treatment is necessary only for patients with severe illness and for those whose medical or social circumstances make treatment at home impossible. Patients with sputum-positive pulmonary tuberculosis need to be placed in a private room with special ventilation. Persons entering the room should wear masks (if the patient is coughing and does not reliably cover his mouth) and a gown if gross contamination of clothing is likely. Patients should be taught to cover the mouth and nose when coughing or sneezing and how to dispose of sputum and secretion-soiled tissues. The need to adhere to the prescribed chemotherapeutic regimen

must be reemphasized repeatedly. Patients who are bacteriologically negative, who do not cough or who are known to be on adequate chemotherapy need not be isolated.

3) Concurrent disinfection: Handwashing and good housekeeping practices should be maintained according to routine policy. There are no special precautions necessary for handling fomites (dishes, laundry, bedding, clothes and personal effects). Microbial decontamination of air by ventilation; this may be supplemented by UV light.

4) Quarantine: None.

5) Immunization of contacts: Preventive treatment of close contacts (see 9A4, above) is indicated. BCG vaccination of tuberculin-negative household contacts, especially infants and children, may be warranted under special circumstances such as continuing exposure to untreated or ineffectively treated patients with sputum-positive pulmonary tuberculosis. (See 9A5, above.)

6) Investigation of contacts: Tuberculin testing of all members of the household and close extra-household contacts. If negative, a repeat skin test should be performed 2–3 months after exposure has ended. Positive reactors at either time should be x-rayed. Preventive treatment is indicated (see 9A4, above) for contacts who are positive reactors and for initially negative reactors, especially young close contacts, until the repeat skin test is shown to remain negative.

7) Specific treatment: Most initial infections heal without treatment; when they are recognized, preventive antimicrobial therapy with isoniazid is indicated to reduce the risk of progressive disease or later reactivation.

Patients with tuberculosis should be given prompt treatment with an appropriate combination of antimicrobial drugs. Currently accepted regimens include isoniazid (INH) combined with one or more of the following: rifampin (RIF), streptomycin (SM), ethambutol (EMB), and pyrazinamide (PZA). INH and RIF is the combination of choice; regimens including these 2 drugs may be given for as short a period as 9 months. Regimens not including both of these drugs should be continued for at least 12 months. If sputum fails to become negative after 3–4 months of regular therapy or reverts to positive after a series of negatives or if clinical response is poor, examination for inadequate drug taking or development of drug resistance is indicated. Drug resistance is usually the result of irregularity in taking drugs, and necessitates a change in regimen; at least 2 drugs to which the organisms are sensitive should be included; a single new drug should never be added to a failing regimen. In areas or populations characterized by a high prevalence of INH-resistance, 3 drugs including INH should be given until the drug susceptibility of the organisms has been determined. Since 12% of organisms from cases in foreign-born Latin Americans and 15% of those from foreign-born Asians have been initially resistant, it is prudent to initiate therapy in Hispanic and Asian patients with a 3–drug regimen and continue this until tests indicate that the organisms are susceptible to INH and RIF when the third drug could be discontinued. All drugs occasionally cause adverse side reactions. Thoracic surgery is rarely indicated.

Current regimens used in developing countries with low financial resources are usually of a year's duration, consisting of 1–2 months of daily INH plus one or two additional drugs, followed by daily or twice-weekly INH plus another drug for the remainder of the year. The two most commonly used companion drugs with INH are streptomycin and thiacetazon. In some countries, rifampin and pyrazinamide have been introduced only in the initial phase to strengthen the regimen without increasing the cost excessively; this also permits shortening the regimen and may thus improve compliance.

C. *Epidemic measures:* Alertness to recognize and treat aggregations of new infections resulting from contact with an unrecognized infectious case and intensive search for and treatment of the source of infection.

D. *Disaster implications:* None.

E. *International measures:* X-ray screening of individuals from high prevalence countries upon immigration. WHO Collaborating Centres (see Preface).

MYCOBACTERIOSES   ICD-9 031

Mycobacteria, other than *M. tuberculosis, M. africanum, M. bovis* and *M. leprae,* are ubiquitous in nature and may produce disease in man. These acid-fast bacilli in the past have been variously termed atypical, or unclassified mycobacteria, and have been separated into four groups by Runyon (Group I, photochromogens; Group II, scotochromogens; Group

III, nonphotochromogens; and Group IV, rapid growers). Of the numerous identified species only about a dozen are recognized as being pathogenic to man. Clinical syndromes associated with the pathogenic species of mycobacteria can be broadly classified as follows: (1) Pulmonary disease resembling tuberculosis—*M. kansasii, M. avium-intracellulare* (the Battey bacillus), *M. avium, M. fortuitum, M. xenopi;* (2) lymphadenitis (primarily cervical)—*M. scrofulaceum, M. avium-intracellulare, M. kansasii;* (3) skin ulcers—*M. ulcerans* (Buruli ulcer), *M. marinum (balnei);* and (4) injury or injection abscesses—*M. fortuitum, M. chelonei.*

The epidemiology of the diseases attributable to these organisms has not been well delineated but the organisms have been found in soil, milk and water; other factors such as host tissue damage or immunodeficiency may predispose to infection. With the exception of organisms causing skin lesions, there is no evidence of person-to-person transmission. A single isolation of these bacilli from sputum, gastric or other specimen is not diagnostic without compatible clinical findings. In general, the diagnosis of disease requiring treatment is based on repeated isolations of many colonies from symptomatic patients with progressive illness. Where human infections with nontuberculosis mycobacteria are prevalent, cross reactions may interfere with the routine skin test for *M. tuberculosis.* Chemotherapy is relatively effective in treating *M. kansasii* disease but may not be effective for the other mycobacterioses. For selection of an efficient drug combination, drug susceptibility tests for all antituberculosis agents should be performed on the isolated organisms. Surgery should be given more serious consideration than in tuberculosis, especially when the disease is limited, as in localized pulmonary disease, cervical lymphadenitis or a subcutaneous abscess; surgical excision is more effective than drug therapy in some of these infections.

TULAREMIA
(Rabbit fever, Deerfly fever, Ohara's disease)

ICD-9 021

1. **Identification**—An infectious zoonotic disease with a variety of clinical manifestations related to the route of introduction and the virulence of the strain. Most often presents as an indolent ulcer, often on the hand, accompanied by swelling of the regional lymph nodes (ulceroglandular type). There may be no apparent primary ulcer but only enlarged and painful lymph nodes which may suppurate. Inhalation of infectious material may be followed by a pneumonic disease or a primary systemic (typhoidal) picture. Ingestion of organisms may produce a pharyngitis, with or without ulceration, intestinal pain, diarrhea and vomiting. The conjunctival sac is a rare route of introduction (oculo-glandular type). Jellison

type A strains of organisms, common in rabbits (cottontail, jack and snowshoe), restricted to N America and frequently of tick origin, are more virulent with a case fatality rate of 5–10%, mainly from typhoidal or pulmonary disease; with appropriate treatment the case fatality rate is negligible. Jellison type B strains, from sources other than rabbits in N America, and strains from all other parts of the Northern Hemisphere from muskrats and water rats, and from rabbits in Japan, are less virulent and, even without treatment, produce few fatalities. Tularemia may be confused with plague.

Diagnosis is made by recovering the infectious agent on special media or by inoculation of laboratory animals with material from lesions, blood or sputum; and by a rise in specific antibodies in the patient's serum; cross agglutinations occur with *Brucella, Proteus,* and heterophile antibody. Examination of ulcer exudate, lymph node aspirates and other clinical specimens with FA may provide rapid diagnosis.

2. Infectious agent—*Francisella tularensis (Pasteurella tularensis, Bacterium tularense).* All isolates seem to be antigenically homogenous but are differentiated epidemiologically and biochemically into Jellison type A and type B strains (see section 1, above).

3. Occurrence—Throughout N America and in many parts of continental Europe, USSR, and Japan. Occurs in the USA all months of the year; incidence may be higher in early winter during rabbit hunting season and in the summer when ticks and deerflies are abundant.

4. Reservoir—Numerous wild animals, especially rabbits, hares, muskrats, beavers and some domestic animals; also various hard ticks.

5. Mode of transmission—Inoculation of skin, conjunctival sac or oropharyngeal mucosa with blood or tissue while handling infected animals, as in skinning, dressing, or performing necropsies; or by fluids from infected flies, ticks or other animals; or through the bite of arthropods including a species of deerfly, *Chrysops discalis* and, in Sweden, the mosquito *Aedes cinereus.* By bite of wood ticks, *Dermacentor andersoni;* dog ticks, *D. variabilis;* and Lone Star ticks, *Amblyomma americanum.* By handling or ingestion of insufficiently cooked rabbit or hare meat; drinking contaminated water; or by inhalation of dust from contaminated soil, grain or hay. Rarely, from bites of coyote, skunk, hog, cat, and dog whose mouth presumably was contaminated from eating an infected rabbit. Also from contaminated pelts and paws of animals. Laboratory infections occur and frequently appear as a primary pneumonia or typhoidal tularemia.

6. Incubation period—Related to virulence of infecting strain and to size of inoculum, 2–10 days, usually 3 days.

7. Period of communicability—Not directly transmitted from person to person. Unless treated, the infectious agent may be found in the blood during the first 2 wks of disease, and in lesions for a month from onset; sometimes longer. Flies are infective for 14 days and ticks throughout their lifetime (about 2 yrs). Rabbit meat constantly frozen at −15°C (5°F) has remained infective longer than 3 yrs.

8. **Susceptibility and resistance**—All ages are susceptible; long-term immunity follows recovery; however, reinfection has been reported.

9. **Methods of control**—

A. *Preventive measures:*

1) Use impervious gloves when skinning or handling animals, especially rabbits. Cook the meat of wild rabbits and rodents thoroughly.
2) Educate the public to avoid bites of flies, mosquitoes and ticks or handling such arthropods when working in endemic areas, and to avoid drinking, bathing, swimming or working in untreated water where infection prevails among wild animals.
3) Prohibit interstate or inter-area shipment of infected animals or their carcasses.
4) Killed vaccines are of no value. Live attenuated vaccines are used extensively in USSR and to a limited extent for occupational risk groups in the USA. Administration of a viable vaccine intradermally by the multiple-puncture method has markedly reduced the incidence of laboratory-acquired disease. This vaccine can be obtained from the CDC, Atlanta (see Preface).
5) Wear face masks and rubber gloves when working with cultures of *F. tularensis.*

B. *Control of patient, contacts and the immediate environment:*

1) Report to local health authority: In selected endemic areas (USA); in many countries, not a reportable disease, Class 3A (see Preface).
2) Isolation: Drainage/secretion precautions for open lesions.
3) Concurrent disinfection: Of discharges from ulcers, lymph nodes, or conjunctival sacs.
4) Quarantine: None.
5) Immunization of contacts: Not indicated.
6) Investigation of contacts: Important in each case, with search for the origin of infection.
7) Specific treatment: Streptomycin is the drug of choice; gentamicin and tobramycin have been reported to be effective; the tetracyclines and chloramphenicol are effective when continued until temperature is normal for 4–5

days but relapses are reported to occur more often. Fully virulent streptomycin-resistant organisms have been described.

C. *Epidemic measures:* Search for sources of infection related to arthropods, to animal hosts, and to water, soil and crops. Control measures as indicated in 9A, above.

D. *Disaster implications:* None.

E. *International measures:* None.

TYPHOID FEVER
(Enteric fever, Typhus abdominalis)

ICD-9 002.0

1. **Identification**—A systemic bacterial disease characterized by insidious onset of sustained fever, headache, malaise, anorexia, a relative bradycardia, splenomegaly, rose spots on trunk, nonproductive cough, constipation more commonly than diarrhea, and involvement of the lymphoid tissues. Many mild and atypical infections occur. Ulceration of Peyer's patches in the ileum can produce intestinal hemorrhage or perforation (about 1% of cases), especially late in untreated cases. Nonsweating fever, a relative bradycardia, mental dullness, slight deafness and parotitis may be observed. The usual case fatality rate of 10% can be reduced to $\leq 1\%$ with antibiotic therapy. Relapse occurs in 5–10% of untreated cases and may be more common (15–20%) following antibiotic therapy. Mild and inapparent illnesses occur, especially in endemic areas.

Typhoid bacilli can be isolated from the blood early in the disease and from urine or feces after the 1st week; in cases who already received antibiotics, isolations from bone marrow may be possible. The agglutination reaction becomes positive during the 2nd week permitting diagnosis by a significant rise in titer in paired sera provided vaccine had not been given recently. However, serology is of limited sensitivity and specificity.

2. **Infectious agent**—*Salmonella typhi,* the typhoid bacillus. Presently 106 types can be distinguished by phage typing, of value in epidemiological studies.

3. **Occurrence**—Worldwide. In the USA the number of sporadic cases has remained relatively constant for several years and, with development of sanitary facilities and detection and treatment of cases and carriers, has been virtually eliminated from many areas; most cases now represent importation from endemic areas. Strains resistant to recommended

antibiotics have appeared in several areas of the world. Multi-resistant strains have been reported from Asia, the Middle East and Latin America.

4. **Reservoir**—Man, both patients and especially carriers. Family contacts may be transient carriers. In most parts of the world fecal carriers are more common than urinary carriers. The carrier state may follow acute illness, or mild or subclinical infection. The carrier state is most common among persons, especially females, infected during middle age. Long-term carriers frequently have a chronic typhoid cholecystitis. Urinary carriers are seen frequently in areas where *Schistosoma haematobium* infections also occur.

5. **Mode of transmission**—By food or water contaminated by feces or urine of a patient or carrier. Shellfish taken from sewage-contaminated beds and raw fruits, vegetables, milk and milk products contaminated usually by hands of carriers or missed cases are important vehicles in some parts of the world. Flies can infect foods in which the organisms may multiply to achieve an infective dose.

6. **Incubation period**—Depends on size of infecting dose; usual range 1–3 wks.

7. **Period of communicability**—As long as typhoid bacilli appear in excreta; usually from the 1st week throughout convalescence; variable thereafter. About 10% of untreated patients will discharge bacilli for 3 months after onset of symptoms; 2–5% become permanent carriers.

8. **Susceptibility and resistance**—Susceptibility is general; it is increased in individuals with gastric achlorhydria. Relative resistance which follows recovery from clinical disease, from inapparent infection or from active immunization is inadequate to protect against ingestion of large numbers of organisms. In endemic areas attack rates usually decline with age.

9. **Methods of control**—

   A. *Preventive measures:*

   1) Sanitary disposal of human feces and maintenance of fly-proof latrines. Provide suitable handwashing facilities. Under field conditions dispose of feces by burial at a site distant and downstream from the source of drinking water.
   2) Protect, purify and chlorinate public water supplies; provide safe private supplies; avoid cross connections between different water supplies and back-flow connections to sewer systems. For individual or small group protection, and while traveling or in the field, water should be treated chemically or, alternatively, boiled.
   3) Control flies by screening, spraying with insecticides, and

using insecticidal baits and traps. Control fly breeding by adequate collection and disposal of garbage.

4) Use scrupulous cleanliness in food preparation and handling; refrigerate as appropriate. Particular attention should be directed to the proper storage of salads and other foods served cold. These provisions apply equally for home and public eating places. If uncertain about sanitary practices, select foods that are cooked and served hot.

5) Pasteurize or boil all milk and dairy products. Sanitary supervision of commercial milk production, storage and delivery.

6) Enforce suitable quality control procedures in all plants preparing food and drink for human consumption. Use chlorinated water for cooling during the canned food processing.

7) Encourage breast feeding throughout infancy; boil all milk and water used for infant feeding.

8) Limit the collection and marketing of shellfish to supplies from an approved source. Boil, or steam for at least 10 minutes, before serving.

9) Instruct patients, convalescents, and carriers in personal hygiene. Emphasize handwashing after defecation and before preparing or serving food (see 9A11, below).

10) Educate the general public, and particularly foodhandlers and attendants in the care of patients or children, and in the need for personal cleanliness.

11) Exclude infected persons from handling food. Identify and supervise typhoid carriers. Sewage culture may help in locating carriers. Chronic carriers should not be released from supervision and restriction of occupation until 3 consecutive negative cultures of authenticated fecal and urine specimens taken at least 1 month apart (see 9B2, below). Fresh stool specimens are preferred to rectal swabs; at least 1 of the 6 consecutive negative specimens should be obtained by purging. In long-term carriers, gallstones frequently are present or there is x-ray evidence of biliary dysfunction; cholecystectomy is the treatment of choice. If there is no evidence of biliary disease, prolonged administration of ampicillin or amoxicillin with probenecid, or TMP-SMX, possibly concomitantly, may be effective.

12) Immunization is not routinely recommended in the USA or for travel to developed areas. Current practice is to vaccinate persons subject to unusual exposure from occupation or travel to endemic areas, those living in areas

of high endemicity and institutional populations where maintenance of good sanitation may be difficult and where typhoid is likely to be introduced. The vaccine is given in a primary series of 2 injections several weeks apart. Periodic single reinforcing injections are desirable, usually at 3–year intervals. Vaccination is protective against only small infecting inocula. Oral live attenuated vaccines are being evaluated and may prove highly useful.

B. *Control of patient, contacts and the immediate environment:*

1) Report to local health authority: Obligatory case report in most states and countries, Class 2A (see Preface).

2) Isolation: Enteric precautions while ill; hospital care is desirable during acute illness. Release from supervision by local health authority should be based on not less than 3 consecutive negative cultures of feces and urine taken at least 24 hours apart and not earlier than 1 month after onset; if any one of this series is positive, repeat at intervals of 1 month during the 12 month period following onset until at least 3 negative cultures are obtained (see 9A11, above).

3) Concurrent disinfection: Of feces, urine and articles soiled therewith. In communities with modern and adequate sewage disposal systems, feces and urine can be disposed of directly into sewers without preliminary disinfection. Terminal cleaning.

4) Quarantine: None.

5) Management of contacts: Routine administration of typhoid vaccine to family, household and nursing contacts who have been or may be exposed to cases or carriers is of doubtful value. Household contacts should not be employed as foodhandlers until at least 2 negative feces and urine cultures, taken at least 24 hours apart, are obtained.

6) Investigation of contacts and sources of infection: The actual or probable source of infection of every case should be determined by search for unreported cases, carriers, and contaminated food, water, milk or shellfish. All members of travel groups in which a case has been identified should be followed up. Presence of Vi-agglutinins in blood of suspected carriers is suggestive of the carrier state. Identification of the same phage type in the organisms isolated from patients and from a carrier suggests the chain of transmission.

7) Specific treatment: Chloramphenicol is the drug of choice

for acute infection; for strains not sensitive to it, other drugs such as ampicillin, amoxicillin or TMP-SMX (co-trimoxazole) are of proven value. All *S. typhi* isolates should be checked for drug resistance; some strains which are chloramphenicol-, ampicillin- and amoxicillin- resistant are sensitive to TMP-SMX. (See 9A11, above, for treatment of the carrier state.)

C. *Epidemic measures:*

1) Intensive search for case or carrier who is the source of infection and for the vehicle (water or food) by which infection was transmitted.

2) Exclude suspected food.

3) Pasteurize or boil milk, or exclude milk supplies or other foods suspected on epidemiologic evidence, until safety is assured.

4) Suspected water supplies should be adequately chlorinated under competent supervision or not used. All drinking water must be chlorinated, treated with iodine or boiled before use.

5) Routine use of vaccine is not recommended.

D. *Disaster implications:* With disruption of usual water supply and excreta disposal and controls on food and water, transmission of typhoid can be expected if there are active cases or carriers in the displaced population; however, in reality, such outbreaks are rarely seen. Efforts to restore safe drinking water supplies and excreta disposal facilities are more appropriate than mass typhoid vaccination. Vaccination of such populations is not recommended unless specifically indicated.

E. *International measures:*

1) Inoculation with typhoid vaccine is advised for international travelers to endemic areas, especially if travel will likely involve exposure to unsafe food and water and close contact with rural areas and indigenous populations. Not a legal requirement of any country.

2) WHO Collaborating Centres (see Preface).

TYPHUS FEVER
I.EPIDEMIC LOUSE-BORNE TYPHUS FEVER   ICD-9 080
(Louse-borne typhus, Typhus exanthematicus, Classical typhus fever)

1. **Identification**—Onset is variable, often sudden and marked by headache, chills, prostration, fever and general pains. A macular eruption appears on the 5th-6th day, initially on the upper trunk followed by spread to the entire body but usually not to the face, palms or soles. Toxemia is usually pronounced and the disease terminates by rapid lysis after about 2 weeks of fever. In the absence of specific therapy, the case fatality rate increases with age and varies from 10–40%. Mild infections may occur without eruption, especially in children and persons partially protected by prior immunization. The disease may recrudesce years after the primary attack (Brill-Zinsser disease ICD-9 081.1); this is milder, has fewer complications, need not be associated with lice, and has a lower case fatality rate.

The IFA test is most commonly used but may not discriminate between louse-borne and murine typhus unless the sera are differentially absorbed with the respective rickettsial antigen prior to testing. Other diagnostic methods are CF with group-specific or washed type-specific rickettsial antigens, toxin-neutralization test, and Weil-Felix reaction with *Proteus* OX-19. Antibody tests usually become positive in the 2nd week. In Brill-Zinsser disease, the initial antibody is IgG and the Weil-Felix test may not be positive.

2. **Infectious agent**—*Rickettsia prowazekii.*

3. **Occurrence**—In colder areas where people may live under unhygienic conditions and are louse-infested; historically a concomitant of war and famine. Endemic foci exist in mountainous regions of Mexico, Central and S America, in central Africa and numerous countries of Asia. In the USA, the last outbreak of louse-borne typhus occurred in 1921. In the USA this rickettsia exists as a zoonosis of flying squirrels *(Glaucomys volans);* there is serologic evidence that at least 33 humans have been infected from this source, possibly by the squirrel flea. Most of these have been in the east coast states but 2 cases were reported from Indiana and 1 each from California, Illinois, Ohio, Tennessee and W Virginia.

4. **Reservoir**—Man is the reservoir and is responsible for maintaining the infection during inter-epidemic periods. The importance of the flying squirrel as a reservoir has not been determined.

5. **Mode of transmission**—The body louse, *Pediculus humanus,* is infected by feeding on the blood of a patient with acute typhus fever. Patients with recrudescent typhus (Brill-Zinsser disease) can infect lice and

may serve as foci for new outbreaks in louse-infested communities. Infected lice excrete rickettsiae in their feces and usually defecate at time of feeding. Man is infected by rubbing feces or crushed lice into the bite or into superficial abrasions. Inhalation of infective louse feces as dust may account for some infections. Transmission from the flying squirrel is presumed to be by the bite of the squirrel flea but this has not been documented.

6. **Incubation period**—From 1–2 wks, commonly 12 days.

7. **Period of communicability**—The disease is not directly transmitted from person to person. Patients are infective for lice during the febrile illness and possibly for 2–3 days after the temperature returns to normal. The louse is infective by passing rickettsiae in its feces within 2–6 days after the infected blood meal; it is infective earlier if crushed. The louse invariably dies within 2 weeks after infection; rickettsiae may remain viable in the dead louse for weeks.

8. **Susceptibility and resistance**—Susceptibility is general. One attack usually confers long-lasting immunity.

9. **Methods of control**—

A. *Preventive measures:*

1) Apply by hand or power blower an effective residual insecticide powder at appropriate intervals to clothes and persons of populations living under conditions favoring lousiness. A lousicide should be used which has been shown to be effective on local lice.

2) Improve living conditions with provisions for bathing and washing clothes.

3) Prophylaxis of persons subject to unusual risk by use of residual insecticide applied to clothing by dusting or impregnation.

4) Immunize susceptible persons or groups of persons entering typhus areas, particularly military or labor forces. No commercially prepared vaccine is available in the USA or Canada. A live vaccine prepared from the attenuated strain E of *R. prowazekii* has shown promise.

B. *Control of patient, contacts and the immediate environment:*

1) Report to local health authority: Report of louse-borne typhus fever required as a Disease under Surveillance by WHO, Class 1A (see Preface).

2) Isolation: Not required after proper delousing of patient, clothing, living quarters and household contacts.

3) Concurrent disinfection: Appropriate insecticide powder

applied to clothing and bedding of patient and contacts; launder clothing and bedclothes; treat hair for louse eggs (nits) with effective chemical agents. Lice tend to leave abnormally hot or cold bodies in search of a normothermic clothed body (see 9A1, above). If death from louse-borne typhus occurs before delousing, delouse the body and clothing by thorough application of an insecticide.

4) Quarantine: Louse-infested susceptibles exposed to typhus fever should ordinarily be quarantined for 15 days; after application of an insecticide with residual effect, these susceptibles may be released.

5) Management of contacts: All immediate contacts should be kept under surveillance for 2 wks.

6) Investigation of contacts: Every effort should be made to trace the infection to the immediate source.

7) Specific treatment: Tetracyclines or chloramphenicol orally in a loading dose followed by daily doses until the patient becomes afebrile (usually 2 days) plus 1 day. A single dose of doxycycline (5 mg/kg) is curative. When faced with a seriously ill patient with possible typhus, suitable therapy should be started without waiting for laboratory confirmation.

C. *Epidemic measures:* The imperative measure for rapid control of typhus is application to all contacts of an insecticide with residual effect. Where infection is known to be widespread, systematic application of residual insecticide to all persons in the community is indicated. If a vaccine is available, it should be administered.

D. *Disaster implications:* Typhus can be expected to be a significant problem in endemic areas if social upheavals and crowding occur in louse-infested populations.

E. *International measures:*

1) Telegraphic notification by governments to WHO and to adjacent countries of the occurrence of a case or an outbreak of louse-borne typhus fever in an area previously free of the disease.

2) International travelers: No country currently requires immunization against typhus for entry.

3) Louse-borne typhus is a Disease under Surveillance of WHO. WHO Collaborating Centres (see Preface).

II. MURINE TYPHUS FEVER ICD-9 081.0
(Flea-borne typhus, Endemic typhus fever, Shop typhus)

1. **Identification**—The course of murine typhus fever resembles that of louse-borne typhus, but is milder. The case fatality rate for all ages is about 2%; it increases with age.

Absence of louse infestation, seasonal distribution and sporadic occurrence of the disease help to differentiate it from louse-borne typhus. For laboratory diagnosis, see I, section 1, above.

2. **Infectious agent**—*Rickettsia typhi (Rickettsia mooseri).*

3. **Occurrence**—Worldwide. Found in areas where people and rats occupy the same buildings and where large numbers of mice live. In the USA, fewer than 80 cases are reported annually. Seasonal peak is in late summer and autumn; cases tend to be scattered, but with a high proportion reported from Texas.

4. **Reservoir**—Infection is maintained in nature by a rat-flea-rat cycle. Rats are the reservoir, commonly *Rattus rattus* and *R. norvegicus;* infection in rats is inapparent.

5. **Mode of transmission**—Infective rat fleas (usually *Xenopsylla cheopis*) defecate rickettsiae while sucking blood and contaminate the bite site and other fresh skin wounds. An occasional case may follow inhalation of dried infective flea feces. Infection occurs in opossums, cats and other wild or domestic animals which is self-limited but these animals may transport infective fleas to humans. The cat flea, *Ctenocephalides felis,* is a possible vector.

6. **Incubation period**—From 1–2 wks, commonly 12 days.

7. **Period of communicability**—Not directly transmitted from person to person. Once infected, fleas remain so for life (up to 1 year).

8. **Susceptibility and resistance**—Susceptibility is general. One attack confers immunity.

9. **Methods of control**—

    A. *Preventive measures:*

        1) Apply insecticide powders with residual action to rat runs, burrows and harborages.

        2) To avoid increased exposure of humans, rodent control measures should wait until flea populations have first been reduced by insecticides. (See Plague, 9B5.)

    B. *Control of patient, contacts and the immediate environment:*

1) Report to local health authority: Case report obligatory in most states and countries, Class 2B (see Preface).
2) Isolation: None.
3) Concurrent disinfection: None.
4) Quarantine: None.
5) Immunization of contacts: None.
6) Investigation of contacts and source of infection: Search for rodents around premises or home of patient.
7) Specific treatment: As for louse-borne typhus. See I, 9B7, above.

C. *Epidemic measures:* In endemic areas with numerous cases, use of a residual insecticide effective against rat fleas will reduce the flea index of rats and the incidence of infection in rats and man.

D. *Disaster implications:* Cases can be expected when man, rats and fleas are forced to co-exist, but murine typhus has not been a major contributor to disease rates in such situations.

E. *International measures:* WHO Collaborating Centres (see Preface).

III. SCRUB TYPHUS   ICD-9 081.2
(Tsutsugamushi disease, Mite-borne typhus fever)

1. Identification—A rickettsial disease often characterized by a primary "punched out" skin ulcer (eschar) corresponding to the site of attachment of an infected mite. The acute febrile onset follows within several days, along with headache, profuse sweating, conjunctival injection and lymphadenopathy. Late in the 1st week of fever a dull red maculopapular eruption appears on the trunk, extends to the extremities and disappears in a few days. Cough and x-ray evidence of pneumonitis are common. Without antibiotic therapy, fever lasts for about 14 days. The case fatality rate in untreated cases varies from 1–60%, according to area, strain of rickettsia and previous exposure to disease. It is consistently higher among older persons.

From cases of a benign mononucleosis-like syndrome seen in some areas of Japan, an organism named *Rickettsia sennetsu* was isolated which was serologically distinct from the organism of scrub typhus; antibodies against this organism have been found in serum collections from Malaysia and from the Philippines. This organism has now been shown to be a member of the genus *Ehrlichia,* and the organism classified as *E. sennetsu.*

Diagnosis is made by isolation of the infectious agent by inoculating the patient's blood into mice. Serological tests are complicated by the antigenic differences of various strains of the causal rickettsia; the IFA test is the preferred technique. Many cases develop a positive Weil-Felix reaction with the *Proteus* OXK strain.

2. **Infectious agent**—*Rickettsia tsutsugamushi (Rickettsia orientalis),* with multiple, serologically distinct strains.

3. **Occurrence**—Central, eastern and SE Asia; from southeastern Siberia and northern Japan to northern Australia and the New Hebrides, as far west as Pakistan and to as high as 10,000 ft above sea level in the Himalayan Mountains. Acquired by man in one of innumerable small, sharply delimited "typhus islands," some covering an area of only a few square ft, where rickettsiae, vectors and suitable rodents exist simultaneously. Occupation greatly influences the sex distribution; restricted mainly to adult workers who frequent scrub, overgrown terrain or other mite-infested areas such as forest clearings, reforested areas, new settlements, or even newly irrigated desert regions. Epidemics occur when susceptibles are brought into endemic areas, especially in military operations in which 20–50% of men have been infected within weeks or months.

4. **Reservoir**—Infected larval stages of trombiculid mites; *Leptotrombidium akamushi, L. deliensis* and related species (varying with area) are the most common vectors for humans. Infection is maintained in mites by transovarian passage.

5. **Mode of transmission**—By the bite of infected larval mites; nymphs and adults do not feed on vertebrate hosts.

6. **Incubation period**—Usually 10–12 days; varies from 6–21 days.

7. **Period of communicability**—Not directly transmitted from person to person.

8. **Susceptibility and resistance**—Susceptibility is general. An attack confers prolonged immunity against the homologous strain of *R. tsutsugamushi* but only transient immunity against heterologous strains. Heterologous infection within a few months results in mild disease, but after a year produces the typical illness. Second and even 3rd attacks of naturally acquired scrub typhus (usually benign or inapparent) occur among persons who spend their lives in endemic areas. No experimental vaccine has been effective.

9. **Methods of control—**

   A. Preventive measures:

   1) Prevent contact with infected mites by personal prophylaxis against the mite vector, achieved by impregnating

clothes and blankets with miticidal chemicals (benzyl benzoate) and application of mite repellents (diethyltoluamide) to exposed skin surfaces.

2) The elimination of mites from the specific sites is best accomplished by application of chlorinated hydrocarbons such as lindane, dieldrin, or chlordane to ground and vegetation in environs of camps, mine buildings and other populated zones in endemic areas.

3) In a small group of volunteers in Malaysia, the administration of 7 weekly doses of doxycycline was an effective prophylactic regime.

B. *Control of patient, contacts and the immediate environment:*

1) Report to local health authority: In selected endemic areas; (clearly differentiate from murine and louse-borne typhus). In many countries not a reportable disease, Class 3A (see Preface).

2) Isolation: None.

3) Concurrent disinfection: None.

4) Quarantine: None.

5) Immunization of contacts: None.

6) Investigation of contacts: None (see 9C, below).

7) Specific treatment: One of the tetracyclines orally in a loading dose, followed by divided doses daily until patient is afebrile (average 30 hours). If treatment is started within the first 3 days, recrudescence is likely unless a 2nd course of antibiotic is given after an interval of 6 days. In Malaysia a single dose of doxycycline was effective when given on the 7th day and in the Pescadores when given on the 5th day; earlier administration was associated with some relapses.

C. *Epidemic measures:* Rigorously employ procedures described in III, 9A1 and 9A2 in the affected area. Daily observation of all persons at risk for fever and appearance of primary lesions; institute treatment upon first indication of illness.

D. *Disaster implications:* Only if refugee centers are sited in or near a "typhus island."

E. *International measures:* WHO Collaborating Centres (see Preface).

WARTS, VIRAL   ICD-9 078.1
(Verruca vulgaris, Common wart, Condyloma acuminata, Papilloma venereum)

1. **Identification**—A viral disease manifested by a variety of skin and mucous membrane lesions. These include the common wart, a circumscribed, hyperkeratotic, rough textured, painless papule varying in size from a pinhead to large masses; filiform warts, elongated, pointed, delicate lesions which may reach 1 cm in length; laryngeal papillomas on vocal cords and epiglottis in children; flat warts, smooth, slightly elevated, usually multiple lesions varying in size from 1 mm-1 cm; venereal warts (condylomata acuminata), cauliflower-like fleshy growths most often seen in moist areas in and around the genitalia which must be differentiated from condyloma lata of secondary syphilis; flat papillomas of the cervix; and plantar warts, flat, hyperkeratotic lesions of the plantar surface of the feet which are frequently painful. Both laryngeal papillomas and genital warts have occasionally become malignant.

The diagnosis is usually based on the typical lesion. If there is doubt, it should be excised and examined histologically.

2. **Infectious agent**—Human papilloma viruses (HPV) of the papovavirus group of DNA viruses (the human wart viruses). At least 24 human papilloma virus types have been identified with probable specific manifestations; HPV types 16 and 18 have been associated with cervical neoplasia, types 6 and 11 with laryngeal papillomata.

3. **Occurrence**—Worldwide.

4. **Reservoir**—Man.

5. **Mode of transmission**—Usually by direct contact, but contaminated floors are frequently implicated. Warts may be autoinoculated, such as by razors in shaving. Condylomata acuminata are usually sexually transmitted. Laryngeal papillomata are probably transmitted during passage of the infant through the birth canal; the viral types in the genital and respiratory tracts are the same.

6. **Incubation period**—About 4 months; range is 1–20 months.

7. **Period of communicability**—Unknown, but probably as long as visible lesions persist.

8. **Susceptibility and resistance**—Common and flat warts are most frequently seen in young children, genital warts in sexually active young adults, and plantar warts in school-age children and teenagers. The incidence of warts is increased in immunosuppressed patients.

9. **Methods of control—**

   A. *Preventive measures:* Avoid direct contact with lesions. Use of a condom probably reduces the transmission of venereal warts.

   B. *Control of patient, contacts and the immediate environment:* Treatment of the affected individual will decrease the amount of wart virus available for transmission.

   1) Report to local health authority: None, Class 5 (see Preface).
   2) Isolation: None.
   3) Concurrent disinfection: None.
   4) Quarantine: None.
   5) Immunization of contacts: None.
   6) Investigation of contacts and source of infection: Sexual contacts of patients with venereal warts should be examined and treated if indicated.
   7) Specific treatment: Verrucae usually regress spontaneously within months to years. If treatment is indicated, freezing with liquid nitrogen for lesions on most of the body surface; salicylic acid plasters and curettage for plantar warts, and 25% podophyllin in tincture of benzoin for readily accessible genital warts except in pregnant females. Surgical removal or laser therapy is required for laryngeal papillomas. Cesarean section should be considered if there is extensive papillomatosis in the genital tract. Clinical trials of interferon in the management of genital and laryngeal warts are in progress.

   C. *Epidemic measures:* Usually a sporadic disease.

   D. *Disaster implications:* None.

   E   *International measures:* None.

YAWS
(Frambesia tropica, Pian, Bouba, Parangi)

ICD-9 102

1. Identification—A chronic relapsing nonvenereal treponematosis characterized by early contagious cutaneous lesions and noncontagious, late, destructive lesions. Typical initial lesion (mother yaw) is a papilloma on the face or extremities which persists for several weeks or months. It proliferates slowly and may form a frambesial (raspberry) lesion, or undergo ulceration (ulceropapilloma), Secondary disseminated or satellite

papillomata appear before or shortly after the initial lesion heals; these lesions occur in successive crops and are often accompanied by periostitis of the long bones, dactylitis and mild constitutional symptoms. Papillomata and hyperkeratoses on palms and soles may appear in both early and late stages; these lesions are very painful and usually disabling. Lesions heal spontaneously but relapses may occur at other sites during early and late phases. The late stage, characterized by destructive lesions of skin and bone, occurs in about 10% of untreated patients, often some years after the early lesions. Unlike syphilis, the brain, eyes, heart, aorta and abdominal organs are not involved. Congenital transmission does not occur and the infection is rarely, if ever, fatal.

Diagnosis is confirmed by darkfield examination of exudates from lesions. Cardiolipin serologic tests for syphilis (VDRL and RPR tests) become positive during the initial stage, remain reactive during the early infection and tend to become nonreactive after many years of latency, even without specific therapy; in some they remain reactive at low titer for life. Treponemal serologic tests (FTA-ABS and MHA-TP) usually remain positive for life.

2. Infectious agent—*Treponema pertenue*, a spirochete.

3. Occurrence—Predominantly a disease of rural children living in warm, humid tropical areas; more frequent in males. Worldwide prevalence was dramatically decreased by mass penicillin treatment campaigns in the 1950–60s, but early yaws has resurged in parts of equatorial and west Africa with scattered foci of infection persisting in Latin America, the Caribbean islands, SE Asia and the South Pacific islands.

4. Reservoir—Man and possibly higher primates.

5. Mode of transmission—Principally by direct contact with exudates of early skin lesions of infected persons. Indirect by contamination from scratching, skin-piercing articles and by flies on open wounds is probable but of undetermined importance. Climate influences the morphology, distribution and infectiousness of the early lesions.

6. Incubation period—From 2 wks to 3 months.

7. Period of communicability—Variable; may extend intermittently over several years while moist lesions are present. The infectious agent is not usually found in late ulcerative lesions.

8. Susceptibility and resistance—No evidence of natural or racial resistance. Infection results in immunity to homologous and heterologous strains; heterologous immunity develops slowly and probably is not complete until after 1 year. Immunity to yaws may partially protect against syphilis.

9. Methods of control—

A. *Preventive measures:* The following are applicable to yaws and to other nonvenereal treponematoses. By present techniques the infectious agents are not differentiable, but it is unlikely the differences in clinical syndromes result only from epidemiologic or environmental factors.

1) General health promotion measures; health education of the public about treponematosis; better sanitation, including liberal use of soap and water, and improvement of social and economic conditions over a period of years to reduce incidence.

2) Organize intensive control activities on a community level suitable to the local problem, clinically examine entire populations, and treat patients with active or latent disease. Treatment of even asymptomatic contacts is justified, and there may be need to treat the entire population within defined areas. Periodic clinical resurveys and continuous surveillance are essential for success.

3) Serological surveys for latent cases, particularly in children, to prevent relapse and development of infective lesions which maintain the disease in the community.

4) Provide facilities for early diagnosis and treatment as a part of a plan in which the mass control campaign (9A2, above) is eventually consolidated into permanent local health services.

5) Treat disfiguring and incapacitating late manifestations.

B. *Control of patient, contacts and the immediate environment:*

1) Report to local health authority: In selected endemic areas; in many countries not a reportable disease, Class 3B (see Preface). Differentiation of venereal and nonvenereal treponematoses, with proper reporting of each, has particular importance in evaluation of mass campaigns and in the consolidation period thereafter.

2) Isolation: None; avoid intimate contact and contamination of the environment until lesions are healed.

3) Concurrent disinfection: Care in disposal of discharges and articles contaminated therewith.

4) Quarantine: None.

5) Immunization of contacts: None.

6) Investigation of contacts: All familial contacts should be treated; those with no active disease should be regarded as latent cases. In areas of low prevalence, treat all active cases, all children, and close contacts of infectious cases.

7) Specific treatment: Penicillin. For patients ≧10 yrs with

active disease or contacts, a single i.m. injection of benzathine penicillin G (Bicillin) 1.2 million units; for patients under 10 yrs, 0.6 million units.

C. *Epidemic measures:* Active mass treatment programs in areas of high prevalence. Essential features are: a high percentage of the population examined through field surveys; treatment of active cases extended to the family and community contacts based on the demonstrated prevalence of active yaws; and periodic surveys made at yearly intervals for 1–3 years, as part of the activities of the established rural public health activities of the country.

D. *Disaster implications:* None.

E. *International measures:* To protect countries against risk of reinfection where active mass treatment programs are in progress, adjacent countries in the endemic area should institute suitable measures against yaws. Movement of infected persons across frontiers may need supervision. (See Syphilis 9E.) WHO Collaborating Centres (see Preface).

YELLOW FEVER   ICD-9 060

1. **Identification**—An acute infectious disease of short duration and varying severity. The mildest cases are clinically indeterminate; typical attacks are characterized by a dengue-like illness, i.e., sudden onset, fever, headache, backache, prostration, nausea and vomiting. As the disease progresses, the pulse slows and weakens, even though the temperature may be elevated; albuminuria, sometimes pronounced, and anuria may occur. Leukopenia appears early and is most pronounced about the 5th day. Common hemorrhagic symptoms include epistaxis, buccal bleeding, hematemesis (coffee-ground or black), and melena. Jaundice is moderate early in the disease and is intensified later. The case fatality rate among indigenous populations of endemic regions is <5%, but may reach 50% among nonindigenous groups or in epidemics.

Laboratory diagnosis is made by isolation of virus from blood by inoculation of suckling mice, mosquitoes, or cell cultures (especially those of mosquito cells), demonstration of viral antigen in the blood by ELISA, and by demonstration of specific IgM in early sera or a rising titer of specific antibodies in paired acute-phase and convalescent sera. Serological cross-reactions occur with other flaviviruses. It is suggested but not proven by demonstration of typical lesions in the liver.

2. **Infectious agent**—The virus of yellow fever, a flavivirus.

3. **Occurrence**—Except for a few cases in Trinidad in 1954, no outbreak of urban yellow fever has been transmitted by *Aedes aegypti* in the Americas since 1942. Urban yellow fever outbreaks are still reported from Africa in areas contiguous to rain forest regions where jungle or sylvan yellow fever is enzootic, the latest being in Burkina Faso (Upper Volta) with at least 250 deaths in 1983. Urban yellow fever, when first introduced into the Americas, attacked both sexes and all ages and races, whereas sylvan yellow fever of tropical America now occurs predominantly among adult males 20–40 years old who are exposed in the forest.

Sylvan yellow fever is enzootic with a few hundred cases each year in northern S America and the Amazon basin, including the Colombian llanos and eastern regions of Peru and Bolivia. Eighteen cases occurred in Trinidad in 1979 in persons exposed in the forest. It has occurred from time to time in all mainland American countries from Mexico to Argentina, with the exception of El Salvador, Uruguay and Chile. In Africa it includes the area between 15°N and 10°S, extending from the Sahara Desert south through Angola, Zaire, and into Zambia, Tanzania, Uganda, Kenya, Ethiopia, the Somali Republic and the Sudan. There is no evidence that yellow fever has ever been present in Asia nor on the easternmost coast of Africa.

4. **Reservoir**—In urban areas, man and *Aedes aegypti* mosquitoes; in forest areas, vertebrates other than man, mainly monkeys and possibly marsupials and forest mosquitoes. Transovarial transmission in mosquitoes may contribute to maintenance of infection. Man has no essential role in transmission of jungle yellow fever or in maintaining the virus.

5. **Mode of transmission**—In urban and certain rural areas, by the bite of infective *Aedes aegypti* mosquitoes. In forests of S America, by the bite of several species of forest mosquitoes of the genus *Haemagogus*. In east Africa, *Ae. africanus* is the vector in the monkey population, while *Ae. bromeliae,* a semidomestic subspecies of *Ae. simpsoni,* a semidomestic mosquito, and probably other *Aedes* species transmit the virus from monkey to man. In large epidemics in Ethiopia, good epidemiological evidence incriminated *Ae. simpsoni* as a person-to-person vector. In west Africa, *Ae. furcifer-taylori, Ae. luteocephalus* and other species are responsible for spread between monkeys and man.

6. **Incubation period**—Three to 6 days.

7. **Period of communicability**—Blood of patients is infective for mosquitoes shortly before onset of fever and for the first 3–5 days of illness. Highly communicable where many susceptible persons and abundant vector mosquitoes coexist. Not communicable by contact or common vehicles. The extrinsic incubation period before *Ae. aegypti* becomes

infective is commonly 9–12 days at the usual summer temperatures. Once infected, mosquitoes remain so for life.

8. Susceptibility and resistance—Recovery from yellow fever is followed by lasting immunity; second attacks are unknown. Mild inapparent infections are common in endemic areas. Transient passive immunity in infants born to immune mothers may persist up to 6 months. In natural infection, antibodies appear in the blood within the 1st week.

9. Methods of control—

A. *Preventive measures:*

1) Urban yellow fever, by eradication or control of *Ae. aegypti* mosquitoes; vaccination when indicated (see 9A3 and 9C1, below).

2) Sylvan or jungle yellow fever, transmitted by *Haemagogus* and forest species of *Aedes,* is best controlled by immunization, which is recommended for all persons in rural communities whose occupation brings them into forests in yellow fever areas, and for persons who intend to visit those areas. Protective clothing, bed nets and repellents are advised for persons not immunized.

3) Active immunization of all persons necessarily exposed to infection because of residence, occupation or travel. A single subcutaneous injection of a vaccine containing viable attenuated yellow fever 17D strain virus, cultivated in chick embryo, is effective. Antibodies appear from 7–10 days after vaccination and may persist for at least 30–35 years, probably much longer, though vaccination or revaccination within 10 years is still required by the International Health Regulations for travel from endemic areas.

B. *Control of patient, contacts and the immediate environment:*

1) Report to local health authority: Case report universally required by International Health Regulations (1969), Third Annotated Edition, 1983, WHO, Geneva; Class 1 (see Preface).

2) Isolation: Blood and body fluid precautions. Prevent access of mosquitoes to patient for at least 5 days after onset by screening the sickroom or by spraying quarters with residual insecticide, or by bed net.

3) Concurrent disinfection: None; the home of patients and all houses in the vicinity should be sprayed promptly with an effective insecticide.

4) Quarantine: None.

5) Immunization of contacts: Family and other contacts and

neighbors not previously immunized should be vaccinated promptly.

6) Investigation of contacts and source of infection: Inquire about all places, including forested areas, visited by patient 3–6 days before onset, to locate focus of yellow fever; observe all persons visiting that focus. Search premises and places of work or visits over the preceding several days for mosquitoes capable of transmitting infection and eradicate them with effective insecticide. Investigate mild febrile illnesses and unexplained deaths suggesting yellow fever.

7) Specific treatment: None.

C. *Epidemic measures:*

1) Urban or *Ae. aegypti*-transmitted yellow fever:
   a) Mass vaccination, beginning with persons most exposed and those living in *Ae. aegytpi*-insected areas.
   b) Spraying all houses in the community with insecticides has shown promise for controlling urban epidemics.
   c) Eliminate or apply larvicide to all actual and potential breeding places of *Ae. aegypti.*

2) Jungle or sylvan yellow fever:
   a) Immediate vaccination of all persons living in or near forested areas or entering such areas.
   b) Avoidance by unvaccinated individuals of those tracts of forest where infection has been localized, and similarly by vaccinated persons for the first week after vaccination.
   c) Aerial spraying has shown promise in control of sylvatic vectors.

3) In regions where yellow fever may occur, a diagnostic viscerotomy service should be organized to collect small specimens of liver from fatal febrile illnesses of 10 days duration or less; many cases and outbreaks otherwise missed are thereby discovered.

4) In Central and S America, confirmed deaths of howler and spider monkeys in the forest are presumptive evidence of the presence of yellow fever. Confirmation by the histopathological examination of livers of moribund or recently dead monkeys or by virus isolation is highly desirable.

5) Immunity surveys by neutralization tests of wild primates captured in forested areas are useful in defining enzootic areas. Serological surveys of human populations are practically useless where yellow fever vaccine has been widely used.

D. ***Disaster implications:*** None.

E. ***International measures:***

1) Telegraphic notification by governments to WHO and to adjacent countries of the first imported, first transferred, or first nonimported case of yellow fever in an area previously free of the disease; and of newly discovered or reactivated foci of yellow fever infection among vertebrates other than man.

2) Measures applicable to ships, aircraft and land transport arriving from yellow fever areas are specified in the International Health Regulations (1969), Third Annotated Edition, 1983, WHO, Geneva.

3) Animal quarantine: Quarantine of monkeys and other wild primates arriving from yellow fever areas may be required until 7 days have elapsed after leaving such areas.

4) International travel: A valid international certificate of vaccination against yellow fever is required by many countries for entry of travelers coming from or through recognized yellow fever zones of Africa and S America; otherwise, quarantine measures are applicable. The International Certificate of Vaccination is valid from 10 days after date of vaccination for 10 years; if revaccinated within that period, valid from date of revaccination for 10 years.

YERSINIOSIS   ICD-9 027.8
(Pseudotuberculosis, Enterocolitis)

1. **Identification**—An acute enteric disease manifested by acute watery diarrhea (especially in young children), enterocolitis, acute mesenteric lymphadenitis mimicking appendicitis (especially in older children), fever, headache, pharyngitis, anorexia, vomiting, erythema nodosum (in about 10% of adults, particularly women), arthritis (Reiter's syndrome), iritis, cutaneous ulceration, hepatosplenic abscesses, osteomyelitis and septicemia caused by either of two bacterial agents, *Yersinia enterocolitica* and *Y. pseudotuberculosis*. *Y. enterocolitica* infections present more commonly with a gastroenterocolitis syndrome, and *Y. pseudotuberculosis* with abdominal pain. Infection with *Y. pseudotuberculosis* in an immunocompromised host has a higher case fatality rate.

Blood cultures are usually positive in generalized infections. With precautions to prevent overgrowth of fecal flora, the organisms can be recovered on usual enteric media. Cold enrichment in buffered saline at

4°C (39°F) for 2–3 weeks selects for some strains of these organisms especially from carriers and may be needed; a new medium (CIN) is highly selective permitting recovery in 24 hours at 32°C (89.6°F) without cold adaptation. Serologic agglutination tests may be useful. Circulating antibodies appear 1–2 weeks after onset, peak at 3–4 weeks and gradually disappear in 2–6 months.

2. **Infectious agents**—*Yersinia pseudotuberculosis* subsp. *pseudotuberculosis* is the official name of this organism and is comprised of 6 serotypes with 4 subtypes; >90% of the infections in man and animal have been O-group I strains. *Y. enterocolitica* is comprised of 57 serotypes and 5 biotypes; most of the strains infecting man have been serotypes 03, 08 and 09 and biotypes 2, 3 and 4. Serotypes causing disease may vary in different geographic areas; types 03 and 09 account for most of the cases in Europe and type 08 in the USA. Some strains of human origin have been invasive in HeLa cell culture; a heat-stable enterotoxin (ST) has been found in some strains.

3. **Occurrence**—Worldwide. *Y. pseudotuberculosis* is primarily a zoonotic disease of wild and domesticated birds and mammals, with man as an incidental host. *Y. enterocolitica* has been recovered from a wide variety of animals without signs of disease; fatal outbreaks have been reported in chinchillas. Since the 1960s the *Yersiniae* have been recognized as etiological agents of gastroenteritis (1–3% of acute enteritis in some areas) and mesenteric lymphadenitis. Approximately two-thirds of *Y. enterocolitica* cases occur among infants and children; three-fourths of *Y. pseudotuberculosis* cases involve 5 to 20 year-olds. Human cases have been reported in association with disease in household pets, particularly with sick puppies and kittens. The number of human cases that are recognized is small and largely dependent on the skill and experience of the microbiologist. The highest isolation rates have been reported during the cold season in temperate climates, especially Scandinavia and N America. Epidemics caused by *Y. enterocolitica* have involved presumed person-to-person spread in hospitals and schools as well as contaminated vehicles such as chocolate milk and tofu. As 20% of these infections in older children and adolescents can mimic acute appendicitis, outbreaks can be recognized by local increases in appendectomies.

4. **Reservoir**—The principal reservoirs for *Yersinia* are domestic animals. *Y. pseudotuberculosis* is widespread among many species of avian and mammalian hosts. *Y. enterocolitica* has been recovered from healthy animals and from primates with acute enteric disease.

5. **Mode of transmission**—Fecal-oral transmission takes place by contact with infected persons or animals, or by eating and drinking fecally contaminated food and water. *Y. enterocolitica* has been isolated from raw milk, ice cream, mussels and oysters, tofu, canned beef, prawns,

beefburger and smoked mackerel paté. It has been recovered from natural bodies of water in the absence of *Escherichia coli* organisms. Nosocomial transmission has been reported.

6. Incubation period—Probably 3–7 days, generally under 10 days.

7. Period of communicability—There is fecal shedding at least as long as symptoms exist. Untreated cases may excrete the organism for 2–3 months; a chronic carrier state probably exists.

8. Susceptibility and resistance—Susceptibility is general, but the disease is more severe in adolescents and older adults. *Y. pseudotuberculosis* exhibits a predilection for male adolescents while *Y. enterocolitica* attacks both sexes equally. Reactive arthritis has a predilection for persons with the HLA-B27 genetic type; the septicemic form generally occurs among persons with underlying illness or on immunosuppressive therapy.

9. Methods of control—

A. Preventive measures:

1) Sanitary disposal of human, dog and cat feces.
2) Protection of water supplies from animal and human feces; appropriate purification.
3) Handwashing prior to foodhandling and eating, and after animal contact.
4) Sanitary preparation of food, especially that to be eaten raw; pasteurization of milk.

B. Control of patient, contacts and the immediate environment:

1) Report to local health authority: Case reporting obligatory in many states and countries, Class 2B, (see Preface).
2) Isolation: Enteric precautions for patients in hospitals. Removal of those with diarrhea from foodhandling, patient care, or occupations involving care of young children. Asymptomatic individuals whose stools are positive should be thoroughly indoctrinated in the need for careful postdefecatory handwashing.
3) Concurrent disinfection: In communities with modern and adequate sewage disposal systems, feces cán be discharged directly into sewers without preliminary disinfection.
4) Quarantine: None.
5) Immunization of contacts: None.
6) Investigation of contacts: Search for unrecognized cases and convalescent carriers among contacts is rarely indicated.
7) Specific treatment: Organisms are sensitive to many antibiotics, but may be resistant to penicillin and its semi-

synthetic derivatives. Therapy may be helpful for gastrointestinal symptoms; definitely indicated for septicemia or other invasive disease. Agents of choice against *Y. enterocolitica* are the aminoglycosides and TMP-SMX. Certain of the 3rd generation cephalosporins are very active in vitro (ceftizoxime, ceftriaxone and moxalactam). *Y. pseudotuberculosis* is usually sensitive to ampicillin, aminoglycosides or tetracycline.

C. **Epidemic measures:**

1) Any group of cases of acute gastroenteritis or appendicitis syndrome should be reported at once to the local health authority, even in the absence of specific identification of the etiology.

2) Investigation of general sanitation and search for common source vehicle; attention to close contacts with animals, especially pet dogs, cats, and other domestic animals.

D. **Disaster implications:** None.

E. **International measures:** None.

ZYGOMYCOSIS
(Phycomycosis)

ICD-9 117.7

Zygomycosis designates all infections caused by fungi of the class Zygomycetes. These include mucormycosis and entomophthoromycosis due to either *Conidiobolus* or *Basidiobolus* spp.

MUCORMYCOSIS

1. Identification—A group of mycoses usually caused by fungi of the family Mucoraceae of the class Zygomycetes. These fungi have an affinity for blood vessels, causing thrombosis and infarction. The craniofacial form of the disease usually presents as nasal or paranasal sinus infections, most often during episodes of poorly controlled diabetes mellitus. Gangrene of the turbinates, perforation of the hard palate, gangrene of the cheek, or orbital cellulitis, proptosis, and ophthalmoplegia may occur. Infection may penetrate to the internal carotid artery or by direct extension to the brain, causing infarction. In the pulmonary form of disease, the fungus causes thrombosis of pulmonary blood vessels and infarcts of the lung. In the gastrointestinal form, mucosal ulcers or thrombosis and gangrene of stomach or bowel may occur.

Diagnosis is confirmed by microscopic demonstration of distinctive broad, nonseptate hyphae in biopsies and by culture of biopsy tissue. Wet preparations and smears may be examined. Cultures alone are not diagnostic because fungi of the order Mucorales are frequently found in the environment.

2. Infectious agent—Some species of *Rhizopus,* especially *R. oryzae* and *R. arrhizus,* have caused most of the culture-positive craniofacial cases of mucormycosis. Probably *Mucor, Rhizomucor* and *Rhizopus* spp. are the chief causes of the pulmonary and gastrointestinal mucormycosis. *Cunninghamella,* and *Absidia* spp. have been reported from a few human cases of mucormycosis.

3. Occurrence—Worldwide. Incidence may be increasing because of longer survival of patients with diabetes mellitus and certain blood dyscrasias, especially acute leukemia.

4. Reservoir—Members of the order Mucorales are common saprophytes in the environment.

5. Mode of transmission—By inhalation or ingestion of spores of the fungal agents by susceptible individuals. Direct inoculation at sites of i.v. catheters and cutaneous burns are seen occasionally.

6. Incubation period—Unknown. Fungus spreads rapidly in susceptible tissues.

7. Period of communicability—Not directly transmitted from person to person or between animals and man.

8. Susceptibility and resistance—The rarity of infection in healthy individuals despite the abundance of the Mucorales in the environment indicates natural resistance. Corticosteroid and immunosuppressive therapy predispose to infection. Malnutrition predisposes to the gastrointestinal form.

9. Methods of control—

A. *Preventive measures:* Optimal clinical control of diabetes mellitus.

B. *Control of patient, contacts and the immediate environment:*

1) Report to local health authority: Official report not ordinarily justifiable, Class 5 (see Preface).

2) Isolation: None.

3) Concurrent disinfection: Ordinary cleanliness. Terminal cleaning.

4) Quarantine: None.

5) Immunization of contacts: None.

6) Investigation of contacts: Ordinarily not profitable.

7) Specific treatment: In the cranial form, clinical control of

diabetes; amphotericin B (Fungizone®) and resection of necrotic tissue have been helpful.

C. *Epidemic measures:* Not applicable, a sporadic disease.

D. *Disaster implications:* None.

E. *International measures:* None

ENTOMOPHTHOROMYCOSIS DUE TO BASIDIOBOLUS

ICD-9 117.7

ENTOMOPHTHOROMYCOSIS DUE TO CONIDIOBOLUS

ICD-9 117.7

These two infections have been recognized principally in tropical and subtropical Asia and Africa, are not characterized by thromboses or infarction, do not usually occur in association with serious preexisting disease, do not usually cause disseminated disease and seldom cause death.

Entomophthoromycosis is a granulomatous inflammation caused by *Basidiobolus haptosporus,* a ubiquitous fungus occurring in decaying vegetation, soil and the gastrointestinal tract of amphibians and reptiles. The disease presents as a firm subcutaneous mass, fixed to the skin, principally in children and adolescents, more commonly in males. The infection may heal spontaneously. Recommended therapy is oral potassium iodide.

Entomophthoromycosis due to *Conidiobolus* (rhinoentomophthoromycosis) usually originates in the paranasal skin or nasal mucosa and presents as nasal obstruction or swelling of the nose or adjacent structures. The lesion may spread to involve contiguous areas, such as lip, cheek, palate or pharynx. The disease is uncommon, occurs principally in adult males. Recommended therapy is oral potassium iodide or i.v. amphotericin B (Fungizone®). The infectious agent, *Conidiobolus coronatus,* occurs in soil and decaying vegetation.

For both forms of entomophthoromycosis, incubation periods and modes of transmission are unknown. Person-to-person transmission does not occur.

DEFINITIONS
(Technical meaning of terms used in the text)

1. **Carrier**—A person or animal that harbors a specific infectious agent in the absence of discernible clinical disease and serves as a potential source of infection. The carrier state may exist in an individual with an infection that is inapparent throughout its course (commonly known as **healthy** or **asymptomatic carrier**), or during the incubation period, convalescence, and postconvalescence of an individual with a clinically recognizable disease (commonly known as **incubatory carrier** or **convalescent carrier**). Under either circumstance the carrier state may be of short or long duration (**temporary** or **transient carrier,** or **chronic carrier**).

2. **Case Fatality Rate**—Usually expressed as a percentage of the number of persons diagnosed as having a specified disease who die as a result of that illness. This term is most frequently applied to a specific outbreak of acute disease in which all patients have been followed for an adequate period of time to include all attributable deaths. The **case fatality rate** must be clearly differentiated from **mortality rate** (q.v.). Synonyms—fatality rate, fatality percentage.

3. **Chemoprophylaxis**—The administration of a chemical, including antibiotics, to prevent the development of an infection or the progression of an infection to active manifest disease. **Chemotherapy,** on the other hand, refers to use of a chemical to cure a clinically recognizable disease or to limit its further progress.

4. **Cleaning**—The removal by scrubbing and washing, as with hot water, soap or suitable detergent or by vacuum cleaning, of infectious agents and of organic matter from surfaces on which and in which infectious agents may find favorable conditions for surviving or multiplying.

5. **Communicable disease**—An illness due to a specific infectious agent or its toxic products which arises through transmission of that agent or its products from an infected person, animal, or inanimate reservoir to a susceptible host, either directly or indirectly through an intermediate plant or animal host, vector, or the inanimate environment (see Transmission of Infectious Agents).

6. **Communicable period**—The time or times during which an infectious agent may be transferred directly or indirectly from an infected person to another person, from an infected animal to man, or from an infected person to an animal, including arthropods.

   In diseases such as diphtheria and streptococcal infection in which mucous membranes are involved from the initial entry of the infectious agent, the period of communicability is from the date of first exposure to a source of infection until the infecting microorganism is no longer disseminated from the involved mucous membranes, i.e., from the period before the prodromata until termination of a carrier state, if the latter develops. Some diseases are more communicable during the incubation period than during actual illness.

In diseases such as tuberculosis, leprosy, syphilis, gonorrhea, and some of the salmonelloses, the communicable state may exist over a long and sometimes intermittent period when unhealed lesions permit the discharge of infectious agents from the surface of the skin or through any of the body orifices.

In diseases transmitted by arthropods, such as malaria and yellow fever, the periods of communicability (or more properly **infectivity**) are those during which the infectious agent occurs in the blood or other tissues of the infected person in sufficient numbers to permit infection of the vector. A period of communicability (**transmissibility**) is also to be noted for the arthropod vector, namely, when the agent is present in the tissues of the arthropod in such form and locus (**infective state**) as to be transmissible.

7.   **Contact**—A person or animal that has been in an association with an infected person or animal or a contaminated environment which might provide an opportunity to acquire the infective agent.

8.   **Contamination**—The presence of an infectious agent on a body surface; also on or in clothes, bedding, toys, surgical instruments or dressings, or other inanimate articles or substances including water and food. **Pollution** is distinct from contamination and implies the presence of offensive, but not necessarily infectious, matter in the environment. Contamination on a body surface does not imply a carrier state.

9.   **Disinfection**—Killing of infectious agents outside the body by direct exposure to chemical or physical agents.

Concurrent disinfection is the application of disinfective measures as soon as possible after the discharge of infectious material from the body of an infected person, or after the soiling of articles with such infectious discharges; all personal contact with such discharges or articles minimized prior to such disinfection.

Terminal disinfection is the application of disinfective measures after the patient has been removed by death or to a hospital, or has ceased to be a source of infection, or after hospital isolation or other practices have been discontinued. Terminal disinfection is rarely practiced; terminal cleaning generally suffices (see Cleaning), along with airing and sunning of rooms, furniture and bedding. Disinfection is necessary only for diseases spread by indirect contact; steam sterilization or incineration of bedding and other items is recommended after a disease such as Lassa fever or other highly infectious diseases.

10. **Disinfestation**—Any physical or chemical process serving to destroy or remove undesired small animal forms, particularly arthropods or rodents, present upon the person, the clothing, or in the environment of an individual, or on domestic animals (see Insecticide and Rodenticide). Disinfestation includes delousing for infestation with *Pediculus humanus,* the body louse. Synonyms include the terms **disinsection** and **disinsectization** when only insects are involved.

11. **Endemic**—The constant presence of a disease or infectious agent within a given geographic area; may also refer to the usual prevalence of a given disease within such area. **Hyperendemic** expresses a persistent intense transmission and **holoendemic** a high level of infection beginning early in life and affecting most of the population, e.g., malaria in some places. (See Zoonosis.)

12. **Epidemic**—The occurrence in a community or region of cases of an illness (or an outbreak) clearly in excess of expectancy. The number of cases indicating presence of an epidemic will vary according to the infectious agent, size and type of population exposed, previous experience or lack of exposure to the disease, and time and place of occurrence; epidemicity is thus relative to usual frequency of the disease in the same area, among the specified population, at the same season of the year. A single case of a communicable disease long absent from a population or the first invasion by a disease not previously recognized in that area requires immediate reporting and epidemiologic investigation; two cases of such a disease associated in time and place are sufficient evidence of transmission to be considered an epidemic. (See Report of a Disease and see Zoonosis.)

13. **Fumigation**—Any process by which the killing of animal forms, especially arthropods and rodents, is accomplished by the use of gaseous agents (see Insecticide and Rodenticide).

14. **Health Education**—Health education is the process by which individuals and groups of people learn to promote, maintain or restore health. Education for health begins with people as they are, with whatever interests they may have in improving their living conditions. Its aim is to develop in them a sense of responsibility for health conditions, as individuals and as members of families and communities. In communicable disease control, health education commonly includes an appraisal of what is known by a population about a disease, an assessment of habits and attitudes of the people

as they relate to spread and frequency of the disease, and the presentation of specific means to remedy observed deficiencies. Synonyms: Education; education for health; education of the public.

15. **Host**—A person or other living animal, including birds and arthropods, that affords subsistence or lodgment to an infectious agent under natural (as apposed to experimental) conditions. Some protozoa and helminths pass successive stages in alternate hosts of different species. Hosts in which the parasite attains maturity or passes its sexual stage are **primary** or **definitive hosts;** those in which the parasite is in a larval or asexual state are **secondary** or **intermediate** hosts. A **transport host** is a carrier in which the organism remains alive but does not undergo development.

16. **Immune individual**—A person or animal that has specific protective antibodies or cellular immunity as a result of previous infection or immunization, or is so conditioned by such previous specific experience as to respond adequately to prevent infection and/or clinical illness following exposure to a specific infectious agent. Immunity is relative; an ordinarily effective protection may be overwhelmed by an excessive dose of the infectious agent or by exposure through an unusual portal of entry; it may also be impaired by immunosuppressive drug therapy, concurrent disease, or the aging process. (See Resistance.)

17. **Immunity**—That resistance usually associated with presence of antibodies or cells having a specific action on the microorganism concerned with a particular infectious disease or on its toxin. **Passive humoral immunity** is attained either naturally by transplacental transfer from the mother, or artificially by inoculation of specific protective antibodies (from immunized animals, or convalescent hyperimmune serum or immune serum globulin (human)); it is of short duration (days to months). **Active humoral immunity,** which usually lasts for years, is attained either naturally by infection with or without clinical manifestations, or artificially by inoculation of the agent itself in killed, modified or variant form, or of fractions or products of the agent. Effective immunity depends on **cellular immunity** which is conferred by T-lymphocyte sensitization, and **humoral immunity** which is based on B-lymphocyte response.

18. **Inapparent infection**—The presence of infection in a host without recognizable clinical signs or symptoms. Inapparent infections are identifiable only by laboratory means or by the development of positive reactivity to specific skin tests. Synonyms: **Asymptomatic, subclinical, occult** infection.

19. **Incidence rate**—A quotient (rate), with the number of new cases of

a specified disease diagnosed or reported during a defined period of time as the numerator, and the number of persons in a stated population in which the cases occurred, as the denominator. This is usually expressed as cases per 1,000 or 100,000 per annum. This rate may be expressed as age- or sex-specific or as specific for any other population characteristic or subdivision (see Morbidity rate and Prevalence rate).

Attack rate, or **case rate,** is an incidence rate often used for particular groups, observed for limited periods and under special circumstances, as in an epidemic, usually expressed as percent (cases per 100). **The secondary attack rate** in communicable disease practice expresses the number of cases among familial or institutional contacts occurring within the accepted incubation period following exposure to a primary case, in relation to the total of exposed contacts; it may be restricted to susceptible contacts when determinable. **Infection rate** expresses the incidence of all infections, manifest and inapparent.

20. **Incubation period**—The time interval between initial contact with an infectious agent and the appearance of the first sign or symptom of the disease in question, or, in a vector, of the first time transmission is possible (**extrinsic incubation period**).

21. **Infected individual**—A person or animal that harbors an infectious agent and who has either manifest disease (see Patient or sick person) or inapparent infection (see Carrier). An **infectious person** or animal is one from whom the infectious agent can be naturally acquired.

22. **Infection**—The entry and development or multiplication of an infectious agent in the body of man or animals. Infection is not synonymous with infectious disease; the result may be inapparent (see Inapparent infection) or manifest (see Infectious disease). The presence of living infectious agents on exterior surfaces of the body, or upon articles of apparel or soiled articles, is not infection, but represents contamination of such surfaces and articles (see Contamination).

23. **Infectious agent**—An organism (virus, rickettsia, bacteria, fungus, protozoa and helminth) that is capable of producing infection or infectious disease.

24. **Infectious disease**—A clinically manifest disease of man or animal resulting from an infection (see Infection).

25. **Infestation**—For persons or animals the lodgment, development and reproduction of arthropods on the surface of the body or in the clothing. Infested articles or premises are those which harbor or give

shelter to animal forms, especially arthropods and rodents.

26. **Insecticide**—Any chemical substance used for the destruction of insects, whether applied as powder, liquid, atomized liquid, aerosol, or as a "paint" spray; residual action is usual. The term **larvicide** is generally used to designate insecticides applied specifically for destruction of immature stages of arthropods; **adulticide** or **imagocide,** to designate those applied to destroy mature or adult forms. The term insecticide is often used broadly to encompass substances for the destruction of all arthropods, but **acaracide** is more properly used for agents against ticks and mites. More specific terms, such as **lousicide** and **miticide** are sometimes used.

27. **Isolation**—As applied to patients, isolation represents separation, for the period of communicability, of infected persons or animals from others in such places and under such conditions as to prevent or limit the direct or indirect transmission of the infectious agent from those infected to those who are susceptible or who may spread the agent to others. In contrast, quarantine (q.v.) applies to restrictions on the healthy contacts of an infectious case. Recommendations which are made for isolation of cases (section 9B2 of each disease) are the methods recommended by CDC (CDC *Guideline for Isolation Precautions in Hospitals,* see Preface) as category-specific isolation precautions. These are divided into 7 categories. Two requirements are common for all 7 categories:

1) *Hands must be washed after contact with the patient or potentially contaminated articles and before taking care of another patient;*

2) *Articles contaminated with infectious material should be appropriately discarded or bagged and labeled before being sent for decontamination and reprocessing.*

The seven categories are:

a) **Strict isolation:** This category is designed to prevent transmission of highly contagious or virulent infections that may be spread by both air and contact. The specifications, in addition to those above, include a private room and the use of masks, gowns and gloves for all persons entering the room. Special ventilation requirements with the room at negative pressure to surrounding areas is desirable.

b) **Contact isolation:** For less highly transmissible or serious infections, for diseases or conditions which are spread primarily by close or direct contact. In addition to the basic requirements, a private room is indicated but patients infected with the same pathogen may share a room. Masks are indicated for those who come close to the patient, gowns are indicated if soiling is likely, and gloves are indicated for touching infectious material.

c) **Respiratory isolation:** To prevent transmission of infectious diseases over short distances through the air, a private room is indicated but patients infected with the same organism may share a room. In addition to the basic requirements, masks are indicated for those who come in close contact with the patient; gowns and gloves are not indicated.

d) **Tuberculosis isolation (AFB isolation):** For patients with pulmonary tuberculosis who have a positive sputum smear or chest x-rays which strongly suggest active tuberculosis. Specifications include use of a private room with special ventilation and the door closed. In addition to the basic requirements, masks are used only if the patient is coughing and does not reliably and consistently cover the mouth. Gowns are used to prevent gross contamination of clothing. Gloves are not indicated.

e) **Enteric precautions:** For infections transmitted by direct or indirect contact with feces. In addition to the basic requirements, specifications include use of a private room if patient hygiene is poor. Masks are not indicated; gowns should be used if soiling is likely and gloves are to be used for touching contaminated materials.

f) **Drainage/Secretion Precautions:** To prevent infections transmitted by direct or indirect contact with purulent material or drainage from an infected body site. A private room and masking are not indicated; in addition to the basic requirements, gowns should be used if soiling is likely and gloves used for touching contaminated materials.

g) **Blood/Body Fluid Precautions:** To prevent infections that are transmitted by direct or indirect contact with infected blood or body fluids. In addition to the basic requirements, a private room is indicated if patient hygiene is poor; masks are not indicated; gowns should be used if soiling of clothing with blood or body fluids is likely. Gloves should be used for touching blood or body fluids.

28. **Molluscicide**—A chemical substance used for the destruction of snails and other molluscs.

29. **Morbidity rate**—An incidence rate (q.v.) used to include all persons in the population under consideration who become clinically ill during the period of time stated. The population may be limited to

a specific sex, age group or those with certain other characteristics.

30. **Mortality rate**—A rate calculated in the same way as an **incidence rate** (q.v.), using as a numerator the number of deaths occurring in the population during the stated period of time, usually a year. A **total** or **crude** mortality rate utilizes deaths from all causes, usually expressed as deaths per 1,000, while a **disease-specific** mortality rate includes only deaths due to one disease and is usually reported on the basis of 100,000 persons. The population base may be defined by sex, age or other characteristics. The mortality rate must not be confused with case fatality rate (q.v.).

31. **Nosocomial infection**—An infection occurring in a patient in a hospital or other health care facility and in whom it was not present or incubating at the time of admission, or the residual of an infection acquired during a previous admission. Includes infections acquired in the hospital but appearing after discharge, and also such infections among the staff and visitors of the facility.

32. **Pathogenicity**—The capability of an infectious agent to cause disease in a susceptible host.

33. **Patient or sick person**—A person who is ill.

34. **Personal hygiene**—Those protective measures, primarily within the responsibility of the individual, which promote health and limit the spread of infectious diseases, chiefly those transmitted by direct contact. Such measures encompass (a) washing hands in soap and water immediately after evacuating bowels or bladder and always before handling food or eating, (b) keeping hands and unclean articles, or articles that have been used for toilet purposes by others, away from the mouth, nose, eyes, ears, genitalia, and wounds, (c) avoiding the use of common or unclean eating utensils, drinking cups, towels, handkerchiefs, combs, hairbrushes and pipes, (d) avoiding exposure of other persons to spray from the nose and mouth as in coughing, sneezing, laughing or talking, (e) washing hands thoroughly after handling a patient or his belongings, and (f) keeping the body clean by sufficiently frequent soap and water baths.

35. **Prevalence rate**—A quotient (rate) obtained by using as the numerator the number of persons sick or portraying a certain condition in a stated population at a particular time (**point prevalence**), or during a stated period of time (**period prevalence**), regardless of when that illness or condition began, and as the denominator the number of persons in the population in which they occurred.

36. **Quarantine**—Restriction of the activities of well persons or animals

who have been exposed to a case of communicable disease during its period of communicability (i.e., contacts) to prevent disease transmission during the incubation period if infection should occur.

a) **Absolute** or **complete quarantine:** The limitation of freedom of movement of those exposed to a communicable disease for a period of time not longer than the longest usual incubation period of that disease, in such manner as to prevent effective contact with those not so exposed (see Isolation).

b) **Modified quarantine:** A selective, partial limitation of freedom of movement of contacts, commonly on the basis of known or presumed differences in susceptibility and related to the danger of disease transmission. It may be designed to meet particular situations. Examples are exclusion of children from school, exemption of immune persons from provisions applicable to susceptible persons, or restriction of military populations to the post or to quarters. It includes: **Personal surveillance,** the practice of close medical or other supervision of contacts in order to permit prompt recognition of infection or illness but without restricting their movements; and **Segregation,** the separation of some part of a group of persons or domestic animals from the others for special consideration, control or observation—removal of susceptible children to homes of immune persons, or establishment of a sanitary boundary to protect uninfected from infected portions of a population.

37. **Repellent**—A chemical applied to the skin or clothing or other places to discourage (1) arthropods from alighting on and attacking an individual, or (2) other agents, such as helminth larvae, from penetrating the skin.

38. **Report of a disease**—An official report notifying an appropriate authority of the occurrence of a specified communicable or other disease in man or in animals. Diseases in man are reported to the local health authority; those in animals to the livestock, sanitary, veterinary or agriculture authority. Some few diseases in animals, also transmissible to man, are reportable to both authorities. Each health jurisdiction declares a list of reportable diseases appropriate to its particular needs (see Preface). Reports should also list suspect cases of diseases of particular public health importance, ordinarily those requiring epidemiologic investigation or initiation of special control measures.

When a person is infected in one health jurisdiction and the case is reported from another, the health authority receiving the report should notify the other jurisdiction, especially when the disease requires examination of contacts for infection, or if food or water or other common vehicles of infection may be involved.

In addition to routine report of cases of specified diseases, special notification is required of all epidemics or outbreaks of disease, including diseases not listed as reportable (see Epidemic).

39. **Reservoir (of infectious agents)**—Any person, animal, arthropod, plant, soil or substance (or combination of these) in which an infectious agent normally lives and multiplies, on which it depends primarily for survival, and where it reproduces itself in such manner that it can be transmitted to a susceptible host.

40. **Resistance**—The sum total of body mechanisms which interpose barriers to the progress of invasion or multiplication of infectious agents or to damage by their toxic products. **Inherent resistance** — an ability to resist disease independent of antibodies or of specifically developed tissue response; it commonly resides in anatomic or physiologic characteristics of the host and may be genetic or acquired, permanent or temporary. Synonym: **Non-specific immunity** (See Immunity.)

41. **Rodenticide**—A chemical substance used for the destruction of rodents, generally through ingestion. (See Fumigation.)

42. **Source of infection**—The person, animal, object or substance from which an infectious agent passes to a host. Source of infection should be clearly distinguished from **source of contamination,** such as overflow of a septic tank contaminating a water supply, or an infected cook contaminating a salad. (See Reservoir.)

43. **Surveillance of disease**—As distinct from surveillance of persons (see Quarantine, b), surveillance of disease is the continuing scrutiny of all aspects of occurrence and spread of a disease that are pertinent to effective control. Included are the systematic collection and evaluation of:
   a) morbidity and mortality reports,
   b) special reports of field investigations of epidemics and of individual cases,
   c) isolation and identification of infectious agents by laboratories,
   d) data concerning the availability, use and untoward effect of vaccines and toxoids, immune globulins, insecticides, and other substances used in control,
   e) information regarding immunity levels in segments of the population, and
   f) other relevant epidemiologic data. A report summarizing the above data should be prepared and distributed to all cooperating persons and others with a need to know the results of the surveillance activities.

The procedure applies to all jurisdictional levels of public health from local to international. **Serological surveillance** identifies patterns of current and past infection using serological tests.

44. **Susceptible**—A person or animal presumably not possessing sufficient resistance against a particular pathogenic agent to prevent contracting infection or disease if or when exposed to the agent.

45. **Suspect case**—A person whose medical history and symptoms suggest that he or she may have or be developing some communicable disease.

46. **Transmission of infectious agents**—Any mechanism by which an infectious agent is spread from a source or reservoir to a person. These mechanisms are:
    a) **Direct transmission:** Direct and essentially immediate transfer of infectious agents to a receptive portal of entry through which human or animal infection may take place. This may be by direct contact as by touching, biting, kissing or sexual intercourse, or by the direct projection (droplet spread) of droplet spray onto the conjunctiva or onto the mucous membranes of the eye, nose or mouth during sneezing, coughing, spitting, singing or talking (usually limited to a distance of about 1 meter or less).
    b) **Indirect transmission:**
       1) Vehicle-Borne—Contaminated inanimate materials or objects (fomites) such as toys, handkerchiefs, soiled clothes, bedding, cooking or eating utensils, surgical instruments or dressings (indirect contact); water, food, milk, biological products including blood, serum, plasma, tissues or organs; or any substance serving as an intermediate means by which an infectious agent is transported and introduced into a susceptible host through a suitable portal of entry. The agent may or may not have multiplied or developed in or on the vehicle before being transmitted.
       2) Vector-Borne—(a) Mechanical: Includes simple mechanical carriage by a crawling or flying insect through soiling of its feet or proboscis, or by passage of organisms through its gastrointestinal tract. This does not require multiplication or development of the organism. (b) Biological: Propagation (multiplication), cyclic development, or a combination of these (cyclopropagative) is required before the arthropod can transmit the infective form of the agent to man. An incubation period (extrinsic) is required following infection before the arthropod becomes **infective.** The infectious agent may be passed vertically to succeeding generations (**transovarian transmission**);

transstadial transmission indicates its passage from one stage of life cycle to another, as nymph to adult. Transmission may be by injection of salivary gland fluid during biting, or by regurgitation or deposition on the skin of feces or other material capable of penetrating through the bite wound or through an area of trauma from scratching or rubbing. This transmission is by an infected non-vertebrate host and not simple mechanical carriage by a vector as a vehicle. However, an arthropod in either role is termed a **vector**.

c) **Airborne**—The dissemination of microbial aerosols to a suitable portal of entry, usually the respiratory tract. Microbial aerosols are suspensions of particles in the air consisting partially or wholly of microorganisms. They may remain suspended in the air for long periods of time, some retaining and others losing infectivity or virulence. Particles in the $1-5\mu$ range are easily drawn into the alveoli of the lungs and may be retained there. Not considered as airborne are droplets and other large particles which promptly settle out (see Direct transmission, above).

1) Droplet nuclei: Usually the small residues which result from evaporation of fluid from droplets emitted by an infected host (see above). They also may be created purposely by a variety of atomizing devices, or accidentally as in microbiology laboratories or in abattoirs, rendering plants or autopsy rooms. They usually remain suspended in the air for long periods of time.

2) Dust: The small particles of widely varying size which may arise from soil (as, for example, fungus spores separated from dry soil by wind or mechanical agitation), clothes, bedding, or contaminated floors.

47. **Virulence**—The degree of pathogenicity of an infectious agent, indicated by case fatality rates and/or its ability to invade and damage tissues of the host.

48. **Zoonosis**—An infection or infectious disease transmissible under natural conditions from vertebrate animals to man. May be enzootic or epizootic (see Endemic and Epidemic).

INDEX

A

459

Note: Bold numbers indicate major reference.